The Guide to
Living with
HIV Infection

The Guide to Living with HIV Infection

Developed at the
Johns Hopkins AIDS Clinic

SIXTH EDITION

John G. Bartlett, M.D.
Ann K. Finkbeiner

The Johns Hopkins University Press
Baltimore

Note to the Reader

This book is not meant to substitute for medical care of people with HIV infection, and treatment should not be based solely on its contents. Instead, treatment must be developed in a dialogue between the individual and his or her physician. Our book has been written to help with that dialogue.

The author and the publisher have taken every step to make the information in this book as up to date as possible.

Drug information: The author and the publisher have made reasonable efforts to determine that the selection and dosage of drugs discussed in this text conform to the practices of the general medical community. The medications described do not necessarily have specific approval by the U.S. Food and Drug Administration for use in the diseases and dosages for which they are recommended. In view of ongoing research, changes in governmental regulations, and the constant flow of information relating to drug therapy and drug reactions, the reader is urged to check the package insert or manufacturer's patient information material of each drug for dosage and for warnings and precautions. This is particularly important when the recommended agent is a new and/or infrequently used drug.

© 1991, 1993, 1996, 1998, 2001, 2006 The Johns Hopkins University Press
All rights reserved. First edition 1991
Sixth edition 2006
Printed in the United States of America on acid-free paper
9 8 7 6 5 4 3 2 1

The Johns Hopkins University Press
2715 North Charles Street
Baltimore, Maryland 21218-4363
www.press.jhu.edu

To purchase additional copies, call 1-800-537-JHUP

Library of Congress Cataloging-in-Publication Data

Bartlett, John G.
   The guide to living with HIV infection : developed at the Johns
Hopkins AIDS Clinic / John G. Bartlett, Ann K. Finkbeiner. — 6th
ed.
      p.   cm. — (A Johns Hopkins Press health book)
   Includes index.
   ISBN 0-8018-8485-3 (hardcover : alk. paper) — ISBN 0-8018-8486-1
(pbk. : alk. paper)
   1. AIDS (Disease)—Popular works.   I. Finkbeiner, Ann K.,
1943– II. Title. III. Series.
   RC607.A26.B376   2007
   362.196'9792—dc22
                                                                    2006009631

A catalog record for this book is available from the British Library.

To Garey Lambert

Contents

The Guide to
Living with
HIV Infection

Introduction:
About This Book

- Medical issues you need to understand first
- Psychological and social issues
- How we know what we know about HIV infection
- About this book

HIV infection puts extraordinary stresses on people's lives. Most of these stresses are unusual, and people are unsure how to handle them. This book guides people through HIV infection, lets them know what they're up against, and helps them deal thoroughly and positively with the medical and emotional problems the infection presents. The book is about how to live with HIV infection, that is, how to live a long and full and satisfying life.

This book will cover the parts of people's lives that HIV infection affects: their physical health, their emotional health and social difficulties, and their financial and legal problems. Sometimes these issues will be kept separate—one chapter is only about medical care, one only about financial and legal problems. Sometimes the issues will be merged—the chapter on what to do when first diagnosed covers both medical and emotional issues.

Medical Issues You Need to Understand First

A few things you need to know right away. Some of these things may not be uppermost in your mind, but you need to know them to protect yourself and others. All these things are discussed in more detail in chapter 1; we include them in this introduction to alert you to their necessity.

1. What HIV infection and AIDS are: AIDS stands for acquired immune deficiency syndrome. *Acquired* means that AIDS is not inherited (many diseases of immune deficiency *are* inherited) but acquired from some substance or microbe outside the body. *Immune defi-*

1

ciency means that the immune system has been weakened. A *syndrome* is not so much a disease as it is a collection of symptoms. In the case of AIDS, the syndrome is evidence of infection by the AIDS virus and either a complication that results from immune deficiency or a test of immune function that indicates susceptibility to such conditions.

AIDS is often used incorrectly as a catch-all term for infection with the AIDS virus. The name of the AIDS virus is HIV, the human immunodeficiency virus, so called because HIV infects the immune system and weakens it.

AIDS is only one stage of a whole series of stages in HIV infection. People with HIV infection do not necessarily have AIDS, and if they are taking drugs against HIV, they may possibly never get it.

When people are first infected with HIV, they show no obvious symptoms for a long period called the *asymptomatic period*. If they are not taking drugs against HIV, they will eventually show symptoms of a weakened immune system, and then are said to be in the *symptomatic period*. When the immune system is weakened severely, people begin having certain specific infections and tumors called *opportunists* or *AIDS-defining diagnoses* (see chapter 6). In this book, we simply call them *complications*. Though AIDS was once defined by the presence of certain complications, it is now defined as HIV infection plus these complications, or HIV infection plus a CD4 count of 200 or less. The CD4 count is a measure of the robustness of the immune system. A count of 200 or less means the body is more susceptible to a complication.

2. What the prognosis is: As far as we know, it's good. It's certainly drastically better than it was ten years ago. Old studies showed that without any treatment whatsoever, half of those with HIV infection would develop AIDS within eight to ten years after becoming infected, and most of the rest would have laboratory evidence of weakened immune systems. The same studies showed that people lived about three and a half years after they were diagnosed with AIDS. These studies were done before any treatment was available.

We now know that with treatment, the whole course of the disease can be slowed down or stopped, and that the statistics from these early studies do not mean much. We also know that new drugs and new treatments are being developed so fast that it is not possible to predict the average time between infection with HIV and the development of AIDS; we know only that the time is longer and may be indefinitely long.

Most people with HIV infection, if untreated, will eventually develop AIDS. Some people progress more quickly to the AIDS stage; others take longer; and some take even longer. This latter group is sometimes called "long-term survivors" or "chronic non-progressors." Medical studies now show that about 2 percent of people with HIV infection will have no symptoms for at least twenty years, even without treatment.

With treatment, that percentage goes much higher; many people seem likely to have good health indefinitely. Although we still have no proof, many (and maybe most) people with HIV infection who are treated aggressively should have a chronic and manageable disease, managed the way diabetes and hypertension are. As of 2005, medical researchers estimated that people currently being treated would live, on average, fifteen more years. We assume that continued progress in research will add substantially to this number.

3. What HAART is: Highly active antiretroviral therapy (HAART) is the term used for the cocktail of drugs you take to treat HIV infection. Because these drugs inhibit the growth of HIV, which is a retrovirus, they are also called antiretroviral agents. HAART is good news and bad news: good news because the drugs are so powerful, killing 90 percent of all HIV in the body within one week and 99 percent within one month; bad news because they cause side effects and require close adherence to what can be a demanding treatment schedule. These drugs are also unforgiving: if you miss doses of a drug, you risk having your HIV become resistant to that drug, and once HIV becomes resistant to a drug or class of drugs, it stays resistant forever.

4. When you can transmit the virus to others: You must consider yourself infectious to others from the time you are infected. Once HIV is in a person's body, it is impossible to become "uninfected." It is possible but unlikely that new drugs not yet available will eventually eliminate the virus. But with the drugs currently available, such cures haven't happened. The current drugs decrease the numbers of the virus by 99.9 percent or more, but they don't completely eradicate it from the body. Having such low numbers of the virus reduces the risk of transmission but doesn't totally eliminate the risk. Once infected, you can transmit the virus for the entire course of the disease.

5. How to avoid transmitting the virus (see chapter 2):
• Have no sex, or have safe sex or safer sex. Safe sex means sex with no exchange of semen, vaginal fluids, or blood, including menstrual

blood; safer sex means intercourse (oral, vaginal, or anal) with a condom.
• If you inject drugs, try to stop. If you cannot, stop sharing needles and works (spoons, cotton, syringes). Some authorities suggest rinsing the needles and works with chlorine bleach after every use, but we don't know whether this helps.
• Do not donate blood, body organs, semen, or other body tissue or fluids.
• To be extra cautious about transmitting HIV through blood, avoid sharing toothbrushes and razors.
• Casual contact—shaking hands, sharing a toilet, living with someone, playing contact sports, sharing eating utensils, sneezing on others—does not transmit the virus.

6. Whom you should notify: You should notify anyone you may have exposed to the virus. That includes anyone with whom you have had unprotected sex (meaning sex without condoms) or with whom you have shared needles or works. If you know when you were infected, tell anyone you may have exposed since then. If you do not know (though no one knows absolutely how far back in time you should go), the common recommendation is to notify anyone you may have exposed in the last one or two years. One reason to do this is that people you may have infected need to be counseled so that they don't themselves unknowingly transmit the virus to others. Another reason is that people you may have infected need health care. If you don't wish to tell them directly, most city and state health departments will tell for you; they will notify the person that he or she may have been exposed and should be tested, but they will not identify you as the source.
You should also tell your physician and dentist of the diagnosis.
Important: Other than sex or needle-sharing partners, and your physician and dentist, you need not tell anyone else. An exception: health care workers who do invasive procedures like surgery may need to notify their supervisors or employers according to local policy, which varies in different institutions.

7. Whether to get medical help: Everyone with HIV infection requires regular medical evaluation. In 1987, when the introduction of AZT offered extended life, medical help was important. In early 1996, with the introduction of protease inhibitors, it became critical. Statistics in the United States indicate that about one-third of people with HIV infection do not know they have it, or they know it and never seek care. This is tragic, because treatment offers health.

Psychological and Social Issues

People affected by HIV infection face greater emotional strain than most people ever do. Furthermore, many face it at an unconscionably young age. Those affected by the disease are shocked or angry or depressed or afraid or guilty or confused or have any number of these emotions at once. They worry about revealing the diagnosis, about expressing sexuality, about relations with the people they love. They worry about the increasingly complicated schedules for taking medication, about the medications' side effects, and about the consequences of missing doses. They worry about the uncertainty of the future. And they worry about the philosophical question common to everyone alive: What is the purpose of my life? The rest of society, not directly affected by the disease, still reacts with fear, prejudice, and pity, making those affected by the disease also feel like outcasts, isolated and lonely.

With time, people come to deal with these worries and emotions, using the same strategies that have worked for them in all their previous periods of difficulty. Their strategies for dealing with their problems are usually effective and usually different. Many of their strategies contradict those used by others. Some people talk out their problems; others work them out alone. Some people immerse themselves in work; others quit and go to Tahiti. Some people refuse to think of themselves as sick; others become AIDS activists. Some contemplate; some act. Some go to mental health professionals; others rely on their friends and themselves. Strategies can be opposite and still be equally effective. People tend to use whatever strategies have worked best in handling past problems. In fact, they use whatever strategies work at all.

Mental health professionals who deal with people affected by HIV infection recommend a few additional guidelines. The first is to protect your physical health. That includes eating healthful foods, cutting alcohol and smoking down or out, and exercising. Before 1996, when HIV infection still progressed inevitably downhill, these changes in lifestyle were not crucial. Now they are. With the treatments, many people with HIV infection have few or no problems with the virus but suffer instead from the consequences of smoking, hypertension, diabetes, and heart disease—all problems affected by behavior, exercise, and diet. In addition, protect the health of others: practice safer sex; don't share needles; avoid passing blood, semen, or vaginal fluids to another person.

The second guideline is to cultivate emotional health. Take care of yourself and be around people who like you. Try to see accurately who you are and what you feel. Find what's necessary to maintain your emotional equilibrium. Enlist your sources of support and try to communicate with them truthfully and thoughtfully. Many people find solace in a support group. If a problem seems too severe or does not go away, or if you are seriously considering suicide, or if you simply want someone to whom you can talk freely, see a mental health professional. Therapy may concentrate on the overwhelming problems people must face and feel they cannot solve: How can I face rejection? How can I deal with my anger? Can I come to feel less guilt? Are there ways to have sex without hurting myself or anyone else? Why me? Why now? What will happen next? What will happen to my kids? My parents? The people I love? Am I a good person?

The third guideline is to take control of your life. In spite of much that is unavoidable or unchangeable, the decisions about your life are yours to make. Consider and accept the consequences of your actions. Once that is done, you know what's best for you. You are in charge.

Satisfy these and any other principles you hold yourself to. Then trust yourself and live the way you feel you must. People affected by HIV infection say the same thing this way: be kind to yourself and others, come to terms with yourself, trust yourself.

How We Know What We Know about HIV Infection

People whose lives are so drastically affected by HIV infection naturally have questions about the disease. But because it is a new disease, medical scientists still have much to learn about its effects on the body and how to treat those effects. What medical scientists know depends on what kinds of studies they have done.

One kind of study examines *virology,* or the virus itself: what genes make it up, how it reproduces, how it attaches to cells, what effect it has on the cell. These studies will ultimately suggest new drugs for controlling or destroying the virus. Another kind of study, called a *clinical trial,* tests drugs to see whether they are effective both against HIV and against the infections that accompany a weakened immune system.

The third kind of study is *epidemiological;* that is, it charts the course of HIV infection through whole populations. In the early 1980s, epidemiological studies were responsible for identifying and defining the disease and for finding out how the disease was transmitted, even before the virus was discovered. Currently, a federal agency, the Centers for Disease Control and Prevention, or CDC, does epidemiological studies that keep track of the spread of the infection. From those studies, we now know the number of cases of AIDS, the populations that are affected, the way the virus is transmitted, the average course of the disease, the most common complications, and the average life expectancy.

To further help epidemiologists keep track of it, AIDS was made a "reportable disease," meaning that health care providers are required to report, by name, all people with AIDS to their state's department of health. (HIV infection is reportable by name in some states but not in others.) Ultimately, the states report these cases to the CDC, but not by name. As a consequence, the CDC has excellent information on AIDS. Information on other stages of HIV infection, however, is much more fragmented and incomplete. Only about half the states report everyone with HIV infection, but even these states' reports are incomplete because most of those infected have never been tested.

In short, the answers to questions about HIV infection are limited by how far medical science has progressed in its studies. Knowledge of how the virus operates in the body depends on the progress made in the virological studies. Knowledge of what drugs are most effective depends on the progress made in the clinical trials. Knowledge of the natural course of the disease in the body depends on the progress made in epidemiological studies. Information coming out of these studies is discussed throughout this book.

As a result, some questions people have about HIV infection can be answered completely and substantially. Other questions will have answers that are, for the present anyway, closer to educated guesses.

About This Book

This book is meant as a reference and a companion. It is unfortunately not a complete guide to living with HIV infection. One subject left out is home nursing care—you can get specific details about this subject from nurses or home health care workers. Another subject omitted is the care of children with AIDS. Both of these topics warrant books of their own. Any other information omitted or dealt with only sketchily is accompanied by a referral to a reliable source for the information.

This book was not written to be read from start to finish. Read the book in whatever order you please: read one chapter at a time, one section at a time; read about whatever problems you face now, or about whatever questions you currently want answered; skip chapters or sections and go back to them when you're ready, or don't go back to them at all. Each chapter is intended more or less to be read as though it stands alone. As a result, some information gets repeated in several chapters. If the repetition is annoying, please forgive us.

The book discusses emotional and social issues in human voices, that is, in the words of the people affected by the infection. The reason is that many of the ways of dealing with those issues come not only from mental health professionals but also from the people affected by HIV. In some of the following chapters are the voices of eight people: their names are Dean Lombard, June Monroe, Steven Charles, Helen Parks, Alan Madison, Rebecca Wolfe, Edward Carroll, and Lisa Pratt. Together, these people are meant to represent the population of people affected by HIV. They are men and women, have different financial resources, are different ages, have different jobs. Those with HIV have become infected a number of different ways. Some are newly infected; some have lived with the virus a long time. Some are doing well on the drugs, some less well. Though their names and certain characteristics are fictional, what they say is not. In every case, the words are quotes of real people affected by HIV; the quotes are nearly verbatim.

This book is full of medical terms, some of them familiar, some complicated and unfamiliar. We explain these terms as they appear. But we also know the reader will not remember every new word or every aspect of its meaning. So at the end of the book is a glossary of all these words, and the reader can refer to it as needed. The glossary includes, among other words, the names of the conditions associated with HIV infection, the tests to diagnose them, and the drugs used to treat them. The drugs usually have two names, the chemical name and (in parentheses) the trade name given by the drug company that discovered it.

And finally, we avoid, where possible, addressing separate groups of readers in separate sections. For the same reason that we avoid separate sections for people with HIV infection and their caregivers, we also avoid having separate sections for women, gay men, or injection drug users. The reason is that most of the issues and problems faced by all these people are the same. Women, gay men, people with hemophilia, transfusion recipients, and injection drug users are surely all concerned about their children. Everyone worries about the legal rights of an unmarried partner. Everyone is made unhappy by social isolation. Condoms should be used during sex regardless of who the partners are. Everyone has an equal chance of responding to treatment, and faces the same challenges of taking the medicines regularly. The prognosis, the laboratory tests, and the complications of the treatments are all the same for everyone.

Some issues, however, are truly unique to one group. Women have medical problems men do not; and they can transmit the virus, through pregnancy and breast-feeding, in ways men cannot. Gay men can face problems because revealing their HIV status can mean also revealing homosexuality; transfusion recipients do not necessarily face a similar problem. Our policy is to discuss issues unique to one group in the section devoted to those issues. So gynecological problems are in the chapter on medical problems; pregnancy and breast-feeding are in the chapter on transmitting HIV; problems of talking about homosexuality are in the section on problems with talking about HIV status.

We also avoid separate sections for people with differing levels of virus. For many people, the new combinations of drugs have boosted their immune systems and reduced the numbers of the virus; for other people, the new drugs are less successful; and for still others, the new drugs are, for various reasons, unusable or unavailable. These groups of people have some concerns that differ, and we try to address the differences. But most concerns of most people are similar. Nearly everyone has bouts of anger and times of depression, frets over the future, and worries about the effect of the infection on people they love.

In short, we're all in this together.

Chapter 1

When First Diagnosed: Understanding and Communicating about HIV

- What you need to know
- Reacting to the diagnosis
- Telling about the diagnosis

The first thing on a person's mind after a positive HIV test is probably not a list of practical things to know and do. Nevertheless, a person with HIV infection should begin doing some things immediately, so this chapter will talk about these things first. After these practicalities are covered, the discussion will turn to the emotional and social concerns people have when first diagnosed.

What You Need to Know

The Accuracy of the Test

The HIV blood test detects and measures the antibodies to HIV (human immunodeficiency virus, sometimes called the AIDS virus). This test, like all tests in medicine, is subject to human and laboratory error. Nevertheless, the standard blood test is one of the most accurate in medicine. The standard test became available in 1985 and has been continually improved. It is still used, but results aren't usually complete for one to two weeks. The more popular test now is a rapid test, so called because it gives the results in twenty to forty minutes. Even more important, the rapid test can be done anywhere—in a clinic, a church, or a civic center—because it needs only a drop of blood and someone who can read the results, which consist of just a red line. The rapid test is as good as the standard test when the results are negative, but it makes rare mistakes when results are positive. For this reason, the rule is that when the result is negative, the person is told it is negative (with limitations noted below). But when the result is positive, the person is told to get further testing and is referred to a place—generally any clinic or laboratory—where the standard test is done. With the standard test, positive results almost always mean you are infected; and negative results almost always mean you are not infected. The likelihood of the standard test reading positive when it is really negative is less than one in 100,000—about the likelihood of winning the lottery.

Occasionally people can't believe a positive blood test and want a second test. This makes sense especially if a person has had no high-risk behaviors. Despite the test having essentially no false positives—results that are positive in people who do not have HIV infection—mistakes from human error or mistakes in labeling or reporting are occasionally made. The best repeat test is a standard blood test.

Further information about the tests and their results is provided in Appendix B, "Understanding Tests for HIV."

The Prognosis

A standard blood test showing the presence of antibodies to HIV means that HIV itself is also in the blood. Unlike antibodies for other infections, the antibodies for HIV cannot kill the virus. This means that once HIV is in the body, it stays in the body.

There have been occasional reports of individuals with positive tests that subsequently became negative—that is, that the virus was once present and then was somehow eliminated. So far, these reports have nearly always turned out to be wrong: further tests show that once the test is positive, it stays positive.

HIV infection, if left untreated, causes the body's immune system to gradually weaken. This process takes years or even decades. For years, the person with HIV infection usually feels entirely well and has no symptoms of infection. We measure the progress of HIV infection by periodically counting the immune system cells that HIV infects, called CD4 cells. The normal CD4 count is usually 500 to 1,500. The count gradually declines, and when it reaches less than 200, people are prone to certain complications or opportunistic infections—infections that a healthy person doesn't get because they are fought off by the immune system. The person is now said to be in the symptomatic stage, or to have AIDS. Studies done before the development of the new drugs indicated that about half the people with positive blood tests for HIV developed AIDS within eight to ten years after being infected, and that after AIDS, people lived a year or longer. This finding was based on studies of people who became infected with HIV in San Francisco as early as 1978.

By 1996, however, changes in treatments were having a revolutionary impact on the prognosis. The most important thing to understand is this: we now know that the disease's progression can be stopped in most people who are getting the right treatment. But the treatment is not easy. Most people require at least three different kinds of pills ("triple therapy" or Highly Active Antiretroviral Therapy or HAART), and the pills have lots of side effects and usually cost about $10,000 to $15,000 a year.

The revolution in treatment resulted from three nearly simultaneous developments in 1995 and 1996. The first development was a series of studies on the virus and how it reproduces. These studies showed that, if untreated, HIV produces billions of new viruses every day in most people throughout the course of infection. The studies made it clear that in most people, the infection is always active. The studies also made it clear that what was needed was to quell the virus.

The second development was the "viral load" test, a test developed in 1996 to measure the amount of virus in the blood. The test is used to determine a person's response to the treatments. Within one day of beginning the new treatments, people had eliminated half the total HIV population in their bodies; and by one month, most people had eliminated 99 percent of the virus. So the test is not only a good indicator of a person's response to treatment, it also suggests that person's prognosis: the larger the amount of virus, the faster the disease progresses.

The third development was the introduction of new drugs. AZT, which has been used since 1987, was the first drug for HIV infection. Between 1991 and 1999, five other HIV drugs in the same class as AZT (ddI, ddC, d4T, 3TC, and ABC) were developed. In late 1995, a second class of drugs, called *protease inhibitors* or PIs (saquinavir, ritonavir, indinavir, nelfinavir, fosamprenavir, atazanavir, tipranavir, and lopinavir/ritonavir), was developed, followed by a third class called *nonnucleoside reverse transcriptase inhibitors* (or NNRTIs: nevirapine, delavirdine, and efavirenz). These second and third classes of drugs were more powerful than AZT and its relatives, but they had to be taken in various combinations to inhibit HIV effectively and prevent HIV from becoming resistant to them. And because lapses in the treatments also result in resistance, people had to adhere to complicated treatment regimens rigidly. Once HIV develops resistance to the drugs, those drugs are less effective, and sometimes, their effectiveness is totally lost forever. But if people stick carefully to the regimens, they can usually count on an indefinite period of good health.

How to Avoid Transmitting the Virus

A positive HIV blood test means that the virus is present and may be transmitted to others. Once infected, people remain infectious to others for the rest of their lives.

In most cases, HIV is transmitted to others by sexual contact or by injection drug use. The blood supply has been screened ever since 1985, so the risk of infection from transfusions is now very low. Extensive studies since then of people who knew how they became infected show that sex, injection drug use, or transmission from mother to fetus have accounted for 99.8 percent of all cases. Some of the remaining 0.2 percent of cases (2 in every 1,000 infected people) are health care workers who had needlestick injuries, people who received organ transplants before routine screening of donors, and the rare people who received infected blood transfusions despite the routine screening of blood.

The point is, it is important for you to know that this virus is not transmitted to others by casual contact—by shaking hands, sharing a toilet, sharing eating utensils, sneezing on others, and the like. Some things about this virus remain mysterious, but the mechanisms of its transmission are now very clear.

The best way to avoid sexual transmission is to abstain from sex. The next best way is to use "safer sex," that is, use condoms for all genital contact, or have the kind of sexual contact that does not involve transferring semen, vaginal fluids, or blood (including menstrual blood) from one person's body into another's. Women with HIV should think carefully through the issues of getting pregnant because of the risk of transmitting the virus to the fetus. Women with HIV who are pregnant and intend to carry the pregnancy to term, who take drugs that reduce HIV in the blood, and who deliver by cesarean section thereby reduce the risk of transmitting HIV to the baby to about 2 percent or less. Women with HIV who have a baby should not breast-feed. The best way for injection drug users to avoid transmission is to stop using drugs. If this is impossible, they must absolutely stop sharing needles and works.

To be extra cautious, avoid sharing toothbrushes and razors. It is also necessary to avoid donating blood, body organs, semen, or other body tissue or fluids. Anyone with HIV infection who has a universal donor card for organ transplantation should destroy this card.

Preventing transmission of HIV is discussed more thoroughly in chapter 2.

Whom to Notify

People with HIV infection have an ethical and, in many places, a legal requirement to notify people whom they may have exposed to HIV. The point of notification is to get these people tested so they can be counseled to prevent further transmission and so they can get the health care that is now life-saving.

Notification can be done directly—you tell the person yourself—or by the contact services of some state or local health departments that notify the person at risk without identifying the source of exposure.

People with HIV infection should notify anyone with whom they have had nonsafe sex (that is, sex without a condom, or sex that involved exchange of semen, vaginal fluids, or blood, including menstrual blood) and with whom they have shared needles or works. This applies to past as well as present and future relationships.

For past relationships, the major problem is knowing how far back in time to go. Most people with HIV do not know when they became infected. Since the infection may be silent for a long time, they may conceivably have been placing others at risk for several years. For practical purposes, most authorities recommend notifying anyone with whom you've had a sexual relationship for the past one or two years. This is the absolute minimum. The person or people with whom you have had sex should get tested right away. The blood test usually takes one to two months after infection to show positive results. This means that people who may have been exposed to HIV recently will not know for sure whether they are infected unless they take the test two to three months after the last exposure. We often recommend a test at six months as well, just to be on the safe side.

People who may have been exposed might also want to ask a physician about the probability of infection, the necessity for medical evaluation beyond simple testing for HIV, and the desirability of subsequent testing (see Appendix B, "Understanding Tests for HIV"). It may be reassuring to know that the virus is not easily transmitted. We know the probabilities of transmission from surveys of discordant couples, couples in which one is infected with HIV and the other is not. The risk of infection without use of condoms is actually less than 1 in 100 for a single sexual contact. The same studies show that even for those who have had regular sexual contact for five years, the risk of infection is less than 50 percent. This includes wives of men with hemophilia, who have infection rates of 10 to 30 percent, despite having had unprotected sex for years. Similar studies have not yet been done for gay men; the risks are probably higher.

In some states, notification of HIV infection is required by law. In

New York State, for example, physicians are required to identify the contacts of their patients with newly detected HIV infection; state authorities will then notify the contacts that they have been placed at risk, without disclosing the source of the risk. Authorities will not notify contacts when such notification is likely to cause domestic violence. This New York law obviously requires the patient to cooperate in identifying contacts. In most states, the role of the physician in notifying people placed at risk by an infected patient is less clear.

There is debate about all this. On the one hand, the patient-physician relationship is privileged, or private. On the other, the physician has an obligation to society. A legal precedent was established with the case of *Tarasoff v. Regents of the University of California,* in which a psychologist who learned of a patient's intent to murder a young woman was held liable for not taking appropriate steps to protect her. This decision established that the physician has what is called a "duty to warn" unsuspecting people whose behavior puts them at risk. As a result, the physician will usually advise a patient to notify people who have been and continue to be placed at risk of infection. If the patient is unwilling to do this, the physician may have the authority and even the responsibility to do it, either directly or through public health authorities.

Abiding by these obligations and notifying others of the possibility of HIV infection is extremely difficult. People who simply cannot do it are advised to discuss their concerns with their physicians. They might also benefit from consulting a psychiatrist or a psychologist, or by participating in support groups, or by talking to friends and relatives. One option is to use a third party, a mutual friend, or a physician (see "Telling about the Diagnosis" in this chapter).

Deciding Whom Else to Tell

Beyond those you must inform, deciding whom to tell and whom not to tell is difficult. For someone who is newly diagnosed, the first advice is to limit the number of people. Tell those who need to know: physicians, dentists, and anyone who has been or will be exposed by sexual contact or shared needles. If you are a health care worker, you should follow local and organizational guidelines about notifying a superior or a medical adviser where you work.

No one else needs to know. Almost all the people who had HIV infection in the early 1980s could recount a seemingly endless array of war stories about how their medical care, employment, and relationships with friends and relatives changed when their diagnoses became known. Since then, society's attitude has become more informed and the war stories have accordingly become less frequent. The stories are, however, by no means gone. So until you have sorted out your own reactions to the diagnosis, and have thought through which people you want to tell and what you want to tell them, you are probably better off not saying anything. Put it off for a while. Limit those you tell.

Finding a Stable and Congenial Source of Medical Care

Everyone with HIV infection requires regular medical care. Medicine cannot yet cure HIV infection, but it can treat it. And the treatments can allow you a nearly normal life for a very long time. (Chapter 6 discusses each complication by symptom; chapter 7 advises how to choose physicians.) Select a physician or a group of physicians or a clinic that you find congenial, that you will continue to visit, and that you can trust. HIV infection is the most rapidly moving field in medicine and requires a physician with experience in and commitment to treating HIV infection.

The best way to find that good HIV physician is through referral by other physicians. Most physicians don't do HIV care; in fact, about 3,000 of the 600,000 physicians in the United States (0.5 percent) provide the care for 80 percent of the people treated for HIV infection. Good HIV physicians follow the journals reporting HIV studies, know the most recent guidelines, go to at least one national conference each year, and have at least fifty patients with HIV infection. So before choosing an HIV physician, ask how many patients with HIV infection the physician has, and whether he or she attends the national HIV conferences. Other physicians in the community usually know who the HIV physicians are. Other patients might be helpful, but be careful, because patients' perceptions of competence are often driven by personality compatibilities. Be leery of advertised medical services and of anyone who claims cures.

The Decision to Become Pregnant

Women who have HIV and then become pregnant can transmit this virus to their babies. Women who become infected with HIV while they are pregnant can also transmit the virus to their babies. Without treatment, the risk of transmission is around 20 percent to 35 percent, meaning that about one-quarter of the babies born to mothers with HIV will also have the virus. A woman who becomes infected with HIV after she has had a baby has less to worry about. Any woman with HIV infection, regardless of when she became infected, must not breast-feed her baby.

HIV infection is different in children than in adults. In children, the disease, unless treated, progresses more rapidly. Most children with HIV infection will have medical problems by age 4 or 5 years, although some children with HIV remain well until they are 10 or 12 years old. Babies and children with HIV infection clearly benefit from treatment, though no one knows much about whether the new drugs, such as protease inhibitors, will also benefit them.

We once thought that women with HIV infection should not become pregnant because the baby had a high risk of being infected, of living for only a few years, or of losing its mother to AIDS. We don't think that any more. Current statistics are much different: the risk of the baby becoming infected is only 2 to 5 percent, and even if the baby is infected, his or her prognosis is much better; and the mother's prognosis, though hard to predict in the long run, is quite good.

For the woman who has HIV infection, the decision to become pregnant should be based on your viral load, how far along you are in the disease, and how willing or able you are to take medications. Women who respond well to treatment have a good long-term prognosis and are unlikely to transmit HIV to their babies. The key issue here is how well the virus is being controlled. If your viral load is low or undetectable, meaning less than 50, the risk of transmission to the baby is nil. If the viral load is less than 1,000, the risk of transmission is still low, less than 2 percent. If the viral load is higher than 1,000, delivering the baby by cesarean section will decrease the risk of transmission to about 2 percent. All these numbers assume that you do not breast-feed.

For the woman who does not have HIV infection but whose sex partner does, the issue of pregnancy is difficult. Getting pregnant requires having unprotected sex, which of course risks transmitting HIV. Artificial insemination is a solution but only if the sperm donor is another, uninfected man. Sperm-washing infected sperm has been done in some countries with reported success, but the process really isn't adequately tested. It appears to be effective, but the services must be done on-site, the procedure is very expensive, and generally the infected man must have no detectable virus. Those interested in sperm-washing should obtain data from clinics where it is done; such data is especially reliable in the United States because of the legal requirements for the consent process.

If a woman has already given birth without prior testing and subsequently learns she has HIV, she should have all her children of preschool age tested. We now know of some older children with HIV infection who have been relatively healthy for up to ten years. So it may be appropriate to have the reassurance of a negative blood test.

Reacting to the Diagnosis

Most people react to learning of their diagnosis of HIV infection with confusion, shock, and disbelief. Steven Charles is 25 years old and infected by HIV but asymptomatic. He is a gay man who lives alone in an apartment. "I got the diagnosis the day after my birthday," he said. "I went for the test, hoping to confirm I was negative. When the doctor told me, I ran out of the office and stood in the hall. I didn't know what my priorities should be."

Lisa Pratt's husband, Glen, a 60-year-old man who had received an infected blood transfusion, would not believe the test results. Like Steven Charles, Lisa's husband reacted to the diagnosis of HIV infection with shock and disbelief: "He kept saying, 'Those idiots don't know what they're doing.' He made them test him again and again," Lisa said later. Some people, because they are gay or use drugs by injection, have anticipated the diagnosis. Others have not. In either case, the diagnosis confronts people, usually for the first time, with all the possibilities of a serious disease.

Serious sickness has no normal place in our lives. We know it might happen, we know other people to whom it has happened, but we live in hope it won't happen to us. No one is ever ready to hear this news, or to assimilate it all at once: "What do you do with that kind of information," said Steven, "that you have this kind of disease?" People continue their lives almost unthinkingly: "For a few days after my diagnosis," Steven said, "if it wasn't automatic, it wasn't getting done." Others say they "freeze up" or "go on hold": Lisa said that for a while, "Glen simply quit getting out of bed, quit eating."

Shock and disbelief are the normal reactions to this diagnosis. So are problems with eating and sleeping. Alan Madison is 35 years old, also infected with HIV, is gay, and lives in a condominium with a long-time partner. "I didn't sleep at first," said Alan. "It was a lot of emotions for one thirty-six-hour period."

With shock and trouble eating and sleeping comes an assortment of related reactions. People blame themselves and lose their good opinion of themselves. They are frightened because they don't know what's coming next. They are agitated and anxious and entirely preoccupied with the diagnosis. They are depressed, sad, unable to enjoy or take pleasure in things. They are afraid no one will like them any more, and at the same time they isolate themselves: "At first," said Alan, "I unplugged the phone and said no visitors. I put up roadblocks on purpose." People first hearing the diagnosis are also furious: "My husband stood in our living room, swearing," said Lisa. "He yelled, 'Damn it, damn it, how did I hit odds that small?'"

Though these feelings are terrible, and though they will recur, their acuteness is short-lived. They last from a few weeks to a few months—typically around six weeks. People deal with these feelings the way they have dealt with all other crises in their lives. They use the same skills, the same strategies they always have. "My husband cried when he told me about it," said Lisa. "I told my husband, 'Don't be sorry. I love you. We'll handle this the way we handle everything else.'"

Strategies for Handling the Feelings

Different strategies for handling the feelings work for different people. In general, people try to fit the infection into their lives, to see what the infection does mean and what it does not mean. Because people are so different, their strategies for coping are different and, in fact, are sometimes completely opposite. Any strategy that allows you to accept the diagnosis and stay emotionally intact is a good one. Use whatever strategies have worked on other problems. Use whatever strategies your needs and personality seem to dictate.

Some people talk about it: "When I got the diagnosis," said Steven, "I called my cousin and she flew in. Then I talked to my parents. My father was hysterical, my mother was in shock. For a while, we were all moderately hysterical together." By sharing news of the diagnosis, people surround themselves with the warmth and comfort of those who care about them. In these surroundings, they find it easier to let the fact of the diagnosis sink in, and easier also then to put that fact into perspective.

Other people want to handle it alone. Lisa used to sit with her head between her knees, giving herself time, she said, to "just feel what I felt" before she had to put a public face on her feelings. The "roadblocks" Alan said he put up between himself and other people gave him time to deal with his own reactions to the diagnosis before taking on anyone else's. If you want the sense of companionship that talking will bring you, talk. If you want time to sort out your feelings alone, don't talk. If you want both, have both.

Some people read books on HIV infection and talk to doctors, to educate themselves about every aspect of the infection. "I went that day to the bookstore, bought a couple of books, found out what I was up against," said Alan. "Then I wrote to organizations. I became very well-read." Being well informed gives people a sense of control over what affects them. Others accept information about the infection bit by bit, as they are ready for it. They want to keep their defenses intact and not feel overwhelmed by the diagnosis.

Some abolish bad feelings: "For a long while now," said Steven, "I've squelched anxiety. I put it out of my mind. I can't worry about craziness." They find that feeling and acting normally helps them accept the diagnosis gradually and stay in control of their feelings. In fact—since human emotions are highly variable—some people seem to have no bad feelings at all. One gay man, in a sustained relationship with his partner who had had HIV for eight years and was currently untreated, became infected with HIV. The partner was so upset he required professional counseling, but the recently infected gay man was unfazed: "It's treatable, right? That's what my partner's doctor tells him, and my partner still looks great. We always knew this was a risk, so I was ready for it even if he wasn't." The man asked his doctor to tell him what to do next, but to "please make it simple because my career is very demanding right now."

Others express the bad feelings—to friends, in a private journal, or alone. They have crying spells. Rebecca Wolfe is 33 and found she had been infected with HIV years before through a former boyfriend; her husband is not infected. "I bawled every day," said Rebecca. Expressing these feelings often seems to dilute them, and they hurt less. Many people alternate between expressing and avoiding their feelings.

Some people, like Steven, talk to other people with HIV infection: "I talked to someone who had HIV infection and asked him a lot of questions," Steven said. "It seemed necessary." Some look up those affected by HIV infection, not to talk about the infection, but simply to socialize: go to the theater, to sports events, out to eat. Many join support groups for people with HIV infection (see section on support groups in chapter 11). In support groups and with friends also affected by HIV infection, they lose their sense of isolation. They no longer feel as alone. They see others handling what seems overwhelming. They hear of new strategies for dealing with the diagnosis and decide what would work for them and what wouldn't.

Many talk to mental health professionals—psychiatrists, psychologists, social workers, counselors, and therapists of all kinds—who help people with HIV infection. Mental health professionals help people understand that their reactions are normal. The professionals often offer advice and alternate strategies, and they can be told anything. Some people can tolerate periods of severe stress much better if they briefly take a tranquilizer. Tranquilizers can be prescribed by any physician; this includes psychiatrists but not psychologists.

Some people turn to their religions: Lisa said her husband became more spiritual, and that she herself was learning "to trust, not my feelings, but God's promise that I'll find peace in the midst of this."

The Turning Point

One way or another, people's strategies usually work, and their acute distress fades. Their sense that life is disrupted gives way to a feeling that life is continuing, but under different circumstances. They come to understand that they can live with the virus. This understanding often comes as a sudden turning point. Alan, after a few days of isolating himself, talked to his mother, who told him to get over it. "That didn't help," he said. "Then the next day in the shower I said to myself, 'This stinks, but I'm stuck with this virus and would rather have my life happy than sad.'"

Lisa's turning point was more religious: "At first, I let the house go. I let junk pile up. After a while, the facts started sinking in. I said to God, 'You've got your work cut out for you. I'm going to turn a lot of this over to you until I can handle it.' Then I went out and bought one hundred narcissus bulbs because I knew we'd need a reminder of the hope of life. And it worked. My husband said, 'They make me feel so good.'"

Of course, not everyone has a turning point; for a lot of people, life just gradually becomes more reasonable. "My first thoughts after diagnosis were, 'I'm damaged goods, no one will want to touch me,'" said Rebecca. "What got me away from those feelings was nothing special, just time."

Occasionally, however, nothing works. Even after a few months, people remain extremely depressed: they are still preoccupied, or think seriously about not wanting to live, or persist in having problems eating and sleeping. This more serious type of depression happens to about 5 percent to 15 percent of people with HIV infection (the same percentages of people who become severely depressed after being told that they have some serious illness). Some people deny they are infected and persist in behavior that puts the health of both other people and themselves at risk. Some people consider suicide, though less than 1 percent of those with HIV infection actually commit suicide. People who experience severe depression, denial, or persistent thoughts of suicide need to get help from a psychiatrist, psychologist, or other mental health professional (see chapter 4). Persistent depression may be best treated with medication, which a psychiatrist can prescribe.

Most people gradually understand and believe that they will get used to the infection and will find answers to their questions. They restabilize, and they continue living. "Life changes, then comes back to normal," said Steven. "I'm no longer sitting around waiting to get sick."

People also understand that living with the virus means taking precautions against infecting other people, and guarding their own health. "I had the universal reactions," said Alan, "but I grew out of it. Now I just try to take care of myself and act responsibly."

This is not to say that under normal circumstances, anxiety or depression or isolation go away and stay away. The feelings almost seem to cycle, to come back in waves over and over again. But with each cycle, the feelings become easier to deal with, and the strategies people use to deal with them become almost automatic. Steven said, "At first, my diagnosis was the only thing on my mind. After a year or so, I still got depressed, but it wasn't the only thing on my mind." Chapters 4 and 11 go into more detail about recurring feelings and about people's strategies for dealing with them.

Telling about the Diagnosis

One of the first practical, concrete problems most people face after their diagnosis is deciding whom to tell. Before telling anyone, however, people generally settle their own feelings. As a general rule, those whom you tell will mirror your own feelings. When you're still feeling angry or scared or guilty about your diagnosis, the people you tell may react with anger, fear, or guilt. When you have figured out where the diagnosis fits in your life, the people you tell are more likely to accept your diagnosis without drama. You can often set the stage for other people's reactions.

Aside from this general rule, however, deciding whom to tell can be tricky. Different people decide differently, depending on the situation, their own personalities, and the personalities of those they might tell. "I told my parents," said Steven. "I learned early in life I put nothing over on them. Everybody around me knows, I tell lots of people." Alan, on the other hand, says he is careful whom he tells: "Only my partner. And my mother, my sister, and my young nephew. No one else." Lisa said, "In the eight months since I've known about my husband, I've told only my daughters, my father, and my stepmother. I have brothers and sisters I have not told." Lisa of course had to be tested for HIV; she is not infected. Later, Lisa became an activist and went public with her and her husband's problems.

Dean Lombard is a 40-year-old gay man with HIV infection. Dean has a son by an earlier marriage and now owns a house with a long-term partner. "I told my partner, my parents, brother, sister, my son, and my pastor," Dean said. "I stopped there. It's hard to explain—I'm extremely close to other people and all my relatives. But I don't want to tell them."

In every case, the decision is a balancing act. Health is a private matter and not generally anyone else's business. "You don't tell everybody everything you know," said Alan. "You don't say, 'Hi, I'm Alan, I'm African American, I work in a bank.' Nothing about me socially is different, there's just something in me I'm battling with." You balance your feelings of privacy against your need for connection. Alan added, "Though it's very fraying keeping it inside. When it's all out on the table, you don't worry about hiding things. But mostly I try to think about myself and my own comfort level." With each person, you balance what you hope they could give you with what their reactions might be.

Whom to Tell and Why

First, decide whom you are obliged to tell. That category includes your doctor and dentist, your sexual partners, needle-sharing partners if you use drugs, the health care institution in which you work (depending on their rules), and, only if you are filing claims for HIV-related conditions, your insurance company.

Otherwise, the decision to "go public" is tough. HIV carries baggage that most illnesses don't, and other people's initial reactions aren't necessarily comforting. Some people still have unrealistic fears of contagion, thinking HIV is transmitted as easily as the flu or colds. Some people seem to think HIV infection invariably makes people sickly and pathetic with a really weird disease. And HIV labels people as having a disease acquired by behaviors that society has historically not accepted—gay sex, injection drugs, or numerous heterosexual lovers. Though much of the labeling is a thing of the past, some of the old biases persist.

So think carefully about whom you would like to tell. Alan's diagnosis was years ago, but "telling is still case by case," he says, "as you get to know people." In general, most people believe they can trust their own inner sense of whom they can tell: "You play it by ear," Alan says. "You know who's right to discuss it with." If you don't know anyone "right to discuss it with," you might try joining a support group for people with HIV infection.

Some people feel that they have a responsibility to tell those they love. They worry that not telling might be seen as lying. Steven and Dean both feel close to their families and do not want to be seen as secret-keepers. They both think their families would want to know something this important. "I couldn't not tell my parents," Dean said, "I owed them at least that."

Many people want to tell those they trust because they need the sympathy and support of these people. "My relatives who knew said, 'Don't tell anyone else,'" said Lisa. "I said, 'I've got to. I can't live alone with this.'" People find it hard to be alone with physical illness or emotional distress. They find that talking to someone alleviates that loneliness. Talking to someone else also makes you present your problems in a logical and understandable way, so that talking eventually makes problems easier to analyze and to solve. And if the problems have no solutions, talking them over makes them easier to live with.

Some people even want to tell everyone—"I'm excruciatingly open," says Steven. They find that going public with their problems helps other, more isolated people. These people write articles and have even begun newspapers and newsletters. Lisa eventually talked to a reporter, she said, "because so many people were hurting. And the article did help people who are alone in this." Once the newspaper article on Lisa was published, the rest of her relatives and friends found out about her husband's diagnosis. Steven gives public talks: "Touching other people in large numbers in one sitting, is why I do it. I'm an expert because I live with it. I have nothing to be ashamed of—I guess it was a way of feeling good about myself."

To decide whom you would like to tell, ask some of the following questions. Who do you feel ought to know? Whom do you love? Who will not run away? Who can see past the infection, and love and value you? Who can keep a confidence? Who can listen to what you have to say? You might also think about which you are more comfortable with: the sense that you have no secrets, or the sense that you take care of your own business.

Lisa initially told her daughters because she baby-sits regularly for one daughter's children and the other daughter is a practical nurse whose help she might need. Steven told his parents partly so they could prepare themselves in case he got sick, and partly because he couldn't put anything over on them. He told his sister so she could help his parents. Alan told his partner, so his partner could get tested and so they could both take precautions. He also told his counselor and a friend, because "it helps when someone knows you other than as a patient." Later, he told a co-worker, who also happened to be infected with HIV, because "he's a positive, 'up' person to talk to. It does good to hear how someone else handles it, someone who has a good outlook." Edward Carroll is a 50-year-old gay man with AIDS. He is increasingly resistant to medication. At the time of his diagnosis, he was politically active in AIDS-related causes. "The people I told were already in this business," he said, "so it wasn't a matter of fear of rejection. I did not tell my parents. They're old and they didn't need that burden, and what could they do? I eventually told them. My father took it with as much aplomb as you can expect, and we had a heart-to-heart talk about how this was my battle, not his."

Sometimes people guess the facts and ask. Perhaps they knew of a person's homosexuality or drug use and had been worrying about the possibility of infection. Alan's partner's father asked Alan's partner, "Alan's been sick a lot. Does he have this AIDS?"

Deciding whom to tell has a complication: telling people about your diagnosis also means telling them how you got the virus. Sometimes that means telling them about a history of blood transfusions or hemophilia, or your spouse's transfusions or hemophilia. Other times, it means telling them things they might find difficult to accept, about sexual habits—"I was worried people would think I'd slept around a lot," said Rebecca Wolfe—or about drug use.

Homosexuality. Information about sexual habits is hard to talk about and hard to hear. Along with learning the diagnosis, some people hear for the first time that their son or brother or husband or lover is gay. As a result, relationships often become unhappy or difficult. One mother, named June Monroe, had found out by accident that her son was gay: "I felt like someone hit me with a claw hammer. It broke my heart. He said, 'I want to explain.' But I didn't want to know. I was bitter. I cried for a month."

One way to resolve the estrangement is to talk about it. One Sunday, June began crying in church and had to leave: "My son followed me outside the church and said, 'Don't you still love me? Am I any different?' I told him I wasn't raised to understand gays. I said I didn't understand it, and he said, 'Mom, I didn't choose my sexuality. And I don't understand you and Dad either.' What bothered me was that I'd miss his marriage and children, but that was just selfish. I had to take the parts of me that were my old beliefs and upbringing and set them aside. I had to come to terms with my son's gayness." Like many people, though, June continued to hope her son would change.

Steven's cousin knew Steven was gay without his telling her: "She said she knew all along," Steven said. "She'd change me if she could. But when I get tired of her arguing about it, I tell her." Steven and his cousin, and June and her son, like many others, discuss their differences, and if they do not understand each other, they agree to let it be. No one in these relationships thinks their differences are as important as their bonds. "Loving is loving," June said. "I've always loved my son. I would have a harder time not loving him than loving him."

Discussion does not always lead to resolution, especially for gay or bisexual men and their wives. Sometimes a couple can discuss the husband's sexuality openly. This sometimes results in divorce, sometimes in friendship, sometimes in an agreement that the man and woman will still help each other out. Other times, the couple has an unspoken agreement to ignore the husband's sexuality; it remains his own private business, and no one asks questions. Sometimes, even after a diagnosis of HIV infection, the husband denies that he is gay and the wife agrees to believe the denial.

All these alternatives work; each couple decides what works best for them. The only resolution that is unhealthy is one in which one person is infected with HIV and the couple does not practice safer sex.

Drug use. Drug users face the same possibility of rejection that gays face. Helen Parks is a divorced, 35-year-old woman with two sons who live with their father. Helen became infected with HIV after using drugs by injection. She said that once she told her father, from then on she had to face his suspicions. "My dad means no harm," said Helen, "but he accuses me of being high when I'm not, like when I'm crying or being easy to get along with. He goes through my things. It plays on my nerves, but I don't resent his suspicions. I've put him through a lot this year."

Drug users are also likely to have to face charges, such as, "So that's where you've been," or "So that's where my money went," or "So that's why you got fired." But in fact, drug users do not usually have to tell their parents or their partners about drug use. Unless drug use is recreational, that is, unless it has not changed the person's life and habits, parents and partners always know before they are told.

Reasons for Keeping Silent

Some people who have made their diagnosis public have compromised their jobs, their ability to get mortgages, and their ability to keep their insurance. All this is much less likely now than it was years ago, but these problems can still pop up unpredictably. For this reason, many advise people with HIV infection to tell as few others as possible: tell those they are obliged to tell, tell those they love and whose support they need, and then tell no others. You are certainly under no obligation to tell your neighbors, your employer, your landlord, or, unless you are filing HIV-related claims, your insurance agent. "I'm not sick, I'm healthy," said Dean. "Nobody has any reason to suspect anything, and I just don't need to talk about this stuff."

The reason most people have for keeping silent is other people's reactions. "I don't make a point of the truth about my son," said June, "but I would answer if asked. So far, no one has. I'm not ashamed of the truth, but it bothers other people." The particular truth of HIV infection does indeed bother people. When Dean first told his mother, she stayed out of church for a long time because she was afraid the other members would not talk to her. Alan worried that his mother would feel guilty, overreact, and make his life more difficult by "asking me questions and giving me orders." Dean worried about how much pain he would cause his relatives.

Other people have related reasons for keeping silent. Helen Parks worried that people would find out without her telling them: she bought the drugs to control her infection in a nearby city so she wouldn't be seen in her local pharmacy. Her sons, she thought, could not keep confidences. She was afraid that those she told would gossip, and she would lose control over who knew and who did not. She worried about having to tell her insurance company. June did not want to tell her mother-in-law, her son's grandmother; the old woman was in failing health, and June did not want to add to her troubles. Dean worried at first that his co-workers would no longer want to work with him; years later, he still has not told them: "If they know, nobody's saying so. As long as I'm doing my job, I don't care and apparently they don't either."

How Others React

Often, these worries are without foundation, and people, when told, react much differently from how we expect them to react. Alan's mother says she feels guilty for not having somehow protected him against the virus, but she is able to talk freely to him. Helen's father, who had always been reserved with her, "dropped his mask," she said, "and changed. He became warm and loving." Steven says not to underestimate your family and friends.

Unfortunately, worries about others' reactions are sometimes justified. Just as sympathy and sensitivity are part of human nature, so are fear, discrimination, and avoidance of illness. Sometimes these unpleasant reactions come from those you most count on. "My best friend I lost," Rebecca said, "because she didn't know what to do or say and so just went into the periphery. When I needed her, she just couldn't be there." During office visits, said Alan, his family doctor "stayed across the room." Dean said, "My dentist told me to go somewhere else. My pastor didn't want me touching anything he had to touch." Helen's stepmother didn't want to visit Helen: "She acted like my house had a plague in it," Helen said, "like it had devils in it."

In some people, these reactions are only temporary: Helen's stepmother stopped worrying about visiting. Steven, who met a man he wanted to date, told about his HIV infection: "He was surprised, shocked," Steven said. "I tried to listen to him, to not react. He was angry. He was afraid he'd get infected. While we were talking about it, he stayed with me, I stayed with him, we didn't shut each other out, we didn't run away from it. And it worked out beautifully."

For other people, these reactions, in spite of being unpleasant, are probably not going to change. Inevitably, you will tell someone who cannot handle the news. This starts a series of reactions in you. You may feel rejected, angry, isolated. Sometimes these feelings are reinforced by other worries: that people are right to reject you, that you brought the virus on yourself, that you are to blame for your diagnosis. This series of reactions is understandable; people are especially vulnerable when the diagnosis is still new.

But these reactions confuse issues that are really separate and unrelated. People who cannot handle your diagnosis are probably not rejecting you personally. In any case, their actions toward you have no bearing on your worth or your good opinion of yourself. Instead, people who reject you are rejecting what they fear. HIV infection reminds them of fears they have—about contagion, illness, sexuality, social isolation—which they cannot face. Rejecting you because you remind them of their fears helps them keep their fears at a distance. They are not thinking about you at all; they are concerned only with their own problems, they are only protecting themselves. "I'll have to do something about telling more people sooner or later, but I'm not ready yet," said Dean. "I don't want to deal with their hysteria. When you first tell people, it's when you most need them and it's when they're least likely to help. Though I suppose everybody's trying to do their best."

Perhaps, while you are still vulnerable to people's reactions, it is best to keep silent. Wait until your feelings stabilize and you feel more sure of yourself. Then decide whom to tell. If you tell someone who disappoints you, the best policy might be to accept them as they are and, if necessary, avoid them.

Alternatives to Outright Telling

Some people ask someone they trust. Rebecca got sick before she went on the new medications and wanted a certain friend to know but didn't have the energy to tell her: "I got another friend to tell her," she said. "And this other friend came back and said, 'You know, it's really hard to say that to people.'"

Sometimes people choose to avoid the problem of whom to tell by finding ways around making the decision. Some people do not tell, but instead let their friends and families ask. These people leave clues: they talk about friends who have HIV infection, leave pamphlets and books on HIV infection where others can find them, say someone at work told them a story about a person with HIV infection, and talk about TV programs on HIV infection and recommend their families watch them. The families and friends sense the truth. Then, if they can handle the information, they will ask; if they can't, they won't.

Some people do trial runs of telling, testing for rejection before telling. One woman was so afraid her children would reject her that she thought she could not tell them without breaking down. So she rehearsed by telling a cousin whose rejection she feared less, and when she finally told her children, she could keep the composure she wanted. Some people, like those who let their friends and families ask, leave clues. Then they judge by reactions to the clues whether telling will be safe or will result in rejection.

Other people find alternatives to the outright facts. If they become sick, they say they have pneumonia or a lung disease, herpes, leukemia, ulcers, meningitis, or hepatitis, or a cancer, or an infection of the nervous system. They choose whatever disease is most appropriate to their symptoms. Helen said, "I read in a medical book about a blood disease that can be either acute or fatal. I'm alive, so I say it's acute."

Chapter 2

Preventing Transmission of HIV Infection: Understanding How HIV Is Spread

- Principles of contagion
- Preventing transmission through sex, drugs, or pregnancy
- Preventing transmission during home care

HIV is a virus that infects white blood cells, primarily those called CD4 cells (also called T4 cells or T-helper cells). CD4 cells are found in several body fluids, but mainly in blood and in genital secretions. HIV is passed, or transmitted, when the CD4 cells from one person's blood or genital secretions get inside the body of another person. Most of the viruses are inside cells, but some may be free in the body fluids as well. Body fluids contain many more cells infected with HIV than they do free HIV. These body fluids are the vehicles for transmission of HIV.

The scientific evidence to support this method of transmission is compelling. What is known about the risk of transmitting HIV has come from two types of scientific studies: partly from studies of the virus, called *virology*; and principally from studies of the people who are infected with the virus, called *epidemiology*. The epidemiological studies came first in time. In 1981, epidemiologists began tracking cases of pneumocystis pneumonia in gay men; by 1983, when HIV was finally discovered, epidemiologists knew most of what was necessary to know about the spread of the disease. They knew that the disease, whatever its cause, was transmitted by sexual intercourse and by blood and by passage from an infected mother to her unborn child. They knew that this sort of transmission suggested that a microbe was responsible (other microbes, including cytomegalovirus and hepatitis B virus, are transmitted in precisely the same ways). In 1983, a French researcher, Luc Montagnier, reported the virology studies that described the virus that came to be called HIV.

But regardless of how compelling the scientific evidence is, misunderstanding of how HIV is transmitted is widespread and causes people a lot of worry. The purpose of this chapter is to discuss, first, what is known and what is not known about the risk of transmitting HIV, and second, how to prevent transmission. In other words, it is about how to avoid giving HIV to someone else and how to avoid getting it yourself.

Most of the public's misconception is based on the belief that HIV is transmitted the way more common viruses, like the influenza virus, are transmitted. We think it is important to emphasize that viruses like the influenza virus and HIV are enormously different, not only in the way they are transmitted, but also in the way they cause disease.

Principles of Contagion

Preventing transmission begins with understanding the principles that govern how infections are transmitted. These principles are called the *principles of contagion*.

Infectious diseases and *contagious diseases* are two different things. Infectious diseases are caused by *microbes;* microbes are viruses, bacteria, fungi, and parasites. Contagious diseases can be spread from person to person. Some diseases, like toxic shock syndrome or Legionnaires' disease, are infectious but not contagious. HIV infection, however, is both infectious (it is caused by a microbe) and contagious (with specific kinds of contact, it can be spread from one person to another). This chapter will begin by comparing HIV infection to another infectious and contagious disease most people know well from firsthand experience: influenza.

The microbe that causes influenza is a virus found in the nose, throat, and lungs of the person who is infected. Influenza is spread when secretions from the nose, throat, or lungs of the infected person are passed to another person. When an infected person coughs or sneezes on another person, or touches another person, these secretions and the virus they carry are transmitted.

People can be either susceptible or not susceptible to an influenza virus. If they have been infected with that particular virus or a closely related one before, or if they have been vaccinated against the virus, they already have antibodies against it, so they are not susceptible and will not get influenza. If they do not have these antibodies, they are susceptible and will get influenza.

Whether susceptible or not, the person will not become infected if the type of contact is wrong. Specific viruses can live only on specific tissues within the body. An influenza virus on the skin of your hand will not give you influenza; the same virus on the membranes of your nose, throat, or lungs will. If the virus is on your hand and you bring your hand to your mouth, however, you may get influenza.

Given susceptibility and the right type of contact, some viruses are more likely than others to be spread from person to person, that is, some viruses are transmitted with greater efficiency than others. Some viruses are difficult to spread; others are easy. For the influenza virus, for example, even very brief contact with a person who is infected is likely to result in transmission. Highly efficient transmission accounts for the annual epidemics of influenza.

The efficiency with which a virus is transmitted also depends on the number of viruses a person is exposed to, or the *inoculum size.* Living with a person with influenza is obviously more likely to result in successful transmission than simply working with that person in the same office. And being sneezed upon poses a greater risk than passing someone in a hallway. In short, how efficiently a virus is transmitted depends on both the number of influenza viruses and the type of contact.

A person, once infected, may continue to feel well for a day or two but, during this time, can still pass the virus to others. This early period between infection and the beginning of symptoms is called the *incubation period.*

HIV, like influenza, follows the same general principles of contagion. An infected person is the source of HIV. HIV is contagious if a person is susceptible and the contact is of the kind necessary for transmission. And HIV has a certain efficiency of transmission and a certain incubation period. There the resemblance ends.

This point deserves emphasis. Much of the misunderstanding about HIV infection has been based on the assumption that HIV is transmitted like other common infectious diseases. It isn't. In brief, for HIV, the types of contact are very specific, transmission is inefficient, and HIV's incubation period is very long.

Sources of HIV

A person with HIV infection is almost the sole source of this infection. The only time a person is not directly the source is in the laboratory when a researcher has taken inadequate precautions and is infected while working with large numbers of the virus. More than a million people have HIV infection, however, and only about three became infected by working with cultures of the virus.

Any person with HIV infection, regardless of symptoms, should be considered capable of transmitting the disease.

Types of Contact

The white blood cells that HIV infects, the CD4 cells, are found in differing numbers in different body fluids. As a result, the numbers of HIV also differ in different body fluids. The numbers of HIV in body fluids—the usual source of transmission—are greatest in semen, vaginal fluid, breast milk, and blood. HIV is unlikely to be in saliva, stool, or tears, though it has been found in these fluids in a minority of people, and then only in very low numbers. HIV has not been found in urine.

In order to cause infection, HIV must travel from the body fluids of an infected person into the bloodstream of an uninfected person. The skin that covers the outside of the body is a formidable barrier. If the skin is intact, simple contact between HIV and the skin will not transmit HIV. The mucous membranes that cover most of the insides of the mouth, vagina, and rectum are also a barrier to the virus. If the skin or a mucous membrane is broken—if it has cuts or sores—the virus can get into the bloodstream. Thus, infected blood (including menstrual blood), vaginal fluids, or semen on intact skin is almost invariably safe. But on skin or mucous membranes that have an open sore or a cut, the same fluids can possibly transmit the virus. Injecting large amounts of infected blood into the body—like a transfusion of blood from an infected person—is the most efficient method of transmission.

We can provide absolute assurance that most types of common contact carry no risk of transmitting the virus. These include a variety of experiences often referred to as "casual contact": shaking hands, hugging, sharing a toilet, sharing eating utensils, closed-mouth kissing, being sneezed on, and so forth. Not only has infection through casual contact not happened, it is biologically unrealistic to suppose it might.

There are three primary types of contact that can result in transmission of HIV:

- Sexual contact, that is, contact with infected genital secretions (semen, vaginal fluids)

- Injection of infected blood through transfusions or needle sharing

- Pregnancy in an infected mother—now rare because of effective preventive treatment

Other kinds of contact more rarely result in transmission of HIV. These are

- Breast-feeding by an infected mother (transmission to baby)

- Breast-feeding by an infected baby (transmission to mother)

- Organ transplantation using organs from infected donors

- Artificial insemination from infected sperm donors

- Needlestick injuries in health care professionals caring for infected people

Oral sex, either cunnilingus (oral sex performed on a woman) or fellatio (oral sex performed on a man), can transmit HIV infection. The greater risk is fellatio: the semen of an infected man has more HIV than the vaginal secretions of an infected woman.

The combined total for these rarer types of contact accounts for about 0.1 percent of U.S. cases, actually amounting to only about 500 of the first 500,000 cases of AIDS reported to the Centers for Disease Control and Prevention (CDC). Transfusions, now screened for HIV, are excluded from this number.

We are sure about what kinds of contact do and do not transmit the virus. More than 500,000 people with AIDS have been studied by the CDC. The types of contact listed above together account for 95 to 97 percent. When researchers went back and looked specifically at the remaining 3 to 5 percent of people not accounted for by these types of contact, they found that most were not problems: many people acknowledged risks when questioned by a more experienced interviewer; some people were so seriously ill at the time of reporting that no reliable medical history could be obtained; and some never had HIV infection to begin with. By the time researchers were done, the type of contact responsible for transmission remained ambiguous in about 0.2 percent of the people. Given the likelihood that people will lie about such sensitive issues as homosexuality and the use of illegal drugs, 2 people out of every 1,000 is an incredibly low figure.

At the same time, we must acknowledge that other types of contact, though unlikely to transmit HIV, might do so at least theoretically. HIV has been found in low numbers in saliva, stool, and tears. HIV has not been found in urine. Although transmission through these fluids is biologically possible, it doesn't seem to happen; the CDC, which tracks all cases of AIDS, has no case in which the only type of contact was clearly through feces or urine or tears. There is one possible case of a bite transmitting HIV, and another case of presumed transmission through deep kissing, but the details of both cases are sketchy. Perhaps the inoculum size—the numbers of the virus—in these fluids is simply too low. In any case, transmission of HIV through these types of contact is extremely inefficient and is not known to happen. Unfortunately, the CDC and other groups continue to talk about "body fluids" as the source of HIV infection. This gives the wrong impression that the source of infection is all body fluids. In fact, the only body fluids that are the source of infection are semen, vaginal fluids, breast milk, and blood, including menstrual blood.

One type of contact that people worry about is mouth contact. Infection by mouth may occur in three ways: breast-feeding, oral sex, or deep kissing. All three are biologically plausible methods of transmission and all three have occurred. The three are enormously different, however, in the level of risk. Breast-feeding results in heavy exposure to infected CD4 cells in breast milk; in African countries, where the major studies have been done, the risk of transmission is 15 to 25 percent. Oral sex, or fellatio, is also a plausible risk for the same reason: semen has a large number of infected CD4 cells. The exact risk with oral sex, however, is hard to quantify because most people practicing oral sex are likely practicing other high-risk behaviors as well. Most researchers suspect that the risk of oral sex is much lower than the risk of breast-feeding but far greater than the risk of deep kissing. Deep kissing is low risk; transmission of HIV through saliva is vanishingly rare, possibly because the numbers of the virus in saliva are low.

Another type of contact people worry about is indirect: becoming infected by a virus on a surface outside the body. To repeat, we are not aware that anyone (except the rare laboratory worker using high concentrations of the virus) has ever become infected by the virus living on a surface outside the body. The reason is that HIV cannot survive outside its host cells, and outside the body, cells die quickly. When host cells die, HIV dies with them. Although HIV can survive outside the body on a surface for up to fifteen days, the numbers of viruses on a surface fall rapidly to levels well below those necessary for infection.

A third possibility that people used to worry about, probably because the news media have paid a lot of attention to it, is that insects, particularly mosquitoes, could conceivably transmit the virus. The argument is that insects transmit other microbes in the blood, such as malaria. But even in Africa, where mosquito-borne diseases like malaria are common, scientists have not been able to find a clear case in which HIV has been transmitted by a mosquito. AIDS in Africa is a disease found almost exclusively in babies of infected mothers and sexually active adults, especially those in cities. Mosquitoes, however, do not select out babies and sexually active adults in cities to bite; mosquitoes are everywhere and bite everyone.

A fourth possibility is that a patient might get HIV infection from an infected health care worker, like a surgeon or dentist. In 1990 a dentist in Florida apparently infected six of his patients, though exactly how the dentist transmitted HIV infection has never been sorted out and never will be. This case raised a new possible mechanism of infection—acquisition from your dentist or possibly from your surgeon, presumably by mixing of blood. A second case involved an orthopedic surgeon in France who is believed to have infected one of the patients he operated on. Ensuing studies show that these two cases were isolated events. Testing of about 20,000 patients who had surgery or dental care from someone with HIV infection failed to turn up a single case of HIV transmission. The paucity of cases has confirmed the incredibly small risk associated with transmission from surgeon to patient.

Efficiency of Transmission

Because the types of contact are so specific and the numbers of the virus in some body fluids are so low, HIV is not transmitted efficiently. Certain kinds of contact transmit HIV more efficiently than others. This section will discuss efficiency of transmission, that is, the likelihood that a given type of contact will transmit HIV. The types of contact that transmit the virus most efficiently are those with the highest risk for infection.

There are four categories of risk for HIV infection, from the kinds of contact that are most likely to transmit the virus to the kinds that are least likely to do so.

1. Very likely risks. These are well-established, common ways to transmit the virus. They account for over 99 percent of cases. The order in which they are discussed below does not imply that there is a hierarchy of risk within this category. All these behaviors pose a high risk of infection.

The first high risk is nonsafe sex—that is, sex without condoms, or sex that involves exchange of body fluids—with people known to have HIV infection, or with people who have a high risk for HIV infection. The risk of getting HIV through nonsafe sex with an infected person is roughly estimated from studies done of discordant couples, couples (usually spouses) in a regular sexual relationship in which one partner has HIV infection and the other does not. These studies show that without condoms and without HIV treatment, the risk of HIV transmission is one per five hundred to one thousand episodes of vaginal sex.

How efficiently HIV is transmitted during sexual intercourse depends on a number of factors. One of the most important is whether the uninfected person has open sores on the genitals. The most common cause of genital sores are other sexually transmitted diseases such as syphilis and chancroid. The most common cause of genital sores in the United States and in the world is genital herpes. Open sores from these or other causes allow the virus to enter directly into the blood. The risk of transmission consequently increases enormously when sores are present on the genitals.

A second factor increasing the risk of transmission is the type of sexual practice. Virtually all sexual contact that has resulted in infection with HIV has been either anal or vaginal intercourse. Studies of transmission of HIV infection among gay men suggest that anal intercourse is an especially efficient means of transmission. During anal intercourse, the thin walls of the rectum are often cut or scraped, exposing blood vessels to infected semen, and the surface area of exposure to the virus is very large. The vaginal wall is thicker and less likely to be cut, and the vagina is short compared to the colon, so transmission is less likely but still distinctly possible. The estimated risk of HIV transmission with a single episode of unprotected anal intercourse is 1 to 3 per 100 (1 to 3 percent); the risk with a single episode of unprotected vaginal intercourse is 1 per 500 to 1,000 (0.1 to 0.2 percent). Although the 1 percent figure for anal intercourse seems low, remember that this is the presumed mechanism of transmission for one-third of all AIDS cases in the United States. In short, any sexual practice that exposes the blood of an uninfected person to the blood (including menstrual blood) or semen or vaginal fluid of an infected person will allow transmission of HIV.

A third factor, and probably the most important, is the numbers of HIV, or the viral load. The idea is simply that infection is more likely if there are more viruses. People have the highest number of viruses—the highest viral loads—in the first three to four weeks after transmission. During this early stage, most people are completely unaware they are infected. Because viral loads are so high and because people are usually unaware they are infected, this early stage of infection actually accounts for an estimated 30 to 40 percent of all sexual transmissions. After three to five weeks, the body develops antibodies to the virus, so the viral load drops and the probability of transmission drops along with it. During the late stage of untreated HIV infection, the viral load increases again, but transmission during this stage is limited because people are sick and less interested in sex. The chances of transmission are about 1 in 100 acts of sexual intercourse in the early stage, 1 in 1,000 acts of sexual intercourse in the chronic stage, and 1 in 500 acts of sexual intercourse in the late stage.

It should be noted that these estimates are based on long-term studies done in Africa of discordant couples without HIV treatment. Since treatment reduces viral load, it should also reduce the probability of transmission; this makes biologic sense, but it is not yet scientifically proved. A concern is that people under treatment who believe their disease is unlikely to be transmitted might practice high-risk behavior: gay men do have high rates of such other sexually transmitted diseases as syphilis and gonorrhea—though the data establishing these rates are restricted to a small number of gay men in specific locations. The bottom line is that regardless of viral load, stage of infection, or treatment status, preventing sexual transmission of HIV requires no sex or safe sex.

A second very likely risk of transmitting HIV infection comes with sharing needles or works (spoons, cotton, syringes) with a person who injects drugs, especially in cities with a high incidence of HIV infection among injection drug users. HIV can be transmitted by blood left on a contaminated needle, or by blood left in the syringe, or by blood on any other components of the works used to prepare the drug for injection. The risk of HIV transmission with needle sharing is estimated at about 3 per 1,000, or 0.3 percent. Factors that influence the efficiency of transmission include the amount of blood, how long the blood has been outside the body before injection, whether the blood is dried, and how many viruses are in the blood. For people who inject drugs, the risk of getting HIV from sharing a needle with a person with HIV infection appears to be about the same as the risk of having sexual intercourse with that person.

A third very likely risk is pregnancy in a woman with HIV infection. An infected mother taking no anti-HIV drugs has a 20 to 35 percent chance of transmitting HIV to her unborn child, unless she delivers her baby by cesarean section. Transmission can take place while the infant is still in the uterus or when the baby passes through the birth canal and is in contact with the mother's genital secretions and blood. When mothers don't take anti-HIV drugs, one-third of transmissions happen in the uterus and two-thirds during birth. When mothers do take anti-HIV drugs, the likelihood of transmission drops; of the transmissions that do occur, about two-thirds happen while infant is still in the uterus and one-third during birth. The lesson here is that when the mother takes drugs to reduce HIV, the infant is less likely to become infected during birth. If the mother's viral load is "undetectable," the risk of transmission to the infant is only 2 percent. If the mother's viral load is not under control, we usually recommend that delivery be done by cesarean section. When delivery is done by cesarean section, the infant's probability of becoming infected is only 2 percent as well.

The bottom line is straightforward. Regardless of how the infection is transmitted, a person with a high viral load is more likely to transmit infection. For instance, someone with a viral load of 100,000 copies of the virus per milliliter is at least ten times more likely to transmit HIV than someone with a viral load of 100. And a low viral load in the blood reduces the risk of transmission but never eliminates it. Furthermore, no one working in this field thinks that the new treatments now being developed will eliminate the risk of transmission. At best, the situation is still much like playing Russian roulette, just with more empty chambers.

2. *Likely risks.* This section discusses the ways in which HIV may possibly be transmitted. The risks are scientifically established, though actual transmission in these ways is rare.

The first likely risk is safer sex with people known to have HIV infection or with people who have a high risk of HIV infection. Safer sex is sex with condoms, or sexual contact that does not involve getting semen, blood, or vaginal fluid from one person's body into another's. Though safer sex is known to be safer, no one believes it is completely safe. The failure rate of condoms—due to breakage or improper use—is 2 to 5 percent. With the proper use of latex and polyurethane condoms, the protection is nearly 100 percent.

The second likely risk is nonsafe heterosexual sex with multiple partners. The risk is higher if partners are anonymous, injection drug users, gay or bisexual men, or prostitutes in cities with high rates of HIV infection. No one knows exactly what the risk of nonsafe sex with multiple partners is; the risk depends entirely on whether your partners are likely to be infected.

The third likely risk is breast-feeding. The risk of transmitting HIV with breast-feeding is high, probably 15 to 25 percent, if done for six to twelve months. The risk appears to diminish with time but never entirely disappears. Drugs to reduce the amount of HIV in the mother and drugs given to the baby to prevent transmission are both effective, but no one knows exactly how effective. Women in developed countries can easily solve the problem of transmitting HIV infection with breast-feeding, simply by avoiding breast-feeding. In developing countries, however, the issues are more complex.

The fourth likely risk is needlestick injury, primarily for health care workers: 1 in 300 needlestick injuries has transmitted the virus to the person stuck when the source of the stick had HIV infection. If the health care worker takes AZT promptly after being exposed, the risk is reduced by 80 percent, to about 1 in 1,500. Of the 4 million health care workers in this country, about 57 have HIV infections from exposures to infected patients. Nearly all of the transmissions were caused by "sharps injuries." A sharps injury is an injury with a sharp instrument like a needle or a scalpel during which the health care worker's blood mixes with the patient's blood. Of every 300 sharps injuries involving patients with known HIV infection, 1 health care worker will become infected. The risk is much higher than 1 in 300 if the injury was deep, if the health care worker was exposed to a lot of infected blood, or if the infected patient's viral load was high. Without these risks, the probability of transmission from an infected patient is much less than 1 in 300. Other kinds of transmission to health care workers are rare. About five health care workers became infected when blood splashed into their eyes, mouth, or skin. This kind of transmission is less than 1 per 1,000 when the blood carries HIV. And it appears that rare patients may acquire HIV infection from infected health care workers as well: we know of one dentist who transmitted HIV to six patients, though just how the transmission occurred is unclear; and we suspect HIV transmission from an infected orthopedic surgeon to his patient during surgery and from a gynecologist to his patient, both in France. These are the only three known cases.

The fifth likely risk is blood transfusion, artificial insemination, or organ transplantation from an infected donor: between 1978, when HIV infection first appeared, and 1985, when the Red Cross began screening all blood for HIV, this was a high risk if the donated blood contained HIV. About 90 percent of the people who received HIV-contaminated blood became infected with HIV. Now the blood supply is almost, but not completely, clear of HIV: it is estimated that about 1 in 500,000 units slips past the HIV screening process. The same scenario held for people with hemophilia, who are treated with a blood product called clotting factor, which is pooled from the blood of several thousand donors. Between 1978 and 1985, about 50 percent of people with hemophilia who were treated became infected with HIV. Currently, not only are all blood donors screened, but the clotting factor is treated so that any HIV that does slip through is destroyed before transfusion. Screening donors and treating blood works very well but not perfectly. Each year in this country, a small number of people get infected with HIV after receiving transfusions with screened blood. During the first three years after screening began, 18 people with hemophilia are known to have become infected from clotting factor; currently, the annual rate is less than 1 per 1,000. And there is one famous case of HIV being transmitted by organ transplantation. A man killed by gunshot donated various organs and tissues to 58 people. Though his blood test was negative, 7 of the recipients became infected. Probably the donor was tested in the "window" between infection and a positive blood test (see Appendix B, "Understanding Tests for HIV"). Note that this is the only case of infection among the 60,000 organs and 1 million tissues transplanted in the United States since 1985. Finally, in the United States, at least 7 women have become infected through artificial insemination, but all these transmissions occurred before 1985, when semen donors began to be screened. Donors are now screened, so this mechanism of transmission appears to be eliminated.

The sixth likely risk is unprotected oral sex. No one knows just how much of a risk unprotected oral sex, or fellatio, is. People have definitely become infected through unprotected oral sex, probably because semen has heavy concentrations of CD4 cells. The problem with figuring out the risk exactly is finding people who have practiced no other risk behaviors except oral sex. Oral sex performed on a woman is much less likely to transmit HIV. Inserting the fingers into the vagina, or fisting, is unlikely to transmit HIV because no body fluid is exchanged. Nevertheless, there is a theoretical risk if the skin on the hand has cuts or abrasions.

The seventh likely risk is biting: there are several reports of people getting HIV infection from human bites, but all save one of these reports were tarnished by the coexistence of other risk factors. One estimate of the risk of transmission when the biter has HIV is 1 in 1,000. One reason for the low rate is that HIV is not usually found in saliva, and when it is, it is in low numbers. A much greater risk is bleeding gums, the apparent cause of a widely publicized case attributed to deep kissing.

The eighth likely risk is home care: people with AIDS often require extensive home care by someone with no training in the methods of controlling the spread of infection. In the hospital, these methods of controlling infection, called "universal precautions," consist of a barrier between the caregiver and such infectious material as blood, stool, or pus. Universal precautions are relatively easy to learn. Most important to know is that now hundreds of thousands of people with AIDS have received home care by loved ones, and we are aware of only eight caregivers who have become infected with HIV as a result of their care. These eight apparently took no precautions.

It is important to emphasize the infrequency of the transmission of HIV in this second category of "likely risks," compared to the first category of "very likely risks." Of the million-plus cases of HIV infection in this country, this second category of "likely risks" accounts for about 0.02 percent, or 1 case in 10,000.

3. Biologically plausible risks, but unlikely and unconfirmed. These types of contact might possibly transmit HIV, but they are unlikely to. They are obviously controversial because they are almost impossible to either prove or disprove. If they do transmit HIV, they do so only rarely. As a matter of fact, there are no established cases in this category at all; these risks are totally theoretical. We include them to pacify the "what-if" crowd, the people who worry about risks that are biologically plausible but have no evidence to support or reject them.

Sharing toothbrushes or razors with an infected person

Exposure to body fluids (tears, urine, feces, saliva, sweat) other than genital secretions or blood

Exchange of saliva with deep kissing

Mosquito transmissions (according to studies, improbable and probably impossible; it is placed in this category simply to be conservative)

4. Transmission that is not biologically possible. Transmitting the virus through the following types of contact is inconceivable. The first lesson learned in medical school is "never to say never": nevertheless, these types of contact not only lack precedent but also appear absurd on the basis of our current scientific knowledge of HIV infection.

Shaking hands

Sharing a toilet

Sharing eating utensils

Being sneezed upon

Living in the same household

Working in the same room or attending the same classroom

Sexual transmission by partners known to be monogamous and un-infected

Any contact with any pet

Closed-mouth kissing

Incubation Period

For most infectious diseases, the incubation period—the period from the time of infection until the person feels the first symptoms—is a few days or weeks. HIV infection is almost unique; its incubation period is five to eight years. This long incubation period accounts for the large reservoir of persons who are infected for years before they are aware of it. Despite not having symptoms, the person infected with HIV is contagious to others throughout the incubation period.

Preventing Transmission through Sex, Drugs, or Pregnancy

Safer Sex

The risk of HIV transmission by sexual contact can be reduced in three ways: (1) reducing the viral load is a theoretically effective method that will probably help reduce transmission but will never be completely effective, because the risk is always relative and never zero; (2) treatment with drugs against HIV after initial exposure works for health care workers with occupational exposures, but the drugs must be taken within hours, and we have no proof that such treatment will also work with sexual exposure; and (3) "safe sex," based on extensive theory and scientific data. Safe sex, to be absolutely safe, means no "exchange of body fluids"; that is, semen, blood (including menstrual blood), or vaginal fluids must not pass from one person's body into another person's. Perhaps, taking human fallibility into account, the better term is "safer sex."

One good way to prevent transmission of HIV during sexual intercourse is to use a barrier against body fluids—that is, use condoms. Condoms should be used during vaginal, oral, or anal sex to prevent exposure not only to HIV but also to all other sexually transmitted diseases, including gonorrhea, syphilis, herpes, and chlamydia.

The Food and Drug Administration inspects condoms for leakage: ten ounces of water are poured into the condom, and the condom is pressed and rolled along blotter paper. If more than 4 per 1,000 condoms leak, the entire manufacturer's lot must be destroyed. The major problems with condoms, however, are not that they leak, but that they are used inconsistently, they break, or they fall off. Surveys show that fewer than 10 percent of Americans use condoms regularly for sexual intercourse. An estimated 2 to 5 percent of condoms tear during use, usually because they are used improperly, not because they are flawed.

The usefulness of condoms in reducing HIV transmission has been established by two studies of discordant couples. In discordant couples, the couple has regular monogamous sex; and one partner has HIV but the other does not. Among the discordant couples who used condoms irregularly, the rate of HIV transmission to the uninfected partner was 10 to 12 percent. Among the couples who used condoms regularly, the rate was 0 to 2 percent. For both groups, the average number of occasions of intercourse was about 120 times per couple. The following suggestions should improve the safety of safer sex:

1. Use latex or polyurethane condoms. They are less porous—that is, they are less likely to have minute holes through which the virus can pass—than condoms made from animal skins. The latex and polyurethane varieties are also substantially less expensive. Condoms manufactured by large companies—Ansell, Inc., Carter-Wallace, Circle Rubber Company, and Schmid Laboratories—are generally more reliable than those from small companies that are sold in novelty shops.

2. Reduce the risk of breakage by leaving the condom in the package until used. Condoms should be stored in a cool and dry place out of direct sunlight. With appropriate storage, most condoms retain their durability for up to three years. Condoms that are in damaged packages or show such signs of age as brittle texture, sticky surface, or discoloration should be discarded. Open the package carefully to avoid tearing the condom. Maintain an adequate supply of condoms.

3. The use of lubricants is encouraged, but oil-based lubricants (like Vaseline, Crisco, baby oil, cooking oil, and skin moisturizers) will dissolve latex and leave microscopic holes and should therefore be avoided. The preferred lubricants are water-based (like K-Y Jelly). Many condoms are supplied with such lubricants as oil, glycerine, or surgical jelly. The lubricant should be placed on the outside of the condom and inside the partner.

4. In 1994, *Consumers' Guide* evaluated 37 brands of latex condoms, 6,500 condoms in all, with air inflation tests that measure breakage potential. The best products were Excita Extra Ultra Ribbed, Ramses Extra Ribbed, and the U.S.-produced version of Sheik Elite. The "best buy" award went to Touch, from Protex, which cost less than 35 cents each.

5. Fewer than 1 percent of people are allergic to latex and experience irritation or burning. This allergy is most common in medical personnel who have extensive contact with latex gloves, catheters, masks, etc. Many of the allergic reactions are actually reactions to the lubricants, spermicides, or materials used in manufacturing; changing the brand of latex supplies is therefore effective. For true allergies to latex, the next best alternative is condoms made from polyurethane (like the Avanti brand).

6. The spermicide nonoxynol 9 rapidly kills both HIV and sperm. It also kills other microbes that cause sexually transmitted diseases like

gonorrhea and chlamydia. Nonoxynol 9 is available as spermicidal creams, jellies, or contraceptive sponges. Nonoxynol 9 was once widely advocated to reduce HIV transmission but has fallen into disfavor because it apparently can cause vaginal irritation and tiny abrasions that actually increase the chance of becoming infected. Current research is now in hot pursuit of other vaginal microbicides that do the job without the irritation.

7. The condom must be put on before any sexual contact, oral or genital or anal. The tip is placed over the erect penis. If the condom has a reservoir tip, first squeeze out the air; if the condom has no reservoir tip, leave about a half-inch space for semen, then squeeze the air out. Unroll the condom down the entire length of the penis.

8. Condoms should be used for vaginal or anal sex and for fellatio (oral sex performed on a man). Rubber or latex dams placed over the woman's genitals should be used for cunnilingus (oral sex performed on a woman). Latex dental dams are available in dental supply stores. There is now a female condom for vaginal intercourse. The female condom looks like a tunnel with two rings at the ends; one ring fits high in the vagina and the other is external. The female condom is expensive and doesn't work as well as male condoms for birth control, and therefore by extension, against HIV transmission. Its main advantage is that it allows women better control.

9. If a condom leaks or breaks, both partners should wash their genitals with soap and water. A spermicide may also be useful for protecting against HIV transmission, but it should be applied rapidly. Douching is not recommended for women because it can force semen up through the cervix. When accidental exposure to HIV has happened, some health services provide a one-month course of anti-HIV drugs. Remember, however, that the drugs must be taken with 48 to 72 hours of exposure, and preferably within 1 to 2 hours. Furthermore, the drugs cause many side effects; the cost of the drugs is $500 to $1,000 for the month's supply, and no one has any evidence that the drugs will prevent transmission.

10. Avoid contact with the menstrual blood of any woman with HIV. Menstrual blood also contains HIV. Use a condom.

Any method of birth control that allows pregnancy will also allow transmission of HIV. Some methods of birth control—rhythm or the pill, for example—prevent pregnancy but allow transmission of HIV.

The alternative to condoms is to have sexual contact that does not exchange body fluids at all. This kind of contact includes body-to-body rubbing, acting out sexual fantasies, or mutual masturbation using disposable latex gloves.

The basic principle of safer sex is to avoid getting the body fluids of a person with HIV infection into the body of another person. That can be accomplished by a barrier—condoms, latex dams, latex gloves—between the body fluids of the person with HIV infection and the other person, or by sexual contact or play that does not involve body fluids at all. For specific safer sex practices, and for alternatives to sex, see the booklet put out by the Gay Men's Health Crisis (GMHC), 129 W. 20th Street, New York, N.Y. 10011, 1–212–807–6655. Even though GMHC specifies gay men in its name, much of its information on safer sex practices applies to heterosexual sexual practices as well.

Avoid Injection Drug Use

The obvious way to avoid transmitting HIV during injection drug use is to stop using drugs that are injected. Many people who use drugs, however, are unable to curb this habit. Some people who would like to stop using drugs may have difficulty finding programs—such as methadone clinics or detoxification centers—that are available. Those who find it impossible to stop using drugs by injection should avoid sharing needles, avoid sharing works, and, of course, practice safer sex.

Anyone who can't avoid sharing should clean the needle and works.

Table 1. Percentage Who Accidentally Become Pregnant in One Year Using Various Birth Control Methods

	Typical Use	Perfect Use
Spermicide only	21%	6%
Rhythm	20	9
Withdrawal	19	4
Diaphragm & spermicide	18	6
Condom	12	3
Pill	3	below 1
Sterilization	below 1	below 1

Source: Adapted from Robert A. Hatcher et al., Contraceptive Technology, 16th rev. ed. (New York: Irvington Publishers, 1994), 113.

Clean needles are often available from needle-exchange programs, which seem to reduce HIV risk without changing the frequency of drug dependency. Another alternative, available in 48 states, is to ask physicians to prescribe needles and syringes and pharmacists to dispense needles and syringes. When re-use is necessary, cleaning between uses makes sense and should work, but there are no guarantees. The few studies that have been done have disappointing results—meaning either that cleaning doesn't work well, or people don't clean often enough or well enough. One problem with cleaning is that it is tedious, and the two-minute wait might seem like two hours. If you decide to clean, then clean needles and syringes by flushing them with household bleach and then rinsing with water, as follows:

1. Use full-strength household bleach.

2. Pour the bleach into a glass, immerse the needle and syringe to cover completely, and then draw the bleach up to fill the syringe. Bleach should probably be left in the syringe not less than two minutes. The two-minute period is absolutely critical.

3. Discharge the bleach and repeat the process.

4. Rinse the syringe by filling and discharging water twice.

5. Alcohol is an adequate substitute for bleach.

The drawback to these ways of preventing transmission of HIV is that using any drugs at all reduces a person's inhibitions. With reduced inhibitions, people are much less likely to practice safer sex and to avoid sharing needles and works, in spite of good intentions. Other substances that reduce inhibitions carry the same danger. This applies to mind-altering drugs that are not necessarily injected, such as alcohol, cocaine, crack, amyl nitrate (poppers), marijuana, barbiturates, and amphetamines (speed).

Think Hard about Pregnancy; Avoid Breast-Feeding

Getting pregnant—as of course people wish to do—without risking transmission of HIV can be done with artificial insemination if the sperm comes from an uninfected man; or if the man's viral load is undetectable, then possibly with sperm-washing. Nevertheless, women with HIV infection may wish to avoid pregnancy. The probability of transmission of HIV to the baby, if the mother takes drugs to reduce HIV, is about 7 percent. This probability varies with the mother's viral load: if her viral load is high at delivery, the probability of transmission is also high; but if her viral load is under 1,000, then the risk of transmission is under 1 percent. Women with higher viral loads have the option of delivering the baby by cesarean section, which reduces the risk of transmission to less than 2 percent. In this case, the cesarean section must be done before the delivery date, at 38 weeks, and before the membranes rupture (before the water breaks). Any woman considering pregnancy or considering an abortion to terminate a pregnancy absolutely must discuss these issues with an obstetrician versed in HIV infection.

To avoid pregnancy, the most reliable method is tubal ligation, or having your tubes tied. The birth control pill is also extremely reliable, 98 percent effective. The rate of failure with condoms is 10 percent, so condoms are considered unreliable. To prevent transmission of HIV infection and other sexually transmitted diseases, use condoms. To prevent transmission and pregnancy, use condoms plus the pill.

If abortion is desired, it is best performed during the first fourteen weeks of pregnancy, when it is considered most safe. Abortions during the period of fourteen to twenty weeks are offered by some specialized clinics, but hospitalization is usually required and the risk to the mother is somewhat greater.

A woman who chooses to continue the pregnancy needs to tell her obstetrician about her HIV infection. In fact, the standard policy is now to give HIV tests to all pregnant women, because the risk of transmitting HIV to the baby can be reduced so effectively with drugs that control HIV and with deliveries by cesarean section. The original study demonstrating the benefit of treatment showed that AZT could reduce the rate of transmission from the mother to the baby from 25 percent to 8 percent. Subsequent studies showed that AZT plus additional drugs could reduce the transmission rate to the baby to 2 to 3 percent. It was then recommended that all pregnant women with HIV infection who decide to continue the pregnancy take standard HAART.

The following are principles for HIV care during pregnancy: (1) The mother should usually receive treatment with multiple drugs, which include AZT because it works. (2) The HIV drug to avoid during pregnancy is efavirenz. (3) The goal of therapy should be to get the viral load as low as possible, both for the mother's health and for reducing transmission to the baby. (4) Consider cesarean section at 38 weeks an option if the viral load is not reduced to less than 2,000. (5) Drugs used to control HIV are often difficult for pregnant women to take because of side effects, especially gastrointestinal problems. Furthermore, different concentrations of HIV drugs are used during pregnancy. Consequently, the pregnant woman with HIV infection needs an obstetrician who specializes in HIV infection.

The safety of the drugs used for HIV infection in pregnant women has been studied for ten years through the HIV Drug Registry, which keeps track of the experiences of pregnant women with all antiretroviral drugs and records the side effects to the unborn child. So far the only unsafe drug found is efavirenz, which causes birth defects in about one in fifty infants exposed to the drug during the first trimester, the first three months of pregnancy. As a result physicians are now warned not to prescribe efavirenz to any woman who is pregnant or likely to become pregnant. Other HIV drugs appear to be safe, but the track record on some of them is still sparse. Obstetricians who specialize in HIV infection stay aware of all the numbers.

The woman who chooses to continue the pregnancy also needs to tell her pediatrician about her HIV infection. The pediatrician will then give the appropriate preventive treatments—usually including AZT for six weeks—to the child. The pediatrician will also know what to look for during the child's medical evaluations, will increase the number of visits, and will decide whether to change the schedule of childhood vaccinations. Many pediatricians do not feel competent to care for children with HIV infection. Nor do many pediatricians know which tests for telling whether the child is infected are currently in vogue; the standard blood test for HIV infection will not give valid results until the child is 15 months old, but alternative tests, including the viral load test, are now commonly used. It might be best to ask your pediatrician to refer you to a pediatrician with a specific interest in HIV infection. You should get this reference immediately, because beginning the treatment early might be critical to the treatment's success.

The woman who continues the pregnancy should also plan not to breast-feed her baby. HIV is found in breast milk, and the baby could also be infected by breast-feeding (see above, page 39).

Women who are already pregnant should take the test for HIV. This testing is for the sake of both the mother and the child. Some obstetricians offer such tests to all pregnant women, some offer the test only to those considered at risk for HIV infection, some do not think of HIV infection at all unless reminded, and some states have laws requiring that HIV tests be offered.

Preventing Transmission during Home Care

Home care means living with or caring for someone with HIV infection. It does not include sexual contact. These guidelines are based on recommendations by the CDC and on extensive experience with home care and hospital care. You should know that these recommendations are intentionally overcautious.

Reality of the Risk

There is no risk associated with simply living in the same household or working in the same office with a person who has HIV infection. This generally involves the types of nonintimate contact previously referred to as "casual contact" (see above, under "Types of Contact"). The type of contact that might involve the risk of transmitting HIV nonsexually usually takes place during medical care in the more advanced stages of disease. Every health care worker who has acquired HIV infection nonsexually has been exposed to the blood or bloody fluids of a person with HIV infection; transmission usually occurs after health care workers inadvertently inject infected blood into themselves.

The type of contact involved in home care of a person with HIV infection carries, in CDC's extensive experience, almost no risk. Only about eight of the tens of thousands of people who provide home care for people with HIV infection have acquired HIV as a result of nonsexual contact. Most of the people who did not become infected provided complete care of people with HIV infection for many months or even years without the benefit of any special training and without any special precautions to prevent HIV infection. Nevertheless, we recommend that caregivers use some simple precautions to be extra safe.

How can we be sure these are the only eight exceptions? We obviously cannot, although most physicians question people with HIV infection for type of contact, and any physician would promptly report contact through home care because of its importance as a public health issue. Testing the blood of people who are caregivers of people with HIV infection answers the question more formally: fourteen studies of well over one thousand caregivers have not identified any additional people who acquired HIV infection by nonsexual contact.

In short, for those who live in the same household and do things that are common for friends and relatives to do, the risk is nil. For those who care daily for people who are seriously ill, the risk is very low, but not zero.

Guidelines for Preventing Transmission of HIV during Home Care

People with HIV infection and those involved in their care will want to lower the already low risk of transmission. This is easily accomplished by using the basic and simple guidelines described below.

Handwashing. Handwashing is an important way to prevent the spread of most infectious microbes, not just HIV. Nevertheless, alcohol wipes are more effective than soap at killing viruses.

Table 2. Sources of HIV Infection in the Estimated 1.5 Million Americans Thought to Have This Disease

How Transmitted	Est. No. in U.S.	Body Fluid	Comments
Sexual contact	1,000,000	Genital secretion	Gay men account for 40% of all AIDS cases, although heterosexual transmission accounts for 29% of new cases in 2002
Injecting drugs	400,000	Blood on shared needles	95% are regular users (more than 1 time/week); 5% are occasional users; together they account for 27% of all new cases reported in 2002
Blood transfusions	40,000	Blood	Largely stopped in 1985 due to screening of blood donors; accounted for 0.2% of new cases in 2001, most of which were infected before 1985
Hemophilia	10,000	Blood products	As above; about 20 documented cases since April 1985 (less than 1/1,000/year)
Infants	8,700	Mother to fetus	Rates substantially reduced due to HIV drugs given to pregnant women; accounted for 90 (0.2%) new cases reported in 2002
Health care workers with exposures in the workplace	57	Blood	These are the only well-established cases reported through 2005; about 130 additional cases are less well established
Organ transplant recipients	38	Blood or organ tissue from donor	This group largely stopped due to screening of donors; the exception is 7 cases from

(*continued*)

Table 2. (*Continued*)

How Transmitted	Est. No. in U.S.	Body Fluid	Comments
			a single donor with a false negative screening test in 1985
Household contact	8	Not known	4 cases were child-to-child transmission; 3 were care providers of people with HIV infection
Artificial insemination	7	Semen	All transmissions before 1985 when donor screening started
Patients with exposures to health care workers	6	Blood	All 6 cases are patients of the Florida dentist; one possible additional case may be a surgeon in France
Unknown	1,000	Not known	About 2 cases in 1,000 (0.2%) that have been adequately investigated have shown no clearly defined risk

Note: Data are based in part on estimates by the U.S. Public Health Service for 2004. The Comments column refers to cases reported since April 1985, the date when the blood test first became available for screening blood and organ donors. The estimated total in the U.S. is 1.5 million people infected with HIV, including 1 million living with HIV infection and 500,000 who have died with AIDS.

Gloves. Wear latex gloves if your hands have any cuts, sores, or torn cuticles. Wear gloves to handle blood or feces or urine, or to clean open sores. Wear gloves for cleaning surfaces that have been soiled by blood or feces or urine. Following use, soiled gloves should be washed with soap and water, then dried, and then discarded in a plastic container such as a trash can lined with a plastic bag.

Disinfectants. No one is known to have become infected from contacting HIV on a surface outside the body. Nevertheless, this virus has been shown to survive on a surface for several days, and it is probably wise to clean up blood or other body secretions on clothing or hard surfaces. Studies show that HIV is killed by heat and by nearly all chemical disinfectants.

The most commonly used disinfectants include household bleach and alcohol (70% isopropyl). Other disinfectants that are effective include hydrogen peroxide, iodophors, phenolics, and quaternary ammonium compounds. These disinfectants are readily available in pharmacies and grocery stores. They are registered with the Environmental Protection Agency (EPA) with directions for use and precautionary information.

The most common disinfectant used is sodium hypochlorite, commonly known as household bleach (the most common brand is Clorox). This is available as a 5.25 percent solution wherever household cleaning products are sold. Household bleach kills a broad range of microbes, including HIV. To clean surfaces contaminated by blood or secretions, use a 1:10 dilution. A 1:10 dilution contains one part of 5.25 percent household bleach and nine parts of tap water (for example, one-fourth cup bleach and two and one-fourth cups water). Leave the 1:10 dilution on the surface for ten minutes, then wipe it off.

If the surface is cleaned before using the bleach, a 1:100 dilution may be used. Some people find it convenient to use the 1:100 dilution of bleach in a spray bottle, to spray on surfaces after they have been wiped clean. Bleach may corrode metals. It may also damage electrical and electronic equipment. Undiluted, it can leave white spots on fabric or eat holes in fabric. Contact with the skin and especially the eyes should be avoided. Use gloves to protect the skin when cleaning and disinfecting with bleach. If bleach comes in contact with skin, eyes, or mouth, the area should be washed or rinsed thoroughly with water. This applies to undiluted bleach and to the 1:10 dilution. Inhaling bleach fumes should also be avoided.

Household bleach may be stored in the original container (or in any opaque container) in a cool area, for up to a year. Bleach in solution is unstable and loses potency when exposed to sunlight, heat, or metal. Diluted bleach solutions should be used within a day or discarded.

Seventy percent isopropyl alcohol is also a very effective disinfectant. One problem with its use on surfaces is that it evaporates quickly. It may also cause skin irritation. This is the usual disinfectant ingredient in waterless handwashing products that are marketed in sealed packets. Isopropyl alcohol need not be diluted before use. Undiluted isopropyl alcohol kills high concentrations of HIV in less than one minute.

Hydrogen peroxide is usually sold in a 3 percent solution, which is too weak to disinfect. Iodine is an adequate skin disinfectant, but it must be used carefully, since it stains fabrics, corrodes metal, cracks plastics, and dissolves rubber.

In summary, the most practical disinfectant to keep on hand is household bleach. Bleach should be properly stored and clearly labeled to avoid misuse or accidental drinking. In addition, 70 percent isopropyl alcohol can be used to clean cuts or other open wounds.

Dishwashing. There is no reason to provide separate dishes, glasses, or silverware for people with HIV infection. Washing dishes in a standard dishwasher or in hot soapy water is adequate.

Laundry. Laundry should be washed with detergent, using the hot cycle. Adding one-third cup of household bleach per ten gallons of wash water will assure disinfection, although it is really not necessary and may damage some fabrics. Fabrics that are soaked with blood or other body secretions should be presoaked and then washed separately. Dry cleaning will disinfect any fabric.

Cuts and other injuries. Any fresh bleeding cut or sore on the caregiver or the person with HIV infection should be wiped free of blood and washed with soap and water or with alcohol (70% isopropyl).

Blood spills. Blood, including menstrual blood, spilled on a surface should be cleaned by a person wearing disposable gloves and using disposable cleaning cloths. After wiping up the blood, clean the area with a disinfectant like household bleach in a 1:10 or 1:100 dilution. Sponges, mops, and fabrics that have blood or body fluids on them may be cleaned with soap and water or with bleach in a 1:10 dilution.

Disposal of waste. Liquid waste that may have HIV in it can be poured into the toilet or sink. This will not contaminate the sewer system: sewage is decontaminated using methods that are clearly adequate to kill HIV and virtually all other microbes as well.

Soiled materials such as bandages, sanitary napkins, disposable gloves, soiled cleaning cloths, and the like should be placed in plastic bags for disposal. This is important primarily when they are soiled with blood. Sharp instruments such as needles, syringes, used razor blades, and broken glass should be placed in containers such as a metal coffee can for disposal. To be extra cautious, some health departments recommend also adding bleach to the container.

To summarize: Caregivers should be cautious and sensible but should not worry excessively. In fourteen years, of all the people who are and have been caregivers, only eight are thought to have become infected by nonsexual contact.

Preventing Transmission of Infections Other Than HIV

People with HIV infection are susceptible to infection by a multitude of other microbes. These microbes cause what are called opportunistic infections or more simply, *complications*. The most common complications are pneumocystis pneumonia, thrush, infection disseminated throughout the body caused by either cytomegalovirus or *Mycobacterium avium* complex, and a brain infection called toxoplasmosis. (These and other complications are discussed at great length in chapter 6.) People commonly want to know whether the caregiver can also be infected by these complications. The short answer is: with rare exceptions, no.

Most of these complications are caused by microbes that we all come in contact with every day. People with HIV infection usually do not develop complications until relatively late in the disease after their immune systems have become profoundly impaired. The caregiver's immune system does not permit such organisms to flourish. In other words, none of these complications can be transmitted from the person to the caregiver either in the home or in the hospital.

Pregnant caregivers are sometimes worried about exposure to people with cytomegalovirus, but most authorities believe these concerns are unjustified (see the section on cytomegalovirus in chapter 6).

In fact, the person with HIV infection is not a significant source of complications even for another person with HIV infection. The reason is that most of these microbes are and always have been everywhere around us, and everyone has been exposed to them for a long time.

Exceptions to the rule.   Some infections *may* be transmitted to the caregiver, and to avoid these infections, the caregiver should use special precautions.

The most important exception is tuberculosis, which is caused by a bacterium called *Mycobacterium tuberculosis. Mycobacterium tuberculosis* is related to another bacterium that people with HIV infection are prone to, *Mycobacterium avium* complex, or MAC, which causes infections throughout the body. MAC is not contagious—that is, it cannot be spread from person to person. *Mycobacterium tuberculosis*, however, *is* contagious.

Tuberculosis has always been recognized as a contagious disease. People with HIV infection are exceptionally vulnerable to infection with tuberculosis, and, once infected, they get the disease severely. Moreover, some of these people are infected with a strain of the TB bacterium called the "multiply drug-resistant strain," that is, a form of the TB bacterium that does not respond to the usual drugs. The multiply drug-resistant strain was a big problem among people with HIV infection, especially in New York City in the early 1990s, but both TB and multiply drug-resistant TB are now much better contained.

All people in the same household as someone with tuberculosis are at special risk. The risk is highest during the period before diagnosis and treatment. This is equally true for people in the household of someone with tuberculosis and HIV infection. People not in the household—visitors, co-workers, casual friends, golf partners, and the like—are not usually considered to be at risk, but this depends to some extent on the type of contact. In any case, people usually become infected by inhaling the droplets in the air after the infected person has coughed.

Whenever a case of tuberculosis is detected, medical authorities evaluate others in the same household. The evaluation starts with a skin test. Because the skin test can take three months to become positive, sometimes treatment is started immediately. And treatment is often started immediately for any children in the household. If the skin test for tuberculosis is positive, the evaluation proceeds to the next step, a chest X-ray. Once tuberculosis is treated with drugs, the infected person rapidly becomes noncontagious. For this reason, the main threat of tuberculosis comes from the person whose tuberculosis has not yet been detected or treated.

People infected with the resistant strain of tuberculosis, which persists in spite of treatment, are an exception. These people require special care and may need to stay in the hospital for prolonged periods. And because the resistant strain of tuberculosis is a major threat to public health, people may even be kept in the hospital against their wishes.

Another infection that is an exception is hepatitis B. Most people with hepatitis B are not aware they have it; they develop antibodies to it and are subsequently protected from infection. However, about 5 or 10 percent of people with hepatitis B will develop a persistent infection, and therefore may infect others for many years. Some people with persistent hepatitis will develop a liver disease called *chronic active hepatitis* that may eventually result in cirrhosis.

The virus that causes hepatitis B is transmitted the same way HIV is: by sexual contact, by blood contact, or by passage from mother to infant. Therefore, the activities that carry a risk of infection with HIV also carry a risk of infection with the hepatitis B virus. People at greatest risk for hepatitis B are men who have homosexual sex, people who use drugs by injection, and men who have hemophilia. Like HIV, hepatitis B may be also transmitted to someone exposed to the blood of an infected person.

Hepatitis B has four features worth emphasizing:

1. Hepatitis B virus is transmitted much more efficiently than HIV. A needlestick injury with blood that contains the hepatitis B virus is

twenty times more likely to transmit hepatitis B than a needlestick injury with blood that contains HIV is to transmit HIV infection.

2. The same guidelines for preventing transmission of HIV through blood and body fluids apply to preventing transmission of hepatitis B.

3. A vaccine can prevent infection by the hepatitis B virus. The hepatitis vaccine is readily available, though it is expensive; it costs about $160 for three injections. Those people who live in the same house as the person with hepatitis B should take the vaccine if they have not already been infected.

4. Hepatitis B can now be treated with several drugs—interferon, lamivudine, adofovir, and entecavir—which all help control the hepatitis B virus. The results of the treatment, however, are quite variable, the medicines (especially interferon) can cause side effects, and the virus may become resistant.

Outside of tuberculosis and hepatitis, the infections that could conceivably be transmitted from the person with HIV to a caregiver are salmonellosis, herpes simplex infection, herpes zoster infection, and cryptosporidiosis. If the caregiver is otherwise healthy, these infections may cause a temporary disease that is not serious.

Salmonellosis is an infection of the intestine by bacteria called *Salmonella*. The main symptom of salmonellosis is diarrhea. Salmonellosis is relatively unusual, and transmission to others is relatively infrequent.

Cryptosporidiosis is also an infection of the intestine but is caused by a parasite. The main symptom of cryptosporidiosis is also diarrhea. It is transmitted by lapses in personal hygiene; that is, small amounts of feces on the hand carry the parasite to someone else's hand, and then to that second person's mouth.

Herpes simplex, usually known as "herpes," causes a blister on the skin, most commonly on the mouth or genitals, though people with advanced HIV infection can also have herpes over much of their bodies. The caregiver can get herpes by touching the blisters, and can avoid transmission easily by wearing gloves when touching the areas with sores until the sores are crusted over.

Herpes zoster, also called shingles, is caused by the virus that causes chickenpox. The virus is transmitted when people inhale it. However, most older children and adults have had chickenpox, even if they don't remember it, and thus are protected by antibodies against the virus. Those who are concerned about herpes zoster are urged to have a blood test to see if they have antibodies to herpes zoster; and to be safe, they should avoid going into the same room as the infected person until the sores are crusted over. They might want to take the new chickenpox vaccine, which is highly effective.

All these infections are discussed in greater detail in chapter 6.

Preventing Transmission of Infections to the HIV-infected Person

Both health care workers and home caregivers are understandably worried that they might transmit infection to the person whose immune system has been damaged by HIV infection. Although this worry sounds rational, in reality it is not much of a problem.

The kinds of infections common in otherwise healthy individuals include upper respiratory tract infections like colds, sinusitis, and pharyngitis; influenza or "flu"; gastroenteritis with diarrhea, vomiting, and fever; and skin infections. Some of these sound like infections, but in reality they are not. Some are infections that are not contagious and cannot be passed from one person to another. And some are contagious diseases in the usual sense. The latter category is the only important one. The most common examples are colds, bronchitis, influenza, and gastroenteritis. Most of these are caused by viruses.

However, people with HIV infection do not get these common contagious diseases any more frequently or any more severely than anyone else. The viruses that cause the common contagious diseases affect a person with HIV the same way they affect other people. The reason seems to be that the part of the immune system that HIV attacks is not the same as the part that defends against colds and flu.

People also worry whether pets can carry infections to people with HIV infection. The most common worry is about the *Toxoplasma gondii* parasite, which causes a brain infection called toxoplasma encephalitis. The parasite is commonly found in the stool of cats. This worry is probably not justified: *Toxoplasma gondii* is one of those microbes that 20–30 percent of all people have in their bodies, and the person with HIV infection who gets toxoplasmosis has probably had this microbe a long time.

If You Think You Have Been Exposed

Persons who think they have been exposed to HIV infection or any of the infections noted above should seek care at a site that offers a treatment called "nonoccupational exposure prophylaxis."

Health care workers who have been exposed to HIV are usually offered two nucleosides. Previous experience with one particular nucleoside reduced the risk of transmission by 80 percent, and other nucleosides are thought to be equally good. A third drug is added if the exposure was to a large amount of virus or if the injury was deep. When the drugs are taken for this reason, they must be started as soon as possible, and certainly within 72 hours of exposure.

We usually start treatment within 2 hours of exposure and think that much of the opportunity to prevent HIV transmission is gone when treatment is delayed over 24 hours. The drugs are taken for one month. HIV blood tests are done before treatment and at three months, and again at six months after exposure. We want to see whether the test turns positive and transmission has indeed taken place.

The CDC's 2005 guidelines for people exposed to HIV by sex or shared needles are based on the experiences of health care workers exposed to HIV occupationally. Basing the guidelines for one group on the experiences of another is not backed by scientific evidence, but it should work anyway. People seeking treatment should have been exposed by sex or needle-sharing with someone who has or probably has HIV infection; and they should be able to begin treatment within 72 hours after the time they were exposed. Treatment begun even sooner is better: health care workers who were exposed occupationally and who received treatment within 2 hours of exposure had an 80 percent reduction in transmission. The treatment regimens recommended are the same as those used for health care workers exposed to HIV. One drug to avoid is nevirapine (Viramune), because of its possible liver toxicity. Another drug, efavirenz (Sustiva), should not be given to pregnant women or women who may become pregnant, because it possibly causes birth defects. People who receive the treatment regimen need to be aware that it has side effects and that it will cost between $500 and $1,200, depending on the regimen. The standard course of treatment takes one month, but the drugs can be stopped immediately if the person who was the source of the exposure is given an HIV test that turns out to be negative.

Chapter 3

HIV Infection and
Its Treatment

- Natural history of HIV infection
- Keeping track of HIV infection
- Treatment of HIV infection
- General advice

Natural History of HIV Infection

What medical scientists call the *natural history* of an infection is simply the chronological story of what the microbe does once in the body, and what the body does in response.

Transmission of HIV

HIV is transmitted—that is, the virus enters the body—almost invariably by sexual contact, by blood-to-blood contact, or through pregnancy. HIV infects cells called *CD4 cells.* The CD4 cell is a white blood cell, or a *lymphocyte,* that belongs to a class of lymphocytes called *T cells,* which, along with B cells, are central components of the immune system. (The CD4 cell is also called a *T4 cell* and a *T-helper cell.*) The CD4 cell's job is to help coordinate the immune system's defense against a variety of infectious diseases.

Once HIV enters the body, it attaches itself to the walls of CD4 cells at certain sites, called *CD4 receptors* (which give CD4 cells their name). After HIV attaches to a CD4 receptor, it enters the cell. At this point, in a complicated series of events, the virus becomes part of the cell's genes. Genes are composed of DNA, the molecule responsible for directing the cell's reproduction. HIV is a virus and has only RNA, a molecule that is actually the mirror image of DNA but which cannot produce new viruses. HIV, however, is a *retrovirus,* meaning that it has a protein called *reverse transcriptase,* which allows the viral RNA to make a mirror image of itself. That is, reverse transcriptase allows viral RNA to turn into viral DNA. The viral DNA then directs the infected cell to produce, not new CD4 cells, but new HIVs instead. The virus eventually destroys the CD4 cell, and the new viruses that have been produced then infect other CD4 cells. The viruses grow rapidly in number, they spread throughout the body extensively, and the destruction they cause is massive. In the first week of infection, concentrations of viruses in the blood reach 1 billion per milliliter, higher than at any other time during the disease. In the first two weeks of infection, about half of all the CD4 cells in the body are infected and killed. The virus spreads widely throughout the body, including the brain; the lymph nodes, which are distributed throughout the body; and the genital tract, which then becomes the source of infection for sexual transmission.

Acute Infection

The first symptoms of HIV infection, sometimes called acute HIV infection or primary HIV infection, occur about 1 to 4 weeks after the virus was transmitted. Probably at least 50 percent and possibly 80 percent of all people with HIV infection have the symptoms of this early, acute HIV infection. Some people, who have the same explosive growth in the number of viruses, have no clearly defined symptoms; they are said to be asymptomatic, and the reason is unknown.

Many of the symptoms of acute infection are nonspecific; that is, they are also symptoms of many common viral infections. Symptoms include fever, sweats, malaise, fatigue, achiness, joint pain, headaches, a sore throat, trouble swallowing, and enlarged lymph glands. Some people have a major illness, somewhat like mononucleosis, with a prolonged fever, night sweats, fatigue, and weight loss of 15 to 20 pounds. Some people have a rash consisting of red spots or splotches over the chest, back, and abdomen. Some have evidence of infection of the brain: severe headaches, mood changes, personality changes, irritability, and confusion. Occasionally, people lose the use of their arms or legs for a short time, then regain use again.

Because some of these symptoms resemble those of infectious mononucleosis, the acute infection stage is sometimes referred to as a mononucleosis-like syndrome. Mononucleosis, however, is caused by an entirely different virus, and with acute HIV infection the blood test for mononucleosis is negative.

Some people with HIV infection have no recollection of an acute infection stage, some mistake it for a common viral infection or flu, and some people feel sick enough to go to a physician. A physician may find a rash, enlarged lymph glands, an enlarged spleen, and an enlarged liver. A blood count will show fewer white blood cells than normal—but then, a low white count accompanies most viral infections. The *CD4 cell count* also decreases (see below), but does not usually decrease much below the lower limits of normal. Liver tests may show changes suggesting mild hepatitis, but many other conditions cause similar changes. A spinal tap to analyze cerebrospinal fluid (the fluid that bathes the brain and spinal cord) may show evidence of meningitis. The usual blood test for HIV, which detects antibodies to HIV, will be negative at this time but will usually become positive within three to six weeks. Blood tests for HIV instead of the antibody to HIV will be positive. The usual test for HIV is the *viral load* test (see below). The viral load test usually shows counts that are very high, often over 100,000 or even several million.

All people recover from acute HIV infection, as a result of their immune responses. The recovery is accompanied by the disappearance of symptoms and a rapid decrease in the viral load.

Acute HIV infection is important to recognize, because it's the time when the concentration of viruses is highest and the risk of transmission is greatest; therefore it should also be the best time to learn about prevention. But acute HIV infection often is not recognized: for it to be recognized, people would have to have symptoms severe enough to see a physician, and the physician would have to be alert enough to the possibility of acute HIV infection to measure the viral load (which is high at this stage) and test for the presence of antibodies to HIV (which are essentially absent at this stage). If acute HIV infection were more easily recognized, this might be the best time to treat HIV. Early treatment would help prevent transmission, and it might favorably alter the progress of the HIV infection: the former is probable, but the latter is completely unknown.

Seroconversion

At the time of acute infection with HIV, the body has not yet made *antibodies* to HIV. Antibodies, proteins produced primarily by certain white blood cells called B lymphocytes, attack substances foreign to the body, including viruses. The fact that symptoms are present even though the blood test to detect antibodies to HIV is negative is not unusual. In most other infections, symptoms precede the body's production of antibodies, and the symptoms disappear once antibodies are produced.

The body usually takes several days or weeks to recognize a foreign substance like a virus, and then it produces antibodies to attack the substance. Six to ten weeks after HIV has entered the body, antibodies to HIV appear in the blood in sufficient concentration to give a positive blood test. Physicians call this appearance of antibodies *seroconversion*. That is, the result of a test for antibodies in the blood serum converts from negative to positive. Over 95 percent of people have positive HIV tests by three months after transmission, and over 99 percent have positive tests by six months.

Antibodies against most viral infections, once they appear, eliminate the virus and then stay in the body to protect against future infections by the same virus. Virtually all people with HIV infection develop antibodies against HIV. These antibodies, along with other immune system mechanisms, reduce the concentration of HIV but do not eliminate HIV. Besides antibodies, the other immune defenses that seem important are the CD8 cells. CD8 cells are lymphocytes that include a subset called CD8-38 cells, which are programmed to attack HIV by hormones called *cytokines* produced by the CD4 cells. This means that a good immune response requires that CD4 cells recognize HIV and then produce cytokines to goose the CD8-38 cells, which then destroy HIV. A goal of early treatment is to preserve this function of the CD4 cells before HIV destroys it. This goal makes sense, but despite extensive study, it has been hard to carry out.

The problem with all this is that most people with acute HIV infection never see a doctor, and even if they do, the doctor does the diagnostic tests only 25 to 30 percent of the time.

Asymptomatic Period

For several years after seroconversion, people with HIV infection feel good. Because they have no symptoms of the infection, this period has been called the *asymptomatic* (meaning "no symptoms") period. During this period the person will be unaware of the HIV infection unless a blood test shows antibodies to HIV. About 70 to 80 percent of the people who presently have HIV infection are in this asymptomatic period.

For many years, we thought that during the asymptomatic period HIV was resting and not reproducing. We now know this is not the case. HIV is reproducing at an amazing rate, every day making an average of 10 billion new viruses, and every day destroying a comparable number of CD4 cells. And every day, the body produces enough new CD4 cells to nearly offset the loss. But the body, in the long run, can't quite keep up. The average net loss of CD4 cells is fifty per milliliter of blood per year, accounting for the gradual decline in CD4 cell counts over the years. Most CD4 cells are in lymph nodes, but we measure their counts in blood because blood is easy to obtain and because the counts in the blood reflect the counts in the entire body. So the CD4 count becomes a good barometer of the immune system.

The actual rate of decline, however, is highly variable. About six months after the virus is transmitted, the amount of HIV in the blood— the viral load—reaches a "set point," a point at which, without treatment, it may stay for several years. If HIV's set point is high, the immune system is not controlling the virus well; the CD4 count falls quickly and the time before AIDS occurs is short. If the set point is low, the CD4 count falls slowly and the time to AIDS is long. This relation between the set point and the progress of the disease makes sense: the viral load is a direct reflection of how fast HIV is multiplying and how well the immune system is controlling it. More viruses mean more CD4 cells are infected and destroyed, so AIDS will be earlier and survival shorter. After years of research, we believe the most critical difference between people whose disease progresses quickly and those whose disease progresses slowly is a difference in their immune responses. The reason for this belief is that two people with the same strain of HIV may have completely different courses of the disease. One may be a "long term non-progressor" who has had no treatment but maintains low viral loads and high CD4 counts for years. Another who also has had no treatment may have high viral loads, a rapidly declining CD4 count, and a diagnosis of AIDS within one or two years. The difference between these people is in immune control, which is probably genetic but is otherwise poorly understood and clearly complex.

We also know that treatment makes a decisive difference in the rate of the infection's progression because treatment resets the set point. The drugs directed against HIV keep the virus from reproducing in the test tube; and the drugs, when given to people, measurably decrease the amount of virus in the blood and do so within hours. In most people who can take treatment successfully, 99 percent of the virus will be eliminated within four weeks; and within four to six months, most of these people will have "no detectable HIV."

Keeping Track of HIV Infection

All people with HIV infection should have regular medical care. Options for medical care will depend to some extent on the resources available (see chapter 7; options for financing this care are discussed in chapter 9). Regular medical care usually includes medical evaluations every three to four months. During the visits, your previous medical problems should be reviewed, and any symptoms or conditions that may or may not be related to HIV infection should be discussed.

During the visits, you should also have a physical examination and any necessary laboratory tests. Your physician should then candidly discuss your health status with you and should recommend subsequent medical care.

The principal laboratory tests are the CD4 cell count and the HIV viral load test. These tests are usually given to all people with HIV infection every three to four months. The purpose of the CD4 count is to evaluate the state of the immune system. The purpose of the viral load test is to evaluate the prognosis based on the rate of viral reproduction. The two tests are complementary. A low CD4 count means vulnerability to complications regardless of the viral load. And the viral load gives the speed of progression regardless of the CD4 count. These tests are critical to making good decisions for treatment: the CD4 count shows how vulnerable the person might be to the complications of HIV, and the viral load shows how well treatment is working.

Viral Load Test

The viral load test, introduced in 1996, measures the number of HIV in a given amount of blood. The terms *viral load* and *viral burden* are used synonymously; the proper scientific term is *quantitative plasma HIV RNA*. The results are reported as "copies per milliliter," meaning the number of viruses per milliliter of blood. Although this test measures the amount of HIV in the blood, over 95 percent of the HIV is in the lymph system. But the total amount of HIV in the body is accurately represented by the amount of HIV in the blood.

The viral load indicates prognosis. The average viral load of someone who has had no treatment is 30,000 to 50,000 copies per milliliter. People who have high amounts of virus, like 100,000 or 1,000,000, and who aren't taking treatment will have a disease that tends to progress rapidly and CD4 cells that decline quickly. They will develop AIDS sooner and live for a shorter time. People who have a low viral load, like 1,000 or 10,000, and who aren't taking treatment will have a disease that progresses relatively slowly and CD4 cell counts that decrease relatively slowly. They will live relatively longer. Therefore, both the CD4 count and the viral load predict the course of the disease. If the CD4 count is low and the viral load is high, the prognosis (without treatment) is poor. If the CD4 count is high and the viral load is low, the prognosis is good.

The viral load is most useful for monitoring people's responses to treatment. When people take antiretroviral treatment, the viral load decreases rapidly and dramatically, at least ten-fold or a hundred-fold and within two to four weeks. For example, a person with a viral load of 100,000 who receives antiretroviral treatment on January 1 will, on February 1, often have a viral load of 10,000 (a ten-fold or one log decrease) or 1,000 (a hundred-fold or two log decrease). The viral load varies, depending on how the test is done. This variation is about three-fold; that is, a result showing 10,000 copies of HIV might really be 3,000 or 30,000 copies. The viral load also varies with different methods of doing the test; so the same laboratory and the same methods should be used for repeated tests over time.

One goal of therapy is to get the viral load down to where it is undetectable, meaning that it's less than the arbitrary threshold of the test, usually less than 50 copies per milliliter. The second goal of therapy is to keep the viral load down as long as possible. When the amount of virus is this low, the virus is reproducing only minimally and the disease does not progress. Fewer viruses also mean fewer mutations—that is, fewer new genes that make the virus resistant to drugs—so the benefit of knocking back the virus is likely to last.

CD4 Cell Count

The CD4 cell count is an indicator of the status of the immune system. The CD4 cell count measures the concentration of CD4 cells in a given amount of blood; for example, a CD4 count of 1,000 means 1,000 CD4 cells per milliliter of blood. The CD4 count for a healthy person is 500 to 1,450; 95 percent of people without HIV infection have counts in this range. Counts above 500 are usually considered normal. Counts of less than 500 mean the immune system has been damaged; counts of less than 350 mean the damage is moderate; counts of less than 200 mean the damage is severe; and counts of less than 50 mean the disease is advanced but not irreparable. Most people do not get the complications of HIV infection until their CD4 counts are less than 200, which is the threshold used to define AIDS. These complications aren't actually common until the CD4 counts are less than 50.

When the new drugs control HIV, people's CD4 counts increase in both number and quality. That is, the CD4 count goes up and the new CD4 cells work like they're supposed to. The average increase, if viral load is low, is about 50 to 100 or 150 the first year, and then about 100 per year thereafter. This means that if a person with a CD4 cell count of 50 started treatment, and the treatment brought the viral load down to undetectable, the CD4 count would increase to 100 to 200 in one year. Many people, even if their counts were well below 50 to start with, have counts that go up in several years to 500 or more.

The relation between viral load and CD4 count, however, is not invariable and differs in different people. Many people whose treatment is not completely controlling the virus still have CD4 counts that go up; the counts, however, don't usually go up as fast or as high as when the virus is completely suppressed. Sometimes physicians call an increasing CD4 count despite persistent high levels of virus the "viral load–CD4 disconnect" or "discordant." We don't know why people with the same degree of viral suppression can have differing responses in their CD4 counts. When the virus is suppressed and the CD4 count doesn't respond, we consider changing regimens. In most cases, however, people continue on the regimen that suppressed the virus. We do know that these people seem relatively well protected from HIV complications.

You need to be cautious in interpreting the CD4 cell count. As with the viral load test, the count can vary with the laboratory technician and the method used to do the test: the same laboratory technician doing the same test twice on the same blood sample can show counts that differ by 30 percent, so that a count of 500, if repeated, might be 350 or 650. Two laboratories working on the same specimen might show results of 70 and 130, or 140 and 260, or 210 and 390, or 280 and 520, and so on.

Other factors alter CD4 counts. The CD4 count is highest in the evening and lowest at noon. It is also lower after heavy exercise or when you have an infectious disease like influenza. We emphasize this because many people have unrealistic expectations of the test and become alarmed when the count decreases slightly. But the CD4 cell count is not particularly fine-tuned, and modest decreases from one test to the next— for example, from 500 to 400—are considered to be "within the error of the test." Repeated tests showing trends over long periods are far more reliable than any isolated sampling. When major decisions about treatment depend on the CD4 count, or when a value for the count doesn't make sense, the usual recommendation is to repeat the count. Almost everyone with HIV infection knows his or her CD4 counts and has them measured at periodic intervals, usually every three to six months.

The cost of the test is usually $40 to $100, and no one seems to know why the charge varies so enormously.

Treatment of HIV Infection

The history of the treatment of HIV is probably one of the most remarkable success stories in the history of medicine. HIV treatment is certainly the most important development in a widespread, serious disease in the last twenty years. This success is based on three factors: (1) the understanding of the virus and how it damages the immune system; (2)

the ability to monitor the disease with tests of the immune function, like the CD4 counts, and tests for the amount of HIV, like the viral load test; and (3) the development of drugs to attack or inhibit HIV.

Right now we have no rigid rules about when to start treatment. The decision to begin treatment should be strongly influenced by your CD4 count and, to a much lesser extent, your viral load. Most important, treatment should start when you are ready to stick with it. Partial treatment is worse than no treatment. In no other disease in medicine is the penalty for noncompliance worse.

We now know that drugs can reverse the loss of CD4 cells, decrease the amount of HIV, and delay or prevent the onset of the complications that accompany HIV infection. Drugs directed against HIV are called antiviral or antiretroviral drugs.

HAART, Highly Active Antiretroviral Therapy

The history of antiviral drugs against HIV infection begins with AZT and a clinical trial whose initial results were spectacular.

A large group of people with HIV infection was given either AZT or an inert pill called a placebo. The results were analyzed by an oversight board, an independent group of scientists who had access to information that the researchers doing the trial did not have. The reason for oversight boards is to find out if the drug is too bad to continue giving it, or too good to continue giving the placebo; either way, the trial will be stopped. In the case of AZT, when the oversight board first reviewed the results, the group getting the placebo had 19 deaths and the group getting AZT had only 1—a person who happened to have stopped taking the medicine. On September 17, 1986, the oversight board had an emergency meeting and stopped the trial. A record-short four months later, the FDA approved AZT as the first drug for HIV infection.

Unfortunately, the benefit from AZT was short-lived, a problem that became painfully clear in the next few years. We now know that HIV became resistant to AZT. But we didn't know that then and we took a decade to prove it. During that decade and the next, drug companies introduced many daughter drugs of AZT. The daughters are sometimes called "D drugs," because of some of their names—ddI, d4T, ddC, 3TC, and ABC—but are more properly called *nucleoside analogs*. All these drugs are chemically related and inhibit the same enzyme, reverse transcriptase, by which HIV turns its RNA into the cell's DNA, thereby producing new viruses. The nucleoside analogs are informally called *nukes*, or *NRTIs* (nucleoside reverse transcriptase inhibitors).

The nucleoside analogs all inhibited the multiplication of HIV, but not enough that they could be used alone. And as HIV continued to multiply, it mutated, changing its genetic structure. Billions of new viruses every day meant millions of mutants; inevitably, a few of the mutants were resistant to the nucleoside analogs. After enough multiplication, the strains of virus vulnerable to the nucleoside analogs were killed off and only the resistant strains were left. These resistant strains of the virus meant that the nucleoside analogs were either less effective or not effective at all. HIV was now multiplying the way it did before AZT existed. Shortly after ddI, the second AIDS drug, was introduced, we tried giving two nucleoside analogs instead of just one—that is, ddI and AZT combined. The combination seemed to work better than when either drug was given alone. But in retrospect, it's difficult to know how much we achieved during the first ten years of the treatment of HIV infection, except that by 1996, we had five drugs that added an estimated six extra months of life.

In 1996 a second class of drugs was introduced, called the *nonnucleoside reverse transcriptase inhibitors,* or *NNRTIs.* As the name suggests, NNRTIs inhibit the same enzyme as the nucleoside analogs but are chemically different. The first NNRTIs were nevirapine, introduced in 1996; delavirdine, in 1997; and efavirenz, in 1998.

Meanwhile in 1996, the FDA also approved a third class of drugs, called *protease inhibitors* or *PIs.* PIs inhibit an enzyme called protease that HIV uses to assemble new viruses. Saquinavir was approved by the FDA in December 1995 and after that, a lot more PIs were approved (see table 3).

So during those next ten years, what did we learn about these treatments? We learned a lot. We learned that the goal of treatment is to inhibit the virus, and the more inhibition, the better. The fewer viruses, the fewer mutations. And the fewer mutations, the less likely the mutations are to confer resistance to drugs. So the rate of resistance mutations depends on the viral load; and a viral load of 50 is better than 500, which is better than 5,000. In fact, with a viral load that's undetectable—that's less than 50—resistance appears to be nil. An undetectable viral load and the absence of resistance mutations result from good adherence to treatment, which should keep people in good health for years, probably decades.

We learned that people need to take two or three active drugs: not one and not four, but sometimes two and usually three. And those drugs are not just any two or three but specific combinations of specific drugs, because we also learned that some combinations work and some do not.

We learned that adherence to the treatment regimen is the key, more important with drugs for HIV than with drugs for most other diseases. First, people need to take at least 95 percent of the prescribed doses to achieve the treatment's goal, which is no detectable virus for a sustained

Table 3. Antiretroviral Drugs Approved by the FDA 1987–2005

Drug Generic Name	Drug Trade Name	Class*	FDA Approval Date
Zidovudine (AZT)	Retrovir	NRTI	March 1987
Didanosine (ddI)	Videx	NRTI	October 1991
Zalcitabine (ddC)	HIVID	NRTI	June 1992
Stavudine (d4T)	Zerit	NRTI	June 1994
Lamivudine (3TC)	Epivir	NRTI	November 1995
Saquinavir (SQV)	Invirase	PI	December 1995
Ritonavir (RTV)	Norvir	PI	March 1996
Indinavir (IDV)	Crixivan	PI	March 1996
Nevirapine (NVP)	Viramune	NNRTI	June 1996
Nelfinavir (NFV)	Viracept	PI	March 1997
Delavirdine (DLV)	Rescriptor	NNRTI	April 1997
Efavirenz (EFV)	Sustiva	NNRTI	September 1998
Abacavir (ABC)	Ziagen	NRTI	February 1999
Amprenavir (APV)	Agenerase	PI	April 1999
Lopinavir (LPV)	Kaletra	PI	September 2000
Tenofovir (TDF)	Viread	NRTI	October 2001
Enfuvirtide (T20)	Fuzeon	EI	March 2003
Atazanavir (ATV)	Reyataz	PI	May 2003
Emtricitabine (FTC)	Emtriva	NRTI	July 2003
Fosamprenavir (FPV)	Lexiva	PI	November 2003
Tipranavir (TPV)	Aptivus	PI	June 2005

*NRTI = nucleoside reverse transcriptase inhibitor
NNRTI = nonnucleoside reverse transcriptase inhibitor
PI = protease inhibitor
EI = entry inhibitor

period. Second, the penalty for not adhering strictly to treatment is harsh. Not only does the virus continue reproducing; it also develops mutations that are resistant to the drugs. The resistant mutations are permanent and limit future options for using these drugs.

We learned that the drugs have side effects. Some side effects were short-term, like allergic reactions and stomach problems. But some were long-term and came as a complete surprise, like the lipodystrophies that change people's blood lipids and appearances.

We learned that many people fail treatment. They fail the first treatment, and when the regimen is changed, they fail that too. And with each failure thereafter, the treatment becomes progressively more complicated and the probability of success progressively less.

We learned—and were surprised—that failed treatment was still better than no treatment. We know this because when people fail treatment and have a high viral load and then stop taking drugs altogether, the viral load immediately jumps even higher and the CD4 count falls faster.

We learned that to improve adherence to treatment, the treatments need to be simplified. People have three problems with adhering to treatment: the pill burden (the total number of pills), the number of times per day the pills have to be taken, and the necessity of taking the pills with or without food. New drug development has focused on these problems. To reduce the pill burden, pills were combined; taking the drugs three times a day became completely antiquated; and the need to take drugs with food was either eliminated or more carefully defined.

We learned that treatment decisions are complicated and require the physician to have substantial skill and experience. The physician has to choose among twenty drugs—and more are coming—that vary substantially in toxicity, potency, and patterns of resistance. The stakes are high and so are the patients' expectations. HIV care has become a specialty. People with HIV infection should be seeing specialists.

From all that we learned in those ten years, we put together certain guidelines for the drugs' use. These federal guidelines are based on good, authoritative sources, experts in the field who laboriously review the data from reports and tests and then write recommendations. Nearly every country in the world has national guidelines for the use of these drugs, and fortunately, they all say the same, or nearly the same, things. (The exception is the World Health Organization guidelines for developing countries, where drug prices drive many of the decisions.) The U.S. federal guidelines are constructed by a panel of about thirty-five experts who communicate by teleconference every month to keep the guidelines up-to-date, in what is clearly the fastest-moving field in medicine. These guidelines (and other federal HIV guidelines for topics like HIV prevention and nonoccupational exposure) are available at www.aidsinfo.nih.gov.

We must acknowledge that guidelines are not rules. Every person with HIV infection is different, and exceptions are normal. Knowing which idiosyncrasies require a detour is the "art" of medicine. This art comes with experience, along with keeping current through a vast array of medical journals, Internet sites, and medical conferences.

When to Start Treatment

The U.S. federal guidelines recommend HIV treatment for all people with an AIDS-defining complication or a CD4 cell count below 200. In fact, all guidelines for Europe, Africa, South and Central America, and Asia make this same recommendation. A CD4 cell count below 200 defines the risk of most complications of HIV infection; it defines AIDS. Taking treatment before the CD4 count goes this low, however, provides a margin of protection and prevents the infrequent complications that occur even when the CD4 cell count is above 200. We often recommend beginning treatment at a CD4 cell count of 350. In short, antiretroviral treatment is a must for a person with a CD4 cell count below 200, and such treatment is seriously considered when the CD4 count is between 200 and 350.

Several issues influence the decision to take treatment when CD4 counts are between 200 and 350. (1) Do you want to be treated? Some people are determined to wipe out that virus as soon as possible; others want to delay the drugs as long as possible. (2) What is your viral load? A high viral load generally means faster progression through the disease and more mutations in the virus. Some experts think that treatment should be considered for anyone with a viral load over 100,000 copies per milliliter. (3) What is your CD4 cell count? A count of 210 is obviously quite different from a count of 340. (4) Are you ready for a complex regimen that requires tenacious adherence? Nonadherence to the regimen takes the risk that your virus will become resistant and tarnish the success of the treatment. (5) What is your CD4 slope? The CD4 slope is the trajectory of the CD4 count over time: a rapid decline is an obvious cause for concern.

For the person with HIV infection, the decision to begin treatment requires a certain amount of introspection, commitment, and realism.

What "No Detectable Virus" Means and Why You Want It

The viral load, which measures the concentration of HIV in the blood, can now be detected at a lower concentration than it could by earlier tests. The lowest level that older tests could detect was 500 copies per milliliter of blood. Newer tests can go down to 20 or 50 copies per milliliter. "Undetectable" means that the concentration of HIV in the blood is lower than the test's limit of detection; in other words, with the older tests, "undetectable" would mean below 500, and with the newer tests, below 50. Most HIV experts now define "undetectable" as below 50 copies per milliliter.

You want no detectable virus because those low concentrations indicate that the virus is reproducing so slowly that drug-resistant mutations are unlikely. The higher the viral load, the more new viruses are made, and with more new viruses the chance of mutations is greater. A person with a viral load of 10,000 has a viral reproduction rate 10 times higher than a person with a viral load of 1,000, a mutation rate 10 times higher, and a resistance rate 10 times higher. A person with a viral load below 50 does not appear to be making enough new viruses to cause clinically meaningful resistance. So a combination of drugs that brings about a viral load of less than 50 should work indefinitely.

You can usually tell soon after treatment starts how well it will work. In the first week, the viral load should drop ten-fold; in 8 to 16 weeks, it should be less than 500; and by 24 weeks, it should be undetectable. Sometimes these goals are achieved more slowly. These early weeks are critical because the first treatment regimen has the highest probability of success.

How to Get "No Detectable Virus"

You have to take all your pills regularly, and that's not easy. The pills can be numerous and toxic, the pill schedule can be demanding, and the side effects are unpleasant. We know that most people find adhering to even simple drug schedules difficult: the average person with high blood pressure, for example, takes only about half the recommended doses. With HIV the difficulties of adherence are much greater. And unfortunately, the consequences of nonadherence are more severe. If HIV is suppressed only incompletely, the remaining virus develops resistance to the drugs. The person with high blood pressure who misses several doses will still, when he or she wants to resume taking pills, have a drug that works. The person with HIV infection who misses pills risks resistance, and once resistance develops, that drug is usually lost to that person forever. Nonadherence might even risk losing the effectiveness of a whole class of drugs for the person.

One study showed that if you take 95 percent of the pills (e.g., 19 out of 20), you'll have an 81 percent chance of getting no detectable virus. If you take only 80 percent of the pills (e.g., 16 out of 20), your chances nose-dive to 30 percent. On the basis of this and other studies, we conclude that occasional missed doses at the 5 percent level probably won't create resistance; resistance might require weeks or months of missed or reduced doses. This risk might be quite different for NNRTIs. So the risk seems to vary with the drug, the viral load, and how many other drugs you've taken.

A few rules are important:

• Always take your medication in full dose, unless your doctor tells you otherwise.

• Understand your regimen. Know what you are taking and when.

If you are unsure, ask. Your resources are your physician, nurse, physician assistant, or pharmacist. They are best if they are affiliated with your care, and best if they are "HIV-savvy." The regimens used generally don't vary. For example, atazanavir (Reyataz) is two 200 mg capsules a day, always with food. "Boosted" atazanavir is two 150 mg capsules a day, with 100 mg of ritonavir (Norvir), again with food. The reason for the ritonavir is to increase the amount of atazanavir in your body by slowing your body's attempt to eliminate it. Ritonavir effectively triples the concentration of atazanavir. The reason for the food is that it increases the amount of drug your gut absorbs by 70 percent; without food, you get about one-third as much drug. We don't make these recommendations simply because they seem to make sense; they are based on facts established by sophisticated pharmacology studies that test people in laboratories, carefully measuring the amount of drug their bodies absorb with and without food, and with and without ritonavir. The standard methods and results of these studies are all part of the one-thousand-page package submitted to the FDA for the drug's approval.

• Know the language. Each HIV drug has a chemical name, a trade name given by the company that manufactures it, and a three-letter abbreviation. For example, efavirenz (chemical name), Sustiva (trade name), and EFV (three-letter abbreviation) are all different names for the same drug. Some clinics and pharmacy books, such as the *Physicians' Desk Reference,* have photographs of the drugs; HIV clinics almost always have wall charts with photographs of the HIV drugs; but because both the books and the clinics have a problem keeping up, you'll often find that one of your drugs isn't pictured because it's too new. The abbreviations are standardized and often used to indicate specific regimens. For example, TDF/FTC/LPV/r means tenofovir, emtricitabine, lopinavir, and low-dose ritonavir; this sounds like a lot of different drugs, but because several drugs are now packaged in one pill, it's actually just Truvada (TDF plus FTC) and Kaletra (LPV plus r).

• Be aware of the side effects. All drugs have them, and they're generally well-known because the FDA requires a drug's toxicity profile before licensing it. With HIV drugs, side effects are important: most studies show that 30 to 40 percent of people need to change regimens because of the drugs' side effects. Some side effects, people know about—nausea, diarrhea, headache. Some are detected primarily by laboratory tests. Some occur immediately; some occur only after months or years of taking the drugs. It's good to know what side effects to expect. Ask.

• Pay close attention to drug interactions, the effect of one drug on another. Drug interactions are common with all PIs and NNRTIs. For example, a person taking ritonavir died from the street drug Ecstasy, because ritonavir increases the blood levels of Ecstasy by up to ten-fold. St. John's Wort can cause severe interactions with all protease inhibitors because it decreases their concentrations to the point where they are useless. Sometimes a cardiologist or an internist is prescribing one set of drugs while the HIV physician prescribes another set. Almost any drug for ulcers is a disaster for atazanavir, which needs stomach acid for absorption. Simvastatin (Zocor), commonly used for blood cholesterol problems, can't be given with any protease inhibitors because the protease inhibitors make the blood levels of Zocor so high that the drug could become toxic. Most of these drug interactions are well worked out and easily found in various charts or on the Internet. The point is, make sure all your physicians know all your medications. You can also look up the drugs you're taking and their interactions on the Internet: some sites allow you to enter two drugs and rapidly learn what drug interaction takes place.

• Pay close attention to instructions to take the drugs with meals or on an empty stomach.

• As a general rule, when you have a problem with part of the regimen, it's best to stop all drugs. Thus, if you stopped one drug of a three- or four-drug regimen because that drug ran out or caused toxicity, you should stop all drugs until a full regimen can be restarted. This recommendation is complicated because two commonly used drugs, efavirenz and nevirapine, last a long time in the body. So when you stop AZT/3TC/EFV immediately, the AZT and 3TC are gone from your body in one day, but the EFV is still there two weeks later. This long period of efavirenz at low levels could possibly trigger resistance. Note that this problem with varying times for clearing a drug out of your body applies only to efavirenz and nevirapine. In any case, HIV physicians deal with these complexities with tricks that are themselves complex, variable, and evolving. In general, then, not stopping the full regimen will inhibit HIV only partially and HIV will become resistant.

• The most important drug regimen is probably the first one taken. The reason is, if you become resistant to one drug, you may also be resistant to other drugs in the same class. This is called cross-resistance, and it happens especially with NNRTIs.

We have worked hard to get treatments that can be taken twice or even once a day, that will be well tolerated, and that will work. Research into adherence shows—as you'd expect—that the best treatments are simple, and that complicated treatments cause confusion and nonadherence.

Research has also been done to learn which patients are most adherent. Being good at taking pills does not appear to be related to gender, race, socioeconomic status, or level of education. Men or women; black, white, or Hispanic; rich or poor; educated or not—we can't predict who will be able to adhere to the HAART regimen. In fact, studies done with AIDS doctors show that most of them cannot adhere to the treatments they regularly prescribe for their patients. The only people who seem predictably bad at adhering to treatment are active substance abusers like alcoholics or injection drug users, people who are mentally ill, and adolescents.

And to make predicting adherence even harder, studies find that most people tend to overstate their adherence. They know their doctors think adherence is important, and they want their doctors to see them as good patients. But research that actually monitors people taking pills reveals that people aren't sticking to the regimen as strictly as they say they are. It's best to be honest.

Sticking to the Regimen

Because the first round of treatment is the best bet for getting no detectable virus, you shouldn't risk failing at it. Under no circumstances should you "give treatment a whirl." Don't start the regimen until you're ready to stick to it. Tell your doctor if you think you can't. This is serious stuff and you may get only a limited number of shots at effective drugs. The following are guidelines that might help adherence:

• People should learn their regimens and those regimens' nuances: which pills and when, which need to be taken with food and which need to be taken while fasting, and what the relevant drug interactions are—can you take the HAART drugs with Prilosec, for example, or with Lipitor?

• Drugstores and clinics have weekly pill boxes with sectioned containers: most pill boxes have seven daily sections, each divided into three to five time compartments. Weekly pill boxes not only remind you of the pills you need to take, but help you keep count of whether you've taken them all.

• In any case, it is a good idea to count out pills weekly and to write down when you missed a dose.

• The dose that's hardest to remember is the midday dose. Pills taken once daily seem easy; twice daily are only a little harder; and three times daily, much harder. Most HIV treatment is now pills taken once or twice daily.

• Try to work pill taking into your daily routine. Pills taken twice a day could be taken when you brush your teeth, and you could remember them by keeping them next to your toothbrush.

• A number of reminder systems are available: watches with alarms, timers, pagers, automatic dialing phone systems. The latter is a system where you program the telephone to ring regularly and deliver a recorded message like "take your pills," or "take two yellow football-shaped tablets and an orange pill." These reminder systems can help, but in general they don't work: because people depend on them, the system fails, and the people miss doses.

• Ask a spouse or colleague or friend to help you remember.

• Some people draw clocks with the names of the pills or colors for each pill marked at the proper times and in relation to meals.

• One common problem with adherence is the drugs' side effects, especially those effects felt immediately, like nausea and diarrhea. (Many people with HIV infection say they didn't feel sick until they got treated.) Try not to stop or miss doses because of trivial side effects. Most side effects are dealt with easily. A few, however, are important indicators of more serious complications, so make sure your health care provider knows every possible side effect you might be having.

• Two major impediments to adherence are depression and substance abuse. If you are depressed or are abusing drugs or alcohol, your health care provider absolutely must know. Both conditions can be treated.

Missing Doses

When HAART fails, the cause is usually poor adherence—people miss too many doses of the drug. Poor adherence not only allows HIV to get out of control, but it also permits resistant viruses to flourish; and resistant HIV limits which drugs will work. Balancing adherence and resistance is a tricky equation and depends on the drugs.

With protease inhibitors, taking most of the doses but not controlling HIV will lead to resistance. Taking even fewer doses—less than half the doses prescribed—will also result in failure to control HIV but will not lead to resistance: in that case HIV can thrive without resorting to resistance. With nevirapine and efavirenz, missing occasional doses is not as dangerous because they last a long time in the body. Missing a lot of doses, however, will cause HIV both to go out of control and to become resistant. With these drugs, you should take every dose, and if stopping is necessary, stop them all at once (unless instructed otherwise).

The general rule, however, is to stick carefully to the regimen but not to panic. Because we pay such enormous attention to adherence, some people worry that a few missed doses will mean harsh penalties. But penalties come not from a few missed doses, but from repeated inconsistencies: taking some drugs but not the whole regimen; or losing the full dosage by taking the drug with food when it should have been taken while fasting. In general, most of the drugs can be taken a few hours late without losing effectiveness. If you forget a dose, you can take it a few hours later. If you've missed by more than a few hours, just wait until the time for the next dose. The exception to this is a pill taken once a day: take it as soon as you notice missing the dose, or you may have a long period with no drug on board. If you have delayed until the time of the next dose, don't "double up"—it is better simply to lose one dose. But do avoid missing a single daily dose consistently. If you have been vomiting, you should stop taking the pills until you can keep them down. If you have diarrhea, take the drugs as usual; diarrhea has little effect on drug absorption.

If you do not take your pills with or without food, whichever is required, you risk the drug not getting into your system. If you have trouble taking the pills with or without food as required, tell your doctor, who can prescribe a more realistic regimen. Treatment may need to be stopped temporarily for many reasons. You may run out of pills, or the pharmacy may run out of them. You may have gastroenteritis or surgery. In general, it's always best to stop all drugs at once. The only drugs that are possible exceptions are efavirenz and nevirapine because they stay in the body a long time. Make no decisions without talking to your doctor.

What Drugs to Treat With

The more we learn about the effects and long-term side effects of the drugs and about the durability of the viral response, the more complicated the treatment of HIV infection has become. But these are the goals of treatment:

1. Suppress the virus as long as possible: we keep track of suppression by measuring the HIV viral load—the concentration of HIV in the blood—usually at three- to four-month intervals.

2. Maintain or get back a good immune system: we keep track by measuring the CD4 cell count, which is the barometer of immune function. Success in keeping the immune system healthy and the CD4 cell count high depends on our ability to suppress the virus, because it is the virus that kills the CD4 cells.

3. Prevent the HIV-related complications: these are the complications, like pneumocystis pneumonia or cryptococcal (fungal) meningitis, that first led to recognition of HIV. These complications virtually never happen when the CD4 cell count is above 200.

4. Avoid the side effects of the drugs used to accomplish goals 1–3. These side effects are summarized below.

5. Maintain as many treatment options as possible: some treatment decisions must balance risk against benefit. A low CD4 cell count risks a major complication, so we need to attack HIV aggressively, even if we have to change treatment many times. With a high CD4 cell count, however, we may have the luxury of going slower, thereby having the benefit of more options down the line. Generalizing about these decisions is difficult because individual risk-benefit calculations are so highly variable.

6. Stop HIV transmission: the likelihood of transmission depends on the risk behavior and the viral load. If we could decrease both, we would be able to slow or stop this epidemic.

HIV treatment has large gray zones and is different for different people. But we do have a consensus, based on vast experience and substantial review, on a few recommended regimens for initial treatment. After making sure the person with HIV infection has realistic expectations of what can be done, the best success for achieving goals 1 to 3 comes from the first regimen.

The usual first regimen is two nucleosides combined with a protease inhibitor, or a boosted protease inhibitor, or a nonnucleoside reverse transcriptase inhibitor. The two nucleosides are sometimes called the "nucleoside backbone," and the drug from the other two classes, a PI or a NNRTI, is just called "the third drug." When a PI is used, it is often "boosted" with ritonavir. Ritonavir is also a PI, but it is used because it increases the blood levels of the other PI, that is, it "boosts" the PI. In this case, the doses of ritonavir are so low that it does not really count as part of the treatment. In short, the first regimen usually consists of three drugs for HIV and is sometimes called "triple therapy."

When to Stop Treatment

Treatment is stopped in three situations. One is when stopping is planned or elective. Sometimes stopping treatment is an option because the person has responded to it so well. For example, when treatment started, the CD4 count was 200 and the viral load was 50,000; four years later, the virus is undetectable and the CD4 count is 800. In a case like this, stopping has generally been safe and effective. The general result is that once the drugs are all stopped, the virus quickly rebounds to pretreatment levels and the CD4 count drops rapidly for two to three months, then levels off. Treatment always needs to be restarted, usually when the CD4 count is down to 300 to 350. Studies of more than 700 patients show that such "drug holidays" can last an average of eight to twelve months and that when treatment restarts, the patients respond well. Just remember that when the viral load is high, transmission becomes a greater risk. And don't be alarmed at the precipitous drop in the CD4 count in the first months.

The other situation in which treatment is stopped is when people feel that it's not working and they want to stop. Many regimens are hard to tolerate or don't control the virus. The viral load is high, and resistance mutations exclude the likelihood that any new combination of drugs will work any better. But even though the drugs cost $10,000 to $15,000 per year, cause side effects, and don't appear to work, they're still working. When the drugs are stopped, the viral load shoots up, usually ten-fold, and the CD4 count drops fast. So even though a treatment appears to fail—assuming no other drug options are better—it should still be continued.

Unplanned drug discontinuations are different and common. These may happen because of gastroenteritis, bad side effects, an operation or surgical procedure, or a pharmacy running out of a drug. In these cases, the best rule is to stop all drugs simultaneously and restart treatment when the full regimen is again feasible. Be sure to let your health care provider know.

When to Change Treatment

The best way to measure the response to treatment is to measure the viral load after the treatment begins. Although we listed six goals for treatment, the most important is number 1, suppressing the virus. The average person with HIV infection, without treatment, produces about 10 billion new HIVs every day. These viruses aggressively invade CD4 cells, multiply inside them, then kill them. We can kill the HIV virus with "triple therapy," but we do not have drugs that reconstitute the CD4 cell count. So the drugs against HIV are the key not only to suppressing the virus, but also to maintaining a good immune system and preventing complications.

The many clinical studies of various treatments have shown that the initial triple therapy will kill about 90 percent of all HIV viruses in the body within one to two weeks, and 99.9 percent within one month. We expect that the viral load will go from an average of about 50,000 to less than 50—that is, to "no detectable virus"—within 16 to 24 weeks. Many studies now indicate that the best predictor of long-term success with treatment is the viral load after 24 weeks of treatment.

When the viral load decreases, the body makes more CD4 cells. The CD4 cell count increases rapidly, often by 40 to 50 in the first two to three months and by an average of 100 to 150 per year thereafter. However, this increase is different in different people. Some people control the virus well, but their CD4 cell response is blunted. Other people have the opposite: a relatively poor control of the virus but a robust jump in the CD4 cell count. These variations are poorly understood, and so far we have few guidelines. In general, we know that killing the virus is critical: killing the virus is the only way we know to raise the CD4 cell count. Controlling the virus also helps prevent HIV-associated complications. But if the virus is under control and the CD4 cell count remains disturbingly low, we sometimes change treatment to see if the CD4 count will rise.

Treatment is changed for two major reasons. The first is "virologic failure," which means the failure to achieve a low viral load, measured at periodic intervals after treatment has started. In the case of one of the recommended treatment combinations, the triple therapy, we have two possible explanations. First, the virus may be resistant to one or more of the drugs. We can conduct a resistance test and get a very good read on why a treatment may not be working. Second, the drugs might not be getting to the places in the body where HIV is found. The most common reason is inadequate adherence. Adherence has always been the most difficult challenge of triple therapy and the most common cause of treatment failure. People with HIV infection hear so much about taking pills as prescribed, more than anyone with any other disease, because the consequences of nonadherence are so punishing.

However, reasons other than poor adherence may cause inadequate drug levels. One reason might be pharmacological—that is, the drug simply is not getting into the system—and this might occur because the drug is taken with food when it should be taken without, or taken on an empty stomach when it needs to be taken with food. We have worked hard to develop treatments that do not have this "food effect," and only a small number of drugs still do. Another reason might be an interaction with another drug: an antibiotic, or a cholesterol pill, or blood pressure medicine may have decreased the concentration of the HIV drug. Drug interactions are most common and most pronounced with the protease inhibitors. And since protease inhibitors also have a marked effect on the concentrations of many non-HIV medications, you should be sure that all the physicians participating in your care are aware of all the drugs you are taking. Sorting this out is extremely complicated—thousands of drugs are currently in the market place—but many computer programs or Internet sites allow you to enter the two drugs and rapidly learn what drug interaction takes place.

If failure to achieve a low viral load—virologic failure—is the most frequent cause for changing treatment, the second most frequent is intolerance of the drugs' side effects. Any of the three drugs you take can have a multitude of side effects. The method of managing the side effects depends on the severity of the reaction—which may have potential long-term consequences. Some side effects are so severe that future use of the drug carries a substantial risk, and the drug can no longer be safely taken. Other drugs are stopped because the side effect is annoying, or gets worse over a period of months or years, or seems intolerable because it makes the quality of life so poor. Such side effects might be severe headaches, uncontrollable diarrhea, or severe nausea. Decisions are simplified because we now have so many drugs: if a regimen, especially the first one, is so awful that it interferes with your usual life activities, it is usually relatively easy to find alternatives. It may get progressively more difficult, though, when you lose the option of taking certain drugs because of either resistance or intolerance.

Long-term studies of people taking triple therapy indicate that about 40 to 50 percent of them will need to change the regimen. About half of these changes are the result of resistance, and the other half arise from drug intolerance. This is not to say that the drugs do not work at all; the drugs do work, but they do not meet our stringent expectations for both keeping the virus controlled and maintaining a good quality of life.

What to Change To

When people encounter virologic failure, the usual alternative is to measure the resistance of the virus to various drugs and then to select drugs based on that "resistance profile." In general, finding alternative regimens after one round of treatment fails is pretty easy; it is a bit harder after two rounds, and it gets more difficult as the number of rounds increases. The reason is that resistance accumulates: you develop resistance to one drug, then another, and so on, and those resistant strains of the virus persist in the body. Sometimes viruses develop "class resistances," meaning they decrease the activity of an entire class of drugs.

How to Test for Resistance

Tests for resistance predict which drugs will work against your strain of HIV. Actually, what the tests do is predict which drugs *won't* work. The two types of resistance tests are phenotypic tests and genotypic tests.

The phenotypic test, done only rarely, checks whether your own strain of HIV has become resistant to a given drug. The test treats your strain of HIV with that drug, then compares the results to another, unmutated HIV, called a "wild type virus," treated with the same drug. If 4 times more of a given drug are needed to inhibit your strain than the wild type, your strain is considered resistant to that drug. If 4 to 10 times more drug are needed to inhibit your strain, your strain is considered very resistant.

The genotypic test is more complicated. HIV is error-prone; when it reproduces, it makes lots of mistakes. Specifically, some of its genes mutate. Some mutations, called resistance mutations, confer resistance to certain drugs.

The convention for reporting resistance mutations is a confusing series of numbers and letters: one is K103N. The number in the middle indicates the particular sequence of amino acids (called a *codon*) on the gene at which the mutation occurs—in this case, codon 103. The first letter refers to the amino acid that is supposed to be at codon 103 (K, here, means lysine). The second letter refers to the amino acid that is actually there as a result of mutation (N means asparagine). So the K103N mutation on the gene for reverse transcriptase means that on codon 103, lysine has been replaced by asparagine. Such changes in the sequence of amino acids can make the virus behave differently.

A virus with a K103N mutation, for instance, won't be affected by efavirenz (Sustiva). Although efavirenz will continue to kill most strains of the virus, it won't kill the strains with a K103N mutation. Those mutated strains will thrive, then gradually predominate. Eventually, the person will have enough HIVs with the K103N mutation that genotypic tests will detect the mutation, showing that efavirenz will no longer lower the person's viral load.

The mutations that affect NNRTIs are often knockouts; that is, the mutations render a drug completely useless: K103N on the reverse transcriptase gene makes the NNRTIs efavirenz and nevirapine (Viramune) useless. The mutations that affect the nucleoside analogs often simply reduce their effectiveness: K65R on the reverse transcriptase gene reduces the effectiveness of didanosine (ddI), tenofovir (TDF), and abacavir (ABC) but has no effect on the effectiveness of zidovudine (AZT).

The mutations that affect protease inhibitors are either signature mutations that affect only specific drugs, or class mutations that affect all protease inhibitors. Class mutations are not usually knockout mutations like those affecting NNRTIs; that is, no single mutation renders the whole class of protease inhibitors completely useless. But several signature mutations, each conferring resistance to specific drugs, can add up so that the whole class of protease inhibitors becomes less effective over time.

In general, as the drugs become less effective, the concentration of resistant viruses increases, and so therefore does the probability of resistance mutations. In a person with a viral load of 20,000, the virus is multiplying ten times faster than in a person with a viral load of 2,000; and the probability of more resistance mutations is ten times greater.

The situation isn't all bad. Although the M184V mutation on the reverse transcriptase gene is a knockout for lamivudine (3TC), the same mutation also seems to injure the virus—the virus simply doesn't reproduce as well. So even though the 3TC isn't killing the virus, it is encouraging the spread of the M184V mutation and thus reducing the virus's ability to reproduce. That is, while people with K103N mutations should no longer take efavirenz or nevirapine, people with M184V mutations often take 3TC.

Resistance mutations are forever. Even though resistant strains seem to disappear when the drug they resist is stopped, they're not really gone. They remain in the body in some sequestered haven, such as the lymph nodes, invisible to resistance tests and ready to rebound when you take that drug again. Say you take 3TC for three years and get the M184V mutation. If you stop 3TC, a resistance test six months later will show that the M184V mutation has disappeared. But M184V is actually still around in low concentrations; it has become what is called a minority species, and resistance tests don't recognize it. If you take 3TC again, the M184V minority species will rebound and soon become a majority again.

The lesson is that decisions about treatment need to consider not only the results of current resistance tests, but also previous resistance tests and previous treatments that have failed.

Side Effects, or Toxicities, of HAART

HAART has been unexpectedly toxic. In fact, much of the research in the field of HIV infection is no longer devoted to the complications of immune suppression but to the complications caused by HAART. People with HIV infection are now faced not with pneumocystis pneumonia or CMV retinitis, but with such side effects as high blood fat, predisposing them to heart disease, and a rearrangement of fat in their bodies.

Most side effects can be described in these three ways:

• Subjective versus objective: Subjective side effects—like gastrointestinal complications, headaches, and weakness, that depend on people's perceptions or feelings—are common and can be debilitating, but their seriousness is often difficult for the physician to assess. Objective side effects are those that cause abnormal laboratory tests; they can be monitored for frequency and tested for confirmation.

• "Deal breakers" versus modifiers: Some side effects are "deal breakers" that rule out the continued use of a drug; others simply mean the regimen needs to be modified or the symptoms need to be treated with another drug.

• Long-term versus short-term: Many of the drugs used for HIV infection have side effects that take months or years to develop and are still poorly understood. This topic is discussed in more detail below. Other side effects become apparent immediately. For example, gastrointestinal side effects are among the most common and usually occur with the first dose; bad dreams with efavirenz, which are quite temporary, are noted with the first night's sleep.

The major side effects associated with individual drugs are noted in table 4. This chapter deals with side effects by category.

Gastrointestinal Intolerance

Symptoms: The usual symptom is nausea, occasionally along with vomiting and abdominal pain. Diarrhea is also common. These side effects are usually noted with the first dose of a drug or drug regimen.

Frequency: The frequency varies greatly, depending on the drug. This type of intolerance is most common with all of the PIs, AZT, and ddI. Diarrhea tends to be particularly frequent with LPV/r (Kaletra) and NFV (nelfinavir).

Treatment: Often tolerance of the drug improves with time. Nausea may improve when the drug is taken with food—though, since some drugs like unboosted indinavir or ddI (didanosine) must be taken on an empty stomach, food is not always an option. Many common medicines for gastrointestinal intolerance, such as Donnagel, Kaopectate, and Pepto-Bismol, are over-the-counter drugs that can be purchased without a prescription. For diarrhea, the standard is Imodium or calcium. These treatments usually clear up or at least improve the gastrointestinal symptoms to the point where they can be tolerated.

Table 4. The Drugs of Highly Active Antiretroviral Therapy (HAART)

Abbreviation and Trade Name	Chemical Name	Dose by Mouth (unless noted otherwise) (adult)	General Comments	Side Effects
The Nucleoside Analogs				
3TC, Epivir	Lamivudine	150 mg twice daily or 300 mg once daily	Great agent—potent and no side effects	Side effects nil
ABC, Ziagen	Abacavir	300 mg twice daily or 600 mg once daily	Potent; problem side effect	Serious allergic reaction with fever, rash, nausea, and vomiting, usually in the first 6 weeks; average at 9 days. Most have fever. If this drug is stopped for hypersensitivity, do not restart.
AZT, Retrovir	Zidovudine	200 mg 3 times/day or 300 mg twice daily	Still a good drug	Anemia, low white blood cell count, nausea, headache, fatigue; lactic acidosis
Combivir, AZT/3TC	Zidovudine + lamivudine	1 tablet twice daily	Combo is easier to take	Side effects of AZT
d4T, Zerit	Stavudine	Over 130 lbs.: 40 mg twice daily; under 130 lbs.: 30 mg twice daily	Good drug for short term, but long-term toxicity	Peripheral neuropathy with painful feet; fat loss—buttocks, legs, and arms; lactic acidosis; blood lipid increases

ddC, HIVID	Zalcitabine	0.75 mg 3 times/day	Rarely used	Peripheral neuropathy with painful feet (rare—pancreatitis, mouth ulcers)
ddI, Videx	Didanosine	Over 130 lbs.: 400 mg once daily; under 130 lbs.: 250 mg once daily	Toxic with long-term use; take on empty stomach	Pancreatitis: abdominal pain, nausea, and vomiting; diarrhea; peripheral neuropathy with painful feet (rare—liver damage); lactic acidosis
Epzicom, ABC/3TC	Abacavir + lamivudine	1 tablet daily	Combo is easier to take	Side effects of ABC
FTC, Emtriva	Emtricitabine	200 mg once daily	Like 3TC	Side effects rare
TDF, Viread	Tenofovir	300 mg once daily	Great drug	Rare—kidney disease
Trizivir, AZT/3TC/ABC	Zidovudine + lamivudine + abacavir	1 tablet twice daily	Combo is easier to take	Side effects of ABC and AZT
Truvada, TDF/FTC	Tenofovir + emtricitabine	1 tablet once daily	Combo is easier to take	Side effects rare
The Protease Inhibitors				
ATV, Reyataz	Atazanavir	400 mg once daily; ATV/RTV: 300 mg/ 100 mg once daily	Requires food; no effect on blood lipids; potent	Gastrointestinal intolerance, jaundice

(continued)

Table 4. (*Continued*)

Abbreviation and Trade Name	Chemical Name	Dose by Mouth (unless noted otherwise) (adult)	General Comments	Side Effects
		The Protease Inhibitors		
FPV, Lexiva	Fosamprenavir	FPV/RTV: 700 mg/ 100 mg twice daily or 1,400 mg/200 mg once daily	Potent	Gastrointestinal intolerance
IDV, Crixivan	Indinavir	400 mg IDV + 400 mg RTV or 800 mg IDV + 100–200 mg RTV twice daily	Needs RTV boosting	Kidney stones, nausea, dry lips and skin; must take large volumes of water to prevent kidney stones
Kaletra, LPV/r	Lopinavir + ritonavir	2 tablets twice daily	Potent; requires food	Gastrointestinal intolerance, especially diarrhea
NFV, Viracept	Nelfinavir	1,250 mg twice daily	Requires food; reduced potency; doesn't boost with RTV	Gastrointestinal intolerance, especially diarrhea
RTV, Norvir	Ritonavir	600 mg twice daily; usually given to boost other PIs in doses of 200–400 mg/day	Rarely used for anti-HIV; used to boost other PIs	Gastrointestinal intolerance, dose-related

Saquinavir	SQV, Invirase	1,000 mg SQV + 100 mg RTV twice daily or 2,000 mg SQV + 100 mg RTV once daily	Potent; requires food; boosting required	Gastrointestinal intolerance
Tipranavir	TPV, Aptiva	TPV/RTV 500 mg/200 mg twice daily	Used only after treatment failure	Gastrointestinal intolerance; liver toxicity; many drug interactions

The Nonnucleoside Reverse Transcriptase Inhibitors

Delavirdine	DLV, Rescriptor	400 mg 3 times/day	Rarely used	Rash
Efavirenz	EFV, Sustiva	600 mg at sleep time	Potent; see side effects	Mental changes during first 2–3 weeks, with bad dreams, confusion, and/or a "disconnected" feeling; rash
Nevirapine	NVP, Viramune	200 mg daily for 2 weeks, then 200 mg twice daily	Potent; see side effects	Rash; severe liver disease, especially with baseline CD4 count over 250 in women

The Entry Inhibitor

Enfuvirtide	T20, Fuzeon	90 mg by injection twice daily	Used only after viral failure	Pain at place where it is injected

Warnings: Abdominal pain along with nausea and vomiting can also be a sign of such very important complications as pancreatitis or lactic acidosis. Pancreatitis is most frequently associated with ddI treatment and can cause severe pain and require hospitalization. If you are taking the drug known to cause this complication and the symptoms began occurring long after the drug was started, you may have pancreatitis. Lactic acidosis can cause weight loss along with the other symptoms; is almost always associated with d4T, ddI, or, less frequently, AZT; and also occurs long after the drug was started (see below for a fuller description).

Lactic Acidosis

Frequency: This is an unusual side effect associated with NRTI drugs, primarily d4T, ddI, and AZT. About 1 percent of people taking these drugs are diagnosed with lactic acidosis each year; the percentage for those on d4T is probably greater. The cause of this syndrome is not clearly defined, but it appears to be the toxic effect on mitochondria, the energy source of cells, when these drugs are used over a long time.

Symptoms: The most common complaints are the slow onset—after months of treatment with the drugs mentioned—of rather nonspecific gastrointestinal and other symptoms, including nausea, appetite loss, stomach pain, vomiting, weight loss, and general fatigue.

Diagnosis: The first step is to suspect the syndrome, because its onset can be subtle and its symptoms nonspecific. The diagnosis can be confirmed with a blood test for lactic acid; it's a standard test and available in most laboratories. The normal level is 2 (2 μmoles); a level of 2–5 is a bit high, 5–10 is serious, and a level over 10 could be regarded as a medical emergency.

Treatment: The usual treatment is to discontinue the drugs that appear to cause the complication and to provide supportive care: intravenous fluid for hydration, and support of various organs that may fail. Lactic acidosis takes a long time to come on, and it also takes a long time to disappear—weeks or months may elapse before the lactic acid levels are back to normal. The future use of drugs after this complication usually is limited to drugs that were not implicated in the first place.

Skin Rash

Frequency: Skin rash is a common side effect of drugs in general and is especially common with nevirapine, efavirenz, fosamprenavir, tipranavir, and atazanavir. About 15 to 25 percent of the people taking these drugs report rashes. Most of the rashes are mild to moderate, and they go away if the drug is continued. In about 2 to 4 percent of the cases, the rash is so severe as to require discontinuing these drugs.

Symptoms: Most mild to moderate rashes consist of blotchy, red spots on the trunk, arms, legs, and face. They may itch. Mild rashes can often be "treated through"; that is, the drug is continued and the rash usually resolves on its own. Treatment may include antihistamines and, occasionally, cortisone ointments. More serious rashes—those associated with blisters, fever, and involvement of the mouth or eyes—mandate immediate medical attention. Any rash that is severe should be seen and managed in a medical-care setting.

Warnings: Two specific skin reactions that include a rash along with other findings indicate a severe and sometimes life-threatening complication, either the abacavir hypersensitivity reaction or the nevirapine liver disease. They are both described below, but we mention them here because a rash may be an important part of the initial side effect. Also, some of the more extensive rash reactions seen with nevirapine or efavirenz, usually in the first sixteen weeks of treatment, may be severe enough to require permanent discontinuation of these drugs.

Liver Disease

Frequency and Description: All antiretroviral drugs may cause liver disease, but the mechanism is quite different for different classes of drugs. And although abnormal liver tests are noted in 5 to 15 percent of all people with HIV infection, most cases are quite trivial: the person has no symptoms and the problem is found by a routine test of liver function. Many or most people do fine with continued treatment. The drug causing liver problems would be stopped only after a judgment call by the physician about how bad the liver test needs to be. This nonthreatening form of liver disease is a side effect of all protease inhibitors but occurs in only 10 to 15 percent of the people taking them. It is also a side effect of the NNRTIs nevirapine and efavirenz, occurring with a similar frequency. The nucleosides may also cause liver disease, but the process is different: the disease results from statosis, or fat deposits in the liver, caused by lactic acidosis.

A further form of liver disease, particularly important to recognize, occurs with nevirapine and is especially common in women who have a CD4 cell count prior to treatment that exceeds 250. This form of liver disease is accompanied by symptoms, usually gastrointestinal symptoms, fever, and/or a rash. The great majority of cases occur during the first 16 weeks of treatment with nevirapine, and the drug must be stopped immediately. Because of this reaction, the standard of care is to test liver function frequently during the first 24 weeks of nevirapine.

Treatment: The treatment of these liver complications is generally restricted to deciding whether they are severe enough, or potentially severe enough, to discontinue the drug. Otherwise, except for supportive care, liver complications have no specific treatment.

Hepatitis and antiretroviral drugs: Some people taking antiretroviral drugs have chronic hepatitis, either hepatitis C or hepatitis B. In these cases, liver disease is commonly associated with the changes in liver function, and it is often impossible to tell whether the cause is the hepatitis virus or the antiretroviral drug. Most HIV care providers, who deal with this on a regular basis, try to determine the cause by using a variety of tests, sometimes a liver biopsy. One form of serious liver disease that is very important is chronic hepatitis caused by the hepatitis B virus. Three of the drugs commonly used for treating HIV are also effective against the hepatitis B virus: tenofovir (TDF), lamivudine (3TC), and emtricitabine (FTC). So the good news is that you can treat both HIV and hepatitis B viral infections with the same drugs. The bad news is that discontinuing any of these drugs may result in a flare-up of the hepatitis virus, a serious complication that requires taking some drug for hepatitis B.

Warnings: The two liver diseases from antiretroviral drugs are the nevirapine (NVP) reaction and the flare-up of the hepatitis B virus. The nevirapine reaction generally occurs during the first 16 weeks of nevirapine treatment and is always associated with symptoms that can be verified by laboratory testing. The flare-up of the hepatitis B virus occurs when one of the three nucleosides that treat hepatitis B is discontinued.

Diabetes

Frequency: Protease inhibitors are associated with something called "insulin resistance," which simply means that the body's insulin operates less effectively. About 3 to 5 percent of the people taking PI-based HAART get diabetes. Nearly all PIs can cause diabetes, but the frequency is variable: diabetes is particularly common with indinavir and infrequent or nil with atazanavir. The change in blood sugar takes place almost immediately after these drugs are given.

Symptoms: The usual symptoms of diabetes are increased appetite, large volumes of urine, and weight loss. In fact, we are usually aware of diabetes long before these symptoms are found. The reason is that a blood sugar is included in most of the standard tests that are done at 3- to 4-month intervals in most people taking HAART. Diabetes is defined by a blood sugar (glucose) level that is over 126.

Treatment: The standard treatment is a diabetic diet along with exercise and weight loss, sometimes supplemented by pills referred to as "oral hypoglycemics." Insulin treatment is rarely necessary unless the person is diabetes-prone as a result of genetics or other factors causing diabetes that are unrelated to antiretroviral treatment. Another option is to switch from the PI implicated to atazanavir or to a NNRTI-based antiretroviral regimen.

Warnings: Diabetes is usually asymptomatic and easily managed with diet and exercise, sometimes supplemented with oral drugs. For people with cardiovascular disease, diabetes is yet another risk factor for a stroke or a heart attack. Other people, particularly those who are diabetes-prone, may have unusual difficulty controlling their levels of blood sugar and may require insulin. These people might do best to change treatment, particularly when they have many options for equally effective antiretrovirals.

Fat Redistribution

Definition: Fat redistribution means a changed distribution of fat and comes in two forms. One, called fat atrophy, is the loss of fat in the arms, legs, and buttocks and in the face only above the upper lip. Fat atrophy is usually a side effect of NRTIs, especially d4T but also ddI and AZT. The other, called visceral fat redistribution, is on the trunk: an accumulation of fat on the back of the neck that looks like a buffalo hump; an increase in breast size in both men and women; and an increase in abdominal fat, particularly on the lower abdomen. Visceral fat redistribution is usually a side effect of protease inhibitors.

Frequency: How often fat redistribution occurs is hard to judge because it is totally subjective. A few laboratory measurements can confirm what we see; but this is a cosmetic issue, and its importance is really in the mind of the person with these changes. The methods to measure the changes are not very useful because they might miss some of the ones that the person thinks are most important and they might emphasize the ones that people will ignore. For example, the appearance of sunken cheeks is easy to see but hard to measure. Nevertheless, those who have tried to define the condition of fat redistribution have reported fat accumulation in 20 to 60 percent of people taking long-term PI-based HAART, and fat atrophy in 30 to 70 percent of people taking long-term d4T.

Significance: Although this is a cosmetic effect, self-image can be a very important factor in the quality of life. The loss of fat in the face may particularly bother people.

Treatment: Sometimes plastic surgery is successful: injections into the area of fat loss in the face, or liposuction of buffalo humps, or breast reduction. These procedures tend to be expensive and are generally not covered by third-party insurance companies. The alternative is "switch therapy"; that is, changing to other drugs. Switch therapy is easiest with d4T, which has many equally effective alternatives from the same class, but the reversal of fat redistribution is very slow and, according to some studies, virtually nil one to two years later. For PI-associated fat accumulation, switching drugs may not be particularly effective. Although the fat changes are commonly ascribed to PIs, they have also been noted with NNRTIs.

Increase in Blood Fats

Definition: Antiretroviral drugs are associated with substantial changes in blood cholesterol and another high-risk fat, triglycerides. The typical changes are an increase in the total cholesterol, the LDL cholesterol (the bad cholesterol), and the triglycerides.

Frequency: These increases have been reported in 40 to 70 percent of people taking protease inhibitors, and they occur within days of beginning treatment. The exception is atazanavir, which is not associated with these changes. An elevated triglyceride finding is also noted with d4T.

Context: The trade-off sounds terrible: the progression of HIV infection is reduced, but the risk of cardiovascular disease rises. But the risks must be viewed from the proper perspective. For a person with a CD4 cell count of 200 and the average risk profile for heart disease, not taking antiretroviral drugs increases the risk of death in the next five years by 50 times. Nevertheless, the increase in blood fats needs attention and can be serious, and it can be treated. Most important is the assessment of other risks for cardiovascular disease. Contributing factors include previous cardiovascular disease with a heart attack or stroke (the greatest risk for a second event), hypertension (high blood pressure), diabetes, smoking, elevated blood cholesterol or triglycerides prior to taking antiretroviral drugs, and genetics. Genetics here means having a first-degree male relative with cardiovascular disease before the age of 45 or a first-degree female relative with cardiovascular disease before the age of 55.

Treatment: The most important treatment is life-style changes, including weight reduction, exercise, diet modification, and discontinuation of smoking. All authorities emphasize the importance of these methods to control the risks, which might exist quite apart from HIV and its treatment. Beyond that, LDL cholesterol can be controlled with drugs, usually statins. However, this advice is complicated by drug interactions between statins and protease inhibitors or NNRTIs. Protease inhibitors increase the levels of some statins to dangerous concentrations; and efavirenz reduces statin concentrations to the point where they may not be particularly effective. These complexities are not too difficult to sort out using the standard guidelines. Triglycerides may also be elevated, also contribute to the risk, and also can be managed with drugs. Another approach is switch therapy, since atazanavir, efavirenz, and nevirapine are relatively free of this side effect.

Neuropathy

Definition: Neuropathy is a side effect of d4T or ddI. It occurs in about 20 percent of people who take these drugs for more than a year and is more common in those who take both drugs together.

Symptoms: The symptoms are pain and tingling in the feet, but continued use of the drugs may result in more pain and involvement of the arms as well. Eventually people might have relatively severe pain, causing difficulty walking and eventually requiring narcotics if the drugs are not stopped. If they are stopped soon enough, the changes go away; if they are continued for a long time, the pain is permanent.

Treatment: There are a variety of treatments, but none are particularly effective. It should be noted that this neuropathy is identical to a neuropathy attributed to HIV infection itself.

Warnings: Peripheral neuropathy will continue to get worse as long as you take the drugs that cause it. Therefore it is important to report this complication as soon as it occurs.

Side Effects Due to Individual Drugs

The side effects reviewed above are "class reactions": they are common to many drugs within a class. Some important side effects, however, occur only with specific drugs.

Abacavir hypersensitivity reaction: About 5 to 8 percent of people taking abacavir have the abacavir hypersensitivity reaction. It is serious. The symptoms are high fever, a rash all over the body, nausea, chills, diarrhea, vomiting, abdominal pain, and sometimes additional symptoms. It typically occurs early in the course of taking abacavir, usually around the ninth day of treatment; 90 percent of the reactions occur in the first six weeks. The drug should be stopped and not started again until the physician is certain that the symptoms were not from an abacavir hypersensitivity reaction. A test dose can result in a much more serious reaction. The concern is that warning people about the seriousness of this reaction and the multitude of symptoms can cause great anxiety. People are tempted to discontinue the drug even when they have only a simple cold, gastroenteritis, or some other common complaint; or when they have side effects from another drug that was taken with abacavir, such as the rash that is seen with nevirapine or efavirenz.

An abacavir hypersensitivity reaction almost always involves two systems. A rash alone (skin only) or cold symptoms alone (respiratory tract only) almost never mean that you have this side effect. The stakes in diagnosing the abacavir hypersensitivity reaction are sizable because if that's what you have, and if you take abacavir again, you may react so severely that you can never take the drug again. One possible approach in difficult cases is to have abacavir administered in a clinic under observation; a characteristic feature of the reaction is that the next administration is always associated with more profound reaction. Some interesting studies suggest a genetic predisposition to the abacavir hypersensitivity reaction, but this information has not yet evolved into a clinically useful tool to predict it or diagnose it.

Efavirenz-associated central nervous system complications: People who take efavirenz often experience an odd complication involving the brain: a "disassociated feeling," along with dizziness, sleepiness, abnormal dreams, difficulty with concentration, or depression. Up to 50 percent of the people who take this drug have this reaction. The good news is that the reaction is generally limited to the first 2 to 3 weeks of treatment. The cause is completely unknown and there is no treatment. Persons taking efavirenz need to be warned about this side effect so that they will know that it is normal and can be expected to simply disappear in 2 to 3 weeks as they continue to use the drug.

Indinavir-associated kidney stones and a dry skin and mouth: Indinavir may form crystals of indinavir in the kidneys and cause a kidney stone. This is actually noted in 15 to 20 percent of the people who take indinavir for a prolonged period. The symptoms are exactly like the symptoms of kidney stone due to other causes. It can be terrifying pain that requires narcotics for relief. This side effect is the reason that large volumes of fluid are required when you are taking this drug. Another odd reaction associated with indinavir is something called "sicca," which involves dry skin, a dry mouth, dry eyes, and possible hair loss. The cause of the sicca syndrome is not known, but most people who take the drug will complain of being "dry."

General Advice

Get Dental Care

The dental problems common to all adults—diseases of the teeth and of the supporting structures of the teeth—seem to occur more frequently and more severely in people with HIV infection. See your dentist regularly. Floss and brush your teeth assiduously. Tell your dentist about your HIV infection: people who are prone to dental problems should probably see the dentist more frequently, and the dentist may change some of his or her normal recommendations.

Follow a Nutritious Diet

Nutrition is important for virtually all people with HIV infection for two reasons. The first is that weight loss is a common symptom of this infection, and during the later stages, many people lose weight excessively. Paying attention to nutrition early in the course of the infection might delay weight loss. The second reason is that good nutrition may help maintain a strong immune system, even apart from HIV infection. It is well established that the immune system functions less well in people who are malnourished, though malnutrition must be severe before immune defects become noticeable.

Malnutrition is more exactly called "protein-calorie malnutrition." Calories come from most food, particularly fats. Proteins come from meat, milk products, poultry, eggs, fish, and dried beans and rice. People need diets that balance calories, protein, and the necessary vitamins. The usual balance for a healthy person is about 50 percent carbohydrate, 20 percent protein, and 30 percent fat, with an ample supply of vitamins. Some people with uncontrolled HIV infection need more calories because HIV infection seems to increase their metabolism: a person with untreated HIV infection requires 2,700 to 3,600 kilocalories per day. People with HIV infection consequently need to eat more. But excessive doses of vitamins, and macrobiotic diets or other fad diets, should be either avoided or undertaken only with the advice of a certified dietitian.

Get Exercise

Exercise programs are widely advocated as a way of staying healthy and of preventing cardiovascular disease. Whether exercise is similarly helpful to people with HIV infection is unknown. "Progressive resistance" exercises, like weight-lifting, when combined with eating enough calories, do increase lean body mass. Exercise will not increase CD4 cell counts, but most people who exercise regularly also feel better both physically and emotionally. There is no reason for a person with HIV infection to avoid regular exercise as long as fatigue or other symptoms do not prevent it. Strenuous exercise like marathon running and Olympic-type training, however, may actually be deleterious to the immune system. For example, Olympic athletes competing in endurance events have more colds and other infections. The implication is that exercise in moderation improves the sense of well-being, while intensive physical training may be hard on the body.

Stop Smoking—How to Do It

Smoking is bad for health in many ways. It is especially bad for the health of people with HIV infection. HIV predisposes people to lung infections; smoking also predisposes people to lung infections; and studies of people with HIV infection show that smoking causes even more lung infections. Before HAART, people often said that smoking was irrelevant because HIV would kill you anyway. HAART has changed that. As people have benefited from HAART and lived longer, they have become more likely to get sick or die from other conditions.

The major risk of smoking is cardiovascular disease. HAART therapy also carries a risk of cardiovascular disease, because of the effect that the drugs—especially the protease inhibitors—have on blood lipids, that is, on LDL cholesterol and triglycerides. These side effects can be measured and treated. Compared to protease inhibitors, smoking is a much greater risk. The second major risk of smoking is lung disease; it's almost a given. The risk of lung cancer increases with time and with the number of packs smoked per year. When you stop smoking, your lung cancer risk begins decreasing immediately and gradually falls to a near-zero increase in risk after about ten years.

Nicotine is one of the strongest addictions, and the effects of its withdrawal are harsh: tension, sleep problems, agitation, and depression. Many of the methods available for stopping are based on the science of nicotine addiction and the psychiatric effects of nicotine withdrawal. The key to stopping is motivation: you have to really want to stop. Many people stop on their own; others need medical help. The treatments come in two forms: nicotine replacement and non-nicotine therapy.

Nicotine Replacement

All of these methods have been reviewed by the FDA, which has determined them to be safe and effective. Which method you choose depends on your own preference.

• Nicotine patch: patches are available in doses based on the person's weight or the number of cigarettes smoked per day. The initial dose is taken for 4 weeks, then decreased every week for the next 4 weeks. The advantages of the patch are that it is easy to use and can be obtained without a prescription. The disadvantage is the lack of good dose control.

• Nicotine gum: doses are 2 mg if you smoke fewer than 25 cigarettes per day, and 4 mg if you smoke more. You chew one piece of gum per hour for 8 to 12 weeks. The advantage is that you can control the dose and you don't need a prescription. The disadvantages are the necessity of chewing correctly, the fact that you can't eat or drink while chewing, and the possibility of dental damage.

• Nicotine lozenge: the dose is a 2 mg lozenge for fewer than 25 cigarettes per day and a 4 mg lozenge for more. The lozenges are taken every 1 to 2 hours while awake for 6 weeks, then every 2 to 4 hours for the next 3 weeks, then every 4 to 8 hours for another 3 weeks, and then when necessary for 3 months. The entire process takes 3 to 6 months. Occasional side effects are headache, heartburn, nausea, and cough.

• Vapor inhaler (Nicotrol Inhaler): Cartridges are inhaled like a cigarette, to simulate smoking. The regimen is 6 to 16 cartridges, used over 3 to 6 months. These may cause throat irritation and cough, and the device is obvious to others when used.

• Nicotine nasal spray (Nicotrol NS): A 1 mg dose of nicotine is taken as a nasal spray, half in each nostril, once or twice an hour over 3 to 6 months. This delivery system replaces nicotine rapidly, and the person using it controls the dose, but it is also the most irritating: it causes irritation in the nose, coughing, sneezing, and tears. Most people learn to tolerate these effects with continued use.

Non-Nicotine Therapy

• Bupropion (Wellbutrin SR or Zyban): This is an antidepressant that has been found to be effective for stopping smoking. It is the only drug in its class approved by the FDA for stopping smoking. Authorities consider it as effective as the nicotine replacement methods. Treatment should start a week before stopping smoking. Use the sustained-release (SR) formulation. The dose is 150 mg per day for 3 days, then 150 mg twice daily. Most people take the drug for 7 to 12 weeks, sometimes as long as 6 months. The advantage of bupropion, compared to the nicotine replacement strategies, is the lack of exposure to nicotine. The disadvantages are the side effects of bupropion: insomnia, nausea, weight loss, dry mouth, and agitation—and, in 1 person in 1,000, seizures that are dose-related and are very rare at these smoking-cessation dosages.

• Nortriptyline (Aventyl, Pamelor) and clonidine: These are two other antidepressants that may be used but have not been reviewed by the FDA for stopping smoking; they are generally considered "second line" treatments.

Keep Working

People with HIV infection should work because working contributes to people's sense of self-worth, to their knowledge that they are contributing members of society. HIV infection should not keep people from working unless fatigue or other symptoms make it impossible. It is unfortunate that the disability laws often mandate not working as a requirement for health coverage. The effectiveness of HAART means that people once disabled can now reenter the workforce, but they may not be able to afford the drugs.

Occasionally employers have used the fact of HIV infection to limit workers' employment or to change their job assignments. The employee has considerable legal recourse as a result of the Rehabilitation Act of 1973, which became law in the United States in July 1992. This law protects every citizen against unfair discrimination based on sex, race, or handicap. Under this law, HIV infection is a handicap, and those who have HIV infection are legally protected. The employer must provide the employee with continued employment in the same job as long as she or he is capable of performing the job. This issue is discussed in more detail in chapter 9.

Know Your Travel and Occupational Risks

Travel Risks. The greatest health risk to people with or without HIV infection is travel in developing countries, where the major problem is microbes that contaminate food and water. Avoid raw fruits and vegetables, raw or undercooked seafood or meat, tap water, ice made from tap water, unpasteurized milk and dairy products, and all food or drink purchased from street vendors. Preferred foods are steaming hot: hot tea or coffee, or meat that's well-cooked. Also safe are peeled fruit, bottled beverages, and anything with alcohol in it. Water may also be treated with iodine or chlorine, but this is not as effective as a rolling boil for one minute.

Most diarrhea in travelers is easily controlled, and access to good health care may be difficult to obtain, so some travelers carry antibiotics to prevent infections during travel to developing countries. Most travelers need not do this, but some people with HIV infection may be considered at high risk. A common recommendation is for ciprofloxacin (Cipro) or a related drug. Travelers to developing countries should take along two types of antidiarrheal medications. One drug, such as loperamide, can control mild diarrhea. The second drug, such as ciprofloxacin, should be taken if the diarrhea is more serious, if it is accompanied by fever, or if there is blood in the stool.

Vaccines are often required or recommended for travel. The general rule for people with HIV infection is that they not receive live virus vaccines. For typhoid fever, get the injected inactivated vaccine, rather than the form taken by mouth. For yellow fever, the only vaccine is a live virus vaccine whose safety in people with HIV infection is uncertain. If you need to travel to an area with yellow fever, you may need to obtain a letter waiving the usual vaccine, and you need to avoid mosquito bites. Killed vaccines—standard diphtheria-tetanus (Dt), rabies, and Japanese encephalitis vaccines—are not a problem.

Travelers need to be aware of the types of infectious diseases in various areas. Many developing countries have high rates of tuberculosis; people with HIV infection are over 100 times more likely to get tuberculosis than people without HIV infection. Many areas also have high rates of malaria: the standard precautions are to avoid insect bites and to take certain preventive drugs that should be no problem for someone with HIV infection. Many tropical countries have visceral leishmaniasis, a disease transmitted by sand flies, that can be a major problem in people with HIV infection. Despite all these warnings, the claim that travel is too dangerous has relatively little support. Even if you are in the late stages of HIV infection, simply take common-sense precautions.

Occupational risks. The occupations that pose risks to people with HIV infection are those in the fields of health care and child care, and occupations that require animal contact. In the health care field, the major risk is of tuberculosis. This risk applies as well to employment in correctional facilities and shelters for the homeless. The amount of risk of tuberculosis depends on the activities of the employee or volunteer and the prevalence of tuberculosis in the community. Among providers of child care, the major risks are of exposure to *Cryptosporidium* and, to a lesser extent, cytomegalovirus, hepatitis A, and giardiasis. These risks may be reduced substantially just by good hygiene.

Occupations requiring animal contact include veterinary work and employment in farms, slaughterhouses, and pet stores. The major risks are of infection by *Cryptosporidium, Toxoplasma gondii, Salmonella, Campylobacter,* and *Bartonella.* There is no good evidence that these occupations carry much of a risk. Only be aware of the risk and use appropriate precautions.

Maintain Mental Health

HIV infection carries a psychological burden, both because of the nature of the disease and because of society's reaction to it. One aspect of this burden is that people are often sensitized to their health and have an understandable tendency to overreact. People with colds may conclude that they have pneumonia, a forgotten appointment may be interpreted as dementia, and a newly discovered freckle raises fear of Kaposi's sarcoma. The fact is, most colds, mood changes, forgotten appointments, and freckles are normal. People with HIV infection have the same trivial medical conditions as anyone else. The average person develops three colds and one case of infectious diarrhea a year; over 90 percent of the general population has occasional headaches. The great majority of these common medical conditions are of no importance to the person with HIV infection. For people with HIV infection, a certain amount of depression is also normal. Most depression is situational; it's the normal psychological response to adverse conditions. Some people, however, become extremely depressed. Their psychological burden becomes incapacitating; some may even consider suicide. These people would do best to consult a psychologist or psychiatrist.

Methods of maintaining mental health will differ with different people. Resources available include mental health professionals (psychiatrists, psychologists, and social workers), support groups, and AIDS-advocacy organizations. Mental health and the methods of maintaining it are discussed in chapter 4 and in chapter 11.

Chapter 4

HIV Infection and Its Effects on the Emotions

- Anger and energy
- Depression and hope
- Fatigue and accommodation
- Fear and realism
- Uncertainty and optimism
- Guilt and self-worth
- Change in perspective

Nearly everyone with HIV infection has, to varying extents and at different times, reacted to the disease with anger, depression, uncertainty, fatigue, fear, and guilt. These feelings do not occur in stages; they come in no order. Some people have several or all of the feelings at once. All the feelings are part of human nature and are reasonable reactions to HIV infection.

They are also more or less unavoidable. That doesn't mean you need to live in the grip of, say, depression. It only means that the emotions are as real as the virus, and that no one has a solid gold, 100 percent rule for curing unpleasant emotions. Though the mental health professionals can be of invaluable help in learning to live with these feelings, the real experts here are the people with HIV infection. Much of this chapter, like chapter 1, is in the voices of those experts.

Anger and Energy

Lisa Pratt: My husband had a lot of anger, which he first directed at me. He criticized, lashed out, once threatened to kill me. At first he refused to use a condom. He said, "Why did some jerk donate blood and now I have to use a condom?" He'd beat his fist on the table.

Alan Madison: I am not particularly angry.

103

Lisa Pratt's husband received an infected blood transfusion in the late 1980s, and like a lot of people could easily admit and express anger. Other people feel anger but do not acknowledge it. Alan Madison was infected by a lover, is doing well on the drugs, and isn't angry at all. Whatever the case, anger is a perfectly reasonable response to HIV infection.

Reasons for Anger

One reason for anger is the unfairness of the situation. In the first place, being singled out by the virus at all is unfair. No one, regardless of how he or she became infected, asked for or deserved this infection. Steven Charles, who became infected through sexual intercourse, said: "Why me? I didn't do anything wrong, I never hurt anyone, I was doing what seemed right to me. I know people who are more promiscuous and they seem to be getting out without a scar." Helen Parks had found a good job in the post office of the small town in which she lives; she had stopped using drugs by injection before she found out she was infected: "I hadn't been getting high any more. I was earning good money," she said. "Why bother to work hard and do good now? I had a rage of fire that wouldn't go out."

In the second place, being sick when you are young is unfair. "I feel gypped," said Rebecca Wolfe, who had been infected by a former boyfriend. "I don't like to dwell on the unlikelihood. I don't like to think about that." Alan Madison became infected with HIV just as he was beginning to reach success and stability in the banking business, and now he wonders whether he should change his long-range goals.

And finally, the social stigma, rejection, and even abandonment this particular virus seems to provoke are unfair. People's anger is particularly intense when they feel they are badly treated by those they thought they could count on most, their ministers and doctors. When Lisa Pratt's priest could not respond to her request for help, she said she was hurt and angry. People are angry that hospital clinics make them wait for hours, that the clinic doctor they felt rapport with last time has been replaced by someone else and the clinic clerks are rude. Edward Carroll's doctor wouldn't believe Edward had pneumonia and couldn't breathe; he told Edward he was hysterical and sent him home. Edward had to go to the emergency room to get treated. "Because of this disease," Edward said, "I've met some great people and some people I wish I'd never met."

Besides unfairness, another reason for anger is frustration at occasionally losing the sense that you're in control of your life. People get angry about having to live with medications that are complicated to take and can have unpleasant side effects. Dean Lombard was taking a drug whose side effect was diarrhea: "Once I messed the bed like a baby. I got so frustrated and angry at not being able to do what I wanted to do, I cried."

And anger at the social service agencies is perennial and universal. People complain that government medical assistance requires that they first become impoverished before they can get help, that they must fill out an amount of paperwork equaled only by the IRS, that even then the outcome is uncertain, and that the clerks are unhelpful and rude. "The workers just mess things up," said Helen. "The people who take your applications are horrible and hateful. They act like they want to keep people from applying for help. It's demeaning and dehumanizing."

Expressing the Anger

Some people express anger directly and openly, usually in private, though Dean has cried in church. "Tremendous anger wells up in me," Dean says. "I cry during hymns, reading those words. At home alone, I lose my temper, bang doors, throw things, yell. It's important to me to release my anger, but I try to be careful not to hurt anything." Rebecca uses almost identical words: "I feel anger building up on a weekly basis. I want to run up and down the road and cry. When I'm really angry, I beat on the bed with a book, which is noisy and very satisfying. Or I go in the bedroom and jump up and down and yell."

Other people express anger more obliquely. "I'd cry every morning and night in the car on the way to and from work," said Helen. "Sometimes I'd have to pull over to the side. And I went through a period where I snapped at my customers in the post office. When they asked why, I'd say, 'Oh, the stupid Xerox machine won't work.'" In fact, people often express anger not at the true causes, at unfairness or at loss of control. Instead, like Helen and the Xerox machine, they get angriest at little things: "My husband expressed a lot of anger about things so small, they were all out of proportion to what he was angry about," said Lisa. "I'd fix him oatmeal, and it was not what he'd wanted, or it wasn't hot enough."

This infection has a lot to be angry about. Some people turn their anger toward the medical system. They say the drugs have unpleasant side effects; tests are painful and invasive, and so are the procedures. Hospitals do not allow a sense of control and privacy. Doctors seem impersonal and inattentive, nurses too slow. The rooms are too hot or too cold. Rebecca got furious at a friend who volunteered with her doing HIV/AIDS education and who got pregnant: "She was single," Rebecca said, "and got pregnant. You know she was having unsafe sex. It's like she thought what happened to me was for nothing."

Some people say they are not particularly angry, and they truly are not. Other people truly are angry but say they are not because they are uncomfortable expressing an emotion that is, after all, overwhelming. They worry that giving in to anger means losing face or losing self-control. Their anger at unfairness and loss of control, however, often has not disappeared. Instead of getting angry at co-workers or the medical system, these people turn their anger on themselves. They feel depressed or guilty or they dislike themselves. Some eat too much: Lisa gained twenty pounds after her husband's diagnosis. Others rely too heavily on alcohol or drugs. Some continue the behavior that put them at risk for the infection in the first place: for a while, though she denied doing it, Helen went back to injecting drugs. In general, when people are depressed, they quit taking care of themselves.

Dealing with Anger

Anger is a justifiable response to this infection. People need to be allowed to be angry. Sometimes directing anger at the wrong target—like Helen at the Xerox machine—just helps you blow off. But sometimes it's ineffectual and at worst harmful. Obviously, it can deprive you of needed friendship and support. "Some people express their anger at everybody and everything else in their lives," said Edward, "and people stay away from them."

Anger turned on yourself is recognized as a form of depression. Those who feel hopeless or isolate themselves or eat or drink too much or continue the behavior that put them at risk for the infection are hurting themselves. Usually people realize they are treating themselves badly; before too long, they stop of their own accord. Sometimes a friend or relative notices that the person is drinking a lot or seems unhappy and recommends getting help. If you do not seem to be stopping on your own, get help from a psychiatrist, psychologist, or social worker. These mental health professionals will help you identify and understand the anger and will help the anger find its proper target. If necessary, they can also recommend alcohol- or drug-treatment programs.

Even anger turned outward can be overwhelming. Certain actions and attitudes help people deal with anger. First, separate the anger from its target. Lisa's husband, after talking to a psychiatrist, understood he was angry at the circumstances, not at Lisa for serving him oatmeal. Steven, who had been furious at the doctors he saw in the clinic, was able to say, "The doctors aren't the people I'm mad at. I can identify the feeling now and separate it out."

Second, find mechanisms that discharge anger. These will be different for different people. Helen screams; she also takes long walks through the fields around her small town. Steven jogs and works out in a gym. Edward writes out his anger in a journal, and talks to his partner, parents, and relatives.

Directing Anger

Much of people's anger about HIV infection is entirely appropriate. After you've figured out what you're truly angry at, after you've separated your anger from its target, you still have to figure out what to do with it. People find ways to direct their anger at its most appropriate targets, and in doing so, sometimes change their whole lives.

Lisa was angry at the social stigma her husband's illness had brought her. She began a newsletter for people in her city with HIV infection, so that others would feel less isolation than she had felt. Steven, who was angry at the medical profession, volunteered for a research study to test drugs. Alan Madison, upset about his career in the banking business, formed an organization that raised money to help local people with HIV infection pay for their rent, medicines, and food. Edward also helped found a money-raising organization for which he single-handedly puts out a newsletter on AIDS research, taught himself immunology, and took over editorship of a local newspaper for which he wrote a regular column on AIDS. "I want to leave behind anger and despair," he said, "and want to keep my desire to spread the word. You teach yourself things and—oh, God—I have so much to learn."

Lisa, Steven, Alan, and Edward are not exceptions. Anger holds an immense amount of energy. All over the country, people affected by HIV have used the energy from their anger to found buddy systems, political action groups, telephone hotlines, newsletters, fund-raising groups, and newspapers. They have successfully influenced medical guidelines and treatments, not to mention the workings of the Food and Drug Administration. Directing anger puts that frightening energy where it will do the most good; it returns to you a sense of control over your own life; it also returns a sense of hope. Sometimes it accomplishes near-miracles.

Depression and Hope

Helen Parks: Sometimes I'm in my room, in my chair, and I think about the people in all the stages of this disease and the people who have left the world with this disease. And I wonder what I'm going to do if I get sicker. I get confused. I get drastic thoughts. I sit in my chair and cry. I get real depressed.

Steven Charles: It feels like I'm caught in a muddy ditch and the walls are mud, there's nothing to grab on to and I can't climb out.

What Depression Feels Like

Depression is one of the most painful feelings a person can have. People say they feel alone and helpless in an indifferent world. They say they lose interest in things, have no energy, feel generally tired. They feel empty and uninterested in things they are normally interested in. They feel lonely and alienated from their friends, relatives, neighbors, co-workers. They doubt themselves or blame themselves or feel they have failed. They quit taking care of themselves. Like Helen, they have "drastic thoughts": they think about dying, sometimes about killing themselves. "When I'm home and completely alone and start dwelling, that's when I'm in trouble," said Edward. "It paralyzes me, I can't do anything. I just lie in bed."

Sometimes depression affects not only the mind, but also the body. Some people report that they cannot think as clearly or quickly as they used to. Some stop eating; others eat too much. Some cannot sleep, especially in the early morning; others sleep too often. In general, people dealing with depression say they are mostly sad and lonely, and they often cry a lot: "For a while, I cried all the time," said Rebecca Wolfe. "I didn't want to cry in front of my husband. I cried when I was alone—in the car, in the shower."

At bottom, depression seems to be the absence of hope. Hope is the sense that life is good, that it holds comforts and delights, that what you do makes a difference, that one way or another things will be all right. Sometimes, for a while, this sense of hope fails you. Faced with hopelessness, people feel helpless. They feel they have no alternative but to continue feeling depressed. They feel they no longer have the power to change how they act or how they feel. They feel that nothing they do matters or ever will matter. Some people, especially early in the course of the infection, consider suicide.

Depression varies in intensity and duration. Sometimes it is a mild feeling of being "down," or devoid of pleasure, or demoralized. Sometimes it is severe, and feels like despair, deep apathy, or true hopelessness. For most people, depression comes and goes: "I get bouts of these depressions," says Steven. The bouts can last a few hours, a few weeks, a few months. Edward, even though he says he has had trouble with depression for much of his life, also says, "I spend a few hours or maybe a day depressed, but that's all."

Causes of Depression

One cause of depression is a sense of being stuck in a frustrating, disheartening situation. Such situations are everywhere in life. Most people at one time or another must face something that they cannot fix, to which they can only adjust. HIV infection is certainly reason for depression: Edward said, "It's in my dreams. It can just percolate—you have this hopelessness. This is not the best thing that ever happened to me." For people facing HIV infection, depression, like anger, is a reasonable response.

Other causes of depression are the inevitable accompaniments of any disease. People get depressed when they go to the clinic for treatment and see other people with HIV infection worse off than they are. "We withdraw when we're sick," said Edward. "We're ashamed when we're sick. And the stigma of HIV isn't gone. It's difficult to stay strong. For a while, friends would call and say 'Let's do something,' and I'd say, 'Why?' If I'd gone to see a therapist, I'd have been diagnosed clinically depressed."

Still other causes of depression are all of life's ordinarily depressing vicissitudes. Steven had a job out of state when, by coincidence and on the same day, two close friends died, one by accident, the other by suicide. "Talk about grief and despair," he said. "I couldn't work, and worked anyway and made mistakes. I was goo, I was slime on the ground. Finally I packed up my dog and drove home and we've been here since. I didn't understand how two people who were young and who I loved could die on the same day. I just worked and took care of the dog, that was my whole life."

Another cause of depression is predisposition: people who have been depressed before their diagnosis might be more likely to be depressed afterward. Another cause is medications: many of the medications used to treat HIV infection and its complications can have depression as a side effect. For example, a small risk of depression is attributed to the long-term use of efavirenz; talk it over with your doctor. Alcohol, which is a depressant, is a particularly treacherous cause of depression because it can start a cycle. To feel better about their depression, people drink, which makes them feel depressed and out of control. So to feel better, they drink some more, get more depressed, and so on and on.

Occasionally, depression may be caused by the virus itself. That is, depression can be a symptom of dementia, a condition that results when the virus enters the brain (see chapter 6).

Finally, depression can be caused by unexpressed anger. Anger is hard to express, especially if it is directed at something as vague as fate, or something as personal as your own body or your behavior. People who do not express such anger either consciously restrain it or unconsciously ignore it. In either case, they unknowingly turn their anger inward on themselves and become depressed.

What to Do about Mild Depression

Depression that is unexpressed anger will disappear if the anger is recognized and dealt with. Depression that is a reasonable response to HIV infection almost always runs its course within days or weeks, and then goes away. For some people, this happens without their intervention. Others need to be more active in dispelling depression. One way to lessen or end depression is with physical activity: get outside, go for walks, cook a wonderful meal, go boating or driving or fishing or bowling, go shopping and buy yourself a little treat. "When I get depressed," said Steven, "I eat Ben and Jerry's coffee Heath Bar crunch ice cream."

Try to accomplish something you want done. A sense of accomplishment can come from doing something small, like cleaning out a closet, writing a letter, or polishing your shoes. No matter how small, a sense of accomplishment is a great weapon against depression. One small accomplishment can give you the hopefulness to embark on the next small accomplishment, and so on until you recover your normal habits of life.

Another way to lessen or end depression is with mental activity: read novels or biographies or philosophy or poetry. Go to the movies or the theater or the opera. Go to an art gallery and really look at the pictures. Talk to your neighbors or friends or family. Play a musical instrument or draw a picture or take some photographs or write a poem. Plan your garden or a trip or a fancy meal. Learn archaeology or medicine or Civil War history or art history. Write your memoirs; write essays about your political opinions or your philosophy of life. The possibilities of emotionally satisfying activities are endless. "I'm not one of those people who immerse themselves in the sickness," said Steven, who is a technician in a scientific laboratory. He takes in stray dogs, operates a ham radio, and reads up on scientific discoveries in astronomy. "I keep my regular life going," he says, "keep on working."

When Helen gets depressed, she has a list of things she does: "I usually notice depression when I hit the house after work. Then I find things to do, to keep my mind relaxed. I dig in the dirt. I walk, anything physical. Clean the closet, walk through the mall and window shop. I take a bubble bath. Read the Bible, help someone else." Lisa's husband did the same: "For months," said Lisa, "my husband sat in a chair and stared. Nothing interested him. Then he got into his workshop and started making crafts, carving wooden ducks." Dean gardens; he says it gives him a great sense of peace and beauty. Edward asks his friends to come visit—"I have a circle of wonderful friends," he said; "they buoy my spirits"—and writes his newspaper column. "I really battle," he said. "I really try to engage myself in something, try to do some work. Work is the answer, it just is."

What such activities do is redirect your attention away from yourself and your very real problems, to other things in life and their very real pleasures. "I do get depressed," said Rebecca. "But I don't set my mind into that. If I sit at home and think, I get depressed. So every day I tell myself, 'Good morning. Have a good day,' and keep myself busy. I go to the museum, go shopping, volunteer at the Aquarium." Alan, who found the clinic depressing, decided to do something about it: "I talk to people at clinic—they feel isolated, too. I've become more of an outgoing individual and I really want people to feel not alone. It's so great to see eyes light up, that they're not the only ones."

These and other activities will not make your life wonderful again, but they do seem to dissolve depression, at least temporarily. Sometimes, during a walk, the balance between hope and hopelessness seems to shift back toward hope, and you feel more yourself again. Don't be too impressed by your depression; you have felt it before and you will feel it again. And when the next bout of depression moves in, you, like Helen, will have your list of accomplishments and activities and distractions and small pleasures handy. "The only thing is to keep busy and find things I want to do," said Edward. "I haven't been put out of commission by worry or anxiety. I have on occasion, I have taken to bed for a day. But next morning I'm right up and at 'em. I think 'Ok, I'm going to take care of this.'"

A lot of people, maybe almost all people, get tired of handling depression on their own. Seeing a mental health worker, like a psychologist, and just talking through thoughts and feelings can be a relief, can reassure you that your problems are more or less normal and you're not going crazy after all.

What to Do about Severe Depression

Sometimes, for some people, depression is too severe or it lasts too long. They feel alienated from everyone, deeply apathetic, profoundly hopeless. Severe, persistent depression is often best treated with medication. Talk to a doctor. If medication taken for another condition is causing depression, the doctor can change the drug or lower the dose. If the depression is part of dementia, the doctor will prescribe medications that ease the symptoms. Most of the persistent depression in people with HIV infection, however, is simply the natural reaction to knowledge of a frightening disease. Depression can be successfully treated with appropriate support and medications. In this case, the doctor will recommend a psychiatrist, who can prescribe medication that restores sleep, appetite, and mood. The drugs currently used for severe depression can be nearly miraculous. They do for depression what penicillin does for pneumonia: about 80 percent of severely depressed people with HIV infection get better, and about 50 percent are cured. For most people, treatment of depression is critical but temporary.

In addition to or instead of medication, you might want professional help. Either the doctor or the psychiatrist might recommend professional psychological help (see the section on mental health professionals in chapter 11). Psychiatrists, psychologists, and social workers can help you talk through whatever is blocking the healing process, though only psychiatrists are trained medically and can prescribe medications. Psychotherapy may concentrate on the overwhelming problems people must face and feel they cannot solve: How can I face rejection? How can I deal with anger? How can I feel less guilty? How can I have sex without hurting myself or anyone else? Why me? Am I a good person? Why now? By helping you confront problems you feel are unsolvable and find new perspectives on those problems, a psychotherapist will help you take control of your life. He or she will help you deny, not the fact of your infection, but your own helplessness and hopelessness in the face of it.

Thoughts of suicide are usually only temporary. When Lisa's husband said he was considering suicide, Lisa asked him to first talk to a psychologist. She also told him she thought he owed it to her not to act without talking to her. He agreed and made those promises. Eventually, he decided against suicide. Like Lisa's husband, many people find their interest in life is stronger than their desire to die. In fact, the suicide rate among people with HIV infection is low. Researchers say that people seem to consider suicide mostly as a means of regaining a feeling of control over their lives. And that makes sense—it is as though people were saying, "This disease does not control whether I live or die, I do." If that choice seems to be in your hands, you feel less helpless, more in control.

Nevertheless, if thoughts about suicide persist, and if thoughts of taking pills become plans to collect specific pills, and if these persistent, concrete thoughts are coupled with an increase in guilt and a sense of punishment, then get help. Call your doctor or psychotherapist.

Fatigue and Accommodation

The Causes of Fatigue

Fatigue for people with HIV infection comes from anything from the stresses of everyday life, to the drugs against the virus, to the virus itself.

Fatigue often accompanies depression: people dealing with depression lose not only a sense of hope but also their physical energy. They are tired, sometimes exhausted, sometimes apathetic. Fatigue can also have physical causes, which can be sorted out by a medical evaluation (see chapter 6, under "Causes of Constitutional Symptoms").

Fatigue is a subjective symptom; it cannot be objectively verified or quantified like a blood count. Fatigue is also common to everyone; up to 25 percent of all people without HIV infection complain of being chronically fatigued. For people with HIV infection, a medical evaluation needs to review factors that cause fatigue but that are treatable: depression, anemia, medicines, and infections. Most people just learn to live with and around fatigue.

The Effects of Fatigue

Although the causes of fatigue may be physical, the effects are psychological. In fact, depression not only causes fatigue but is also caused by it. Dean said he has good days and bad days. On the good days, he has more energy. After a rough night and diarrhea, he will be tired the next day: he said, "Those are the crying days."

Another psychological effect of fatigue is irritation. Lisa Pratt's husband "had always been a go-getter," she said, and resented his fatigue. "My husband," Lisa said, "had to give up little things he liked because he had no stamina. For years, he had been an actor in our local community theater. He couldn't keep up with the rehearsal schedule and thought he was going to have to quit. It hurt to not go. And it made him mad to give in." Dean said that until he learned to pace himself, he regularly worked fourteen hours a day running a small newspaper, came home angry, then "got the blues."

Accommodating to Fatigue

Whether its cause is psychological or physical, fatigue cannot be ignored. First, talk to your doctor so that what's treatable can be treated. After that, the best way to deal with fatigue may be to accept it and go on from there. Decide what you want to do most, be sure it is possible, plan it out, and pace yourself. Lisa's husband stayed in the community theater but tried out only for small roles. Dean kept his job but cut back his hours and tried to have meetings in his office rather than in offices across town.

In general, try to find ways to accomplish what you want with less energy. Lisa's husband's fatigue also affected their social life: "Socially, we didn't go out as much. But then we redefined 'socially.' Instead of going out drinking and dancing, we entertained at home. Our social life didn't disappear." People who find driving tiring can often take public transportation. When they want to buy clothes or household supplies or presents, they order from catalogs or the Internet. To buy groceries, they find a store that delivers, or ask their friends. They get their medication from pharmacies that deliver.

Do what you can; don't give up before you need to. Steven says, "I keep pushing myself. I do wake up tired and don't like that. I make myself get up. I get out of that bed." If you know you've done your best, then relax and rest. Try not to let fatigue affect your good opinion of yourself. You've done what you could. Just take care of yourself.

Fear and Realism

Alan Madison: I'm scared as hell at different periods. I wake up at night and cry a little.

People fear what they do not understand and cannot control. People who are feeling good on the new combinations of drugs fear that the drugs may stop working and worry about the results of each blood test. They worry about their finances: the drug regimens are expensive and they worry about whether they'll be able to continue to afford the drugs. People worry about symptoms that may or may not be serious. They fear being a patient in a hospital, or undergoing painful medical tests and procedures. They fear rejection: Alan was afraid that people would treat him as though he had leprosy; Helen said she was fearful of telling her sons. Rebecca said she'd gotten past her initial fears of being damaged goods, but still "I get little echoes of it when I disclose my HIV status. I hate that conversation." People with HIV infection are afraid they will give someone else the virus.

All these fears are realistic. The point is not to live without fear, only to live without being unduly troubled or hindered by fear.

Sometimes what people feel is not fear but anxiety. That is, they have feelings of fear that are unrealistic. People who are anxious say they feel as if something terrible were about to happen. They cannot say what exactly they fear, only that they have a sense of underlying uneasiness. They feel restless and uncomfortable wherever they are. They are irritable, tense, and preoccupied with their bodies. They have trouble breathing, are nauseated, break out into cold sweats, have racing pulses. Some have periods of feeling panicky.

People whose feelings of anxiety persist too long or are too severe should see a mental health professional or a doctor who might in turn recommend a visit to a psychiatrist. Persistent anxiety takes a tremendous amount of energy, and it is often curable. Psychiatrists can prescribe medication to relieve anxiety. Mental health professionals can teach techniques that help you relax. Physical relaxation usually makes people feel calmer and more themselves again.

Dissipating Fear with Information

Many fears do not hold up in the cold light of reality:

If you fear sickness, find out which symptoms you should see your doctor about and which you should ignore (see chapter 6). "I found out what's what," said Alan, "and now I don't worry about every little cough."

If you fear medications, tests, and procedures, educate yourself about them. Read what you can find, ask your doctor, ask people who have had the experience. Learn about drugs and their side effects. Talk to someone who's had a bronchoscopy, who's gone through a scanner, who's had a lumbar puncture. The fear of such things is often much worse than the things themselves.

Put the fear into perspective. Alan said, "I went to a therapist for a while. Then I had a big gigantic turning point. I was taking a shower and realized that all my problems were coming from the fear itself. Fear was creating all the problems, even the fear. Realizing that made the fear dissipate in a gush. Of course, it came back again, but it kept going away again too."

Uncertainty and Optimism

Everyone with HIV infection faces uncertainty about the future whether they've been sick and didn't improve until the triple therapy was introduced, or whether they've been well on the triple therapy all along. For those who were sick, the drugs work wonders physically: people feel well and energetic. "I look good," said Dean. "My muscle tone is back, it's great to look in the mirror and not cry. That's a real wonderful thing. But there's a whole new game to play here and it's not all that easy." Dean's test results are good; his CD4 counts have been climbing and the virus in his blood—his viral load—is at undetectable levels. But he worries about the next round of tests: "I've had a year now of undetectable virus. As long as I can keep it that low. But it's like a time bomb—you're always waiting for something to happen."

Reasons for Uncertainty

Everyone taking the new drugs feels this disconcerting mixture of uncertainty and hope. Both feelings are accurate reflections of the reality: at the present, the drugs restore people to health; for the future, the drugs could hold HIV in check forever or they could lose their effectiveness. This kind of fundamental uncertainty about sickness and health is not like anxiety, which is an unrealistic response or a response to something unreal. This uncertainty is entirely realistic. HIV infection, in the virulence of the virus and effectiveness of the medical response, has been a remarkable disease, and we are at a remarkable point in its history. The only certainty is, the situation is infinitely better than it once was.

The uncertainty is all the more nagging because many people with HIV infection know exactly what they're up against. "A year ago I was preparing my funeral," Alan said. "I had pancreatitis, couldn't take drugs, was grey, my skin was hanging in folds. My CD4 count was 180 and viral load was 650,000. Now my CD4 is 1,115 and I'm undetectable. I'm 12 years out, alive and kicking and working full-time. But in a way, it's easier to resign yourself to dying than to living."

Rebecca had nearly the same experience: "My counts started going up and my doctor was bouncing out of his skin. I said, 'Forget it. I mean, great, I'm going to live a long life. But what am I going to do with it?' Though I feel like an ungrateful patient. I say to myself, 'It could be worse.' But you know, it really might *get* worse."

Adding to the uncertainty is the scrupulousness with which people have to take the new drugs. "I recently missed a dose," said Rebecca. "One day I was busy and the dish was full as if I hadn't taken a dose. I'll take blood work in a couple weeks. My doctor said, 'Did you miss a whole day?' I didn't, only the morning dose. He said, 'I really don't think you'll have to worry.' But after the test, I'll know how exacting I have to be."

For Helen Parks, the drugs aren't working well; her viral load is down but not undetectable. "My biggest issue is," she said, "will I be spared? My doctor says he doesn't know, he doesn't have a crystal ball. If my viral load were undetectable, if the pills were actually working as they were supposed to according to the newspapers, I'd be feeling better."

Managing Uncertainty

People manage uncertainty partly by accepting it and partly by investing, cautiously, in the future. People who have been extremely sick and have faced the possibilities others only fear, are particularly aware, not only of the uncertainty but also of the investment. Alan, who said that living might be harder than dying, added, "My partner and I just bought a house with a 30-year mortgage."

They do what could be called "bracketing": suspending consideration of sickness, living in the present, planning for the future. "It's possible to separate yourself from having AIDS now," says Steven. "I'm not thinking about it as much." They remain scrupulous about their drug regimens and their doctor appointments. And like Edward and Alan, they make plans, pursue friendships, fall in love. They think about what to do next. "I also want to start a college course in theater," said Alan. "I was always interested and never did anything about it. Also watercolor lessons. And piano lessons again—I used to play." Rebecca would like to have children: "I hope to, when this is all over. I want an end to this. I'm looking forward to my future." They work hard at being ready for the positive alternative, being ready if the drugs keep HIV down forever, being ready to return to life's normal uncertainties. "I live my life like everything's normal," said Steven, "like I'm going to do everything I planned to do. I bury myself in work. It helps."

Some people have to decide whether to work. Their decisions depend on their individual circumstances. "For now, I'm ok financially," said Dean, "but what am I going to do? Start working? Give up disability? I had friends who sold their life insurance and now they have to start over. My family says, 'You're healthy, why don't you go back to work? Why don't you?' I think when my doctor says, 'It's a cure, there's no HIV left,' then I'll go off disability."

Rebecca, who is also on disability, volunteers at several jobs; she's thinking about going off disability and seeing if one of her jobs will hire her full-time. Alan had friends who stopped putting money into retirement funds and who passed up promotions. Alan himself qualified for disability at one point, but when the new drugs gave him more energy, he went back to his banking job. "AIDS is not your whole life now," he said. "It's there and you're worried about it. But it's not everything." Alan decided he'd take the risk of going off disability, even though he worried about what would happen if he got sick again. "I guess I'd rather die with my boots on," he said. "I mean, how disabled would I let myself be?"

Guilt and Self-Worth

What People Feel Guilty About

One of the many peculiarities of HIV is the amount of guilt it seems to inspire. People feel guilty for having become infected. They feel they are somehow to blame for having gotten the virus, that they brought it on themselves. "I feel a little guilt," said Steven. "I should have known to practice safer sex, even though at the time I got infected, no one even knew the virus was around. I know how stupid that sounds, but I feel guilty anyway." They feel guilty about bringing HIV infection into the lives of other people: about putting their partners or spouses at risk, about telling their children they have HIV infection, about distressing their parents, their families, and their friends.

Many people also feel guilty about the behavior that put them at risk in the first place. "I felt guilty over my period of promiscuity when I first came out as gay," said Edward. "I justified it at the time, but I knew it was wrong." The behaviors that exposed most people to the virus—gay lovemaking and injection drug use—are behaviors of which society often disapproves. For many people, social disapproval is distressing, and they feel isolated and punished. Sometimes they unconsciously take social disapproval on themselves as guilt. "A lot of us took society's view," said Dean, "and felt guilty about being gay." The same is generally true for injection drug users: "I was real upset with myself," said Helen. "This disease makes me feel like I've been a dirty person, and I'm not. I'm a clean person."

Even those whose exposure to the virus came through conditions society does not disapprove of—blood transfusions, hemophilia—still feel guilty. Even people whose infection came through heterosexual sex worry about social disapproval: "I got infected by an old boyfriend," said Rebecca, "but I worry that people will think I had been a slut." They feel they are to blame for involving their families in a disease that is socially isolating, and for putting their spouses at risk. Lisa said her husband had been afraid their daughters would say, "What did you do to our family?" "I felt guilty when I was diagnosed," said Dean. "I thought 'I killed my partner.'" Like Dean's partner, Rebecca's husband remains uninfected, but Rebecca worries about the consequences to him if her infection becomes public: "I cannot let my husband be hurt by this. His career would be jeopardized by them finding out about me. Maybe they'd be understanding, but I can't take that risk."

Even caregivers feel guilty. Steven's mother feels that if she had been a better mother, Steven would not have been gay and come in contact with the virus.

Causes of Guilt

Guilt does not necessarily have a cause. Guilt, like fear, is a feeling that may or may not have anything to do with the facts. Some people knowingly did something they should not have done. Perhaps they knew they ran a risk when they became infected. Others are accepting blame for something over which they had no control. Perhaps they knew nothing about the virus or they thought they were taking appropriate steps to avoid infection or they unknowingly received infected blood.

Guilt, like all other reactions to this infection, is a natural human feeling. Sooner or later in their lives, most people feel guilty about something, sometimes justifiably, sometimes not. Alan, for instance, remembers stealing a plastic toy from a dime store when he was seven years old, and though he does not feel like a criminal, he does feel a vague sense of shame and is not able to forget the incident.

Perhaps guilt comes from a sense that good behavior deserves reward and bad behavior deserves punishment, and since the virus feels like a punishment, they must have behaved badly. Perhaps social disapproval operates the same way: people feel isolated and punished, so they feel they must have done something wrong to deserve it. Both of these possibilities are built on bad logic and are just plain wrong.

What to Do about Guilt

First, separate the virus from a sense of punishment. Lisa states: "What I say is, it's a virus, not a punishment. I didn't get the virus and my husband did. Does that make me good and him bad? That's ridiculous. Everyone got this virus like my husband did: being in the wrong place at the wrong time."

The virus does not set out to "get" anyone. It has no brain, no judgment, no ability to pick out who is worthy and who is not. The virus has nothing whatever to do with punishment. Nor does anyone set out to get infected with the virus. The conditions that put most people at risk for the virus—homosexuality and drug addiction—may well be directed by biology and, in any case, are not the result of a conscious intention. No one makes a conscious, informed decision that they will become gay or will use drugs.

Understand that guilt, except when it keeps you from repeating mistakes, is a remarkably useless emotion. Feeling guilty means worrying about something you cannot change. Whether people knowingly ran a risk or not, the past is beyond anyone's power to change. Guilt keeps people captured in the past and prohibits them from doing what they can to improve the present. Guilt uses emotional energy that would be better used on the real problems of life.

Balance guilt by understanding your own worth. Ask yourself, outside my worries, who am I? A pastor who has had experience with people with HIV infection asks people, "What else besides the things you feel guilty about are you? What do your friends like about you? They tell me 'that I helped them move the piano, that I had some good kids, that I was a good friend.'" Steven told himself, "You just have to focus. You're worth something. You're not scum, you can make a difference."

In the process of focusing on your own worth, guilt usually fades away. People come to like themselves for who they are. Some people speed up the process by getting help from a therapist. During therapy, they deal with the attitudes and behavior, often left over from childhood, that make them feel guilty. They learn to feel comfortable with themselves and free themselves of their old, useless burden of guilt.

Sometimes, however, guilt is not particularly personal, that is, people aren't feeling punished or ashamed or responsible or bad. Their worry is more general, more religious or philosophical. They're trying to make sense of their HIV infection, to fit it into their mental worlds, to understand why they got infected.

Helen is an eloquent example. The drugs are less effective with her, her viral load is detectable, and she has trouble not taking it all personally. "So what did I do wrong?" she said. "I can't make it out, to tell you the truth. If it's true that bad things happen to bad people, I'm ruined. People say to me, 'How could this happen? You're such a good person?' I guess maybe I'm not. Or maybe I'm not really a bad person and I'll be spared. For me, usually, reading, getting involved in stories, is a great way to stop worrying. The problem is, in most stories, bad things happen to bad people—it's just there all the time. I don't know how to get around it, even though I'm convinced in my deepest core it's wrong. You can see I've thought about it."

For Helen and others, guilt actually seems to be the first step in making sense of their new lives. Their reasoning goes like this: Why did I get this virus? Did I do something wrong? If I didn't and the virus isn't a punishment, if it's simply a random biological fact that's affecting my life, then what do I do? How do I make sense of that? The question has been addressed by every theologian and philosopher since the Book of Job. The answer is going to be deeply felt, carefully thought out, unique to everyone, and completely beyond the scope of this book or the expertise of its authors.

Change in Perspective

Often the answer to questions like Helen's and Job's involves a change in perspective on life. "Change in perspective" is a vague term that everyone uses and no one defines; it probably means something like, "When you stand in a different place, you see things differently." HIV infection is certainly a different place, and after years of adjusting to these changes, people come to see their lives differently.

"Before I got sick," said Rebecca, "the world was normal. I knew I had a virus in me, but I was living the life I wanted to lead. I was dating, having fun, being me. But when I got sick, I prepared to die. I wrote my last will and testament, made funeral arrangements, did a living will, and fixed up my house to die in—I wanted a pretty place to die in. I had 12 CD4 cells, PCP, esophageal thrush, anemia, had lost over 10 percent of my body weight, and my hair fell out. So I know what it's like to be sick." But Rebecca improved drastically on the medications, and once again, her life changed. "Life before I got sick was very good. I got sick and it all changed. For a long time I thought I should never have taken the meds. I should have just let it go. It almost pissed me off not to be able to die gracefully and beautifully. I don't really want to live. I don't want to die either. So I'll make the best of it. You don't just resume life. And you don't have any hope of ever resuming your life. It's changed. The hand I hold is totally different now, and I have to play this hand I'm dealt."

Faced with their new knowledge, people change their priorities. Accordingly, some people begin thinking how they might change their lives. Rebecca will go back to school, to go into social work. Alan is a banker, but his training was in music, and now he thought he would like to go back to playing the clarinet. Steven, who worked as a technician for a scientific laboratory, had always wanted to teach, and volunteered as a teacher in a community adult education course.

Many people now place greater priority on other people. "When I almost died," said Rebecca, "I realized at that time the most important thing is my relationships. With my time now, I want to spend time with the people I love." Some people begin tidying up relationships: Lisa's husband called his brother more often, and they began going to ball games together.

Somehow or other, such changes in priorities answer people's deep questions about whether life makes sense, whether it has meaning, whether it's good. Dean volunteers at a hospice, and explains himself this way: "Before I got this virus, I had this feeling about God, that I lived a charmed life, that God looked out for me. And this was a wake-up call. I couldn't believe in God the way I did. I thought, 'There's no orchestrating force in life, it's just random. I've spent my life in the best way I can, doing as little harm as possible. Nothing justifies this.' So I had to think where I had ever found meaning before, where I ever had a sense of God. I realized these times were when I cared about someone as much as myself. I needed to get that back. If I could care for those people at the hospice, I could come back. My conception of God has changed. I do see the world as more random. And whoever I was before is gone. But I'm trying to find where God was and where there's meaning. And that's in caring for someone. That's what keeps me going."

Chapter 5

HIV Infection and Its Effects on Interpersonal Relations

- Helplessness, dependency, and control
- Feelings about sex
- Relationships with your children
- Relationships with drug users

We accept as a standard truth that we are separate from all other people: we are alone, we are individuals, we are each one of a kind. We never truly understand what other people feel, nor do they truly understand our feelings. We are on our own, responsible for our own decisions and for solutions to our own problems. We protect ourselves first, and at almost any cost. We live our own lives and die our own deaths.

We accept as just as much a standard truth the opposite: that we are also interconnected. What happens to a friend seems to some extent also to happen to us. When friends are lonely or worried or in pain, we cannot simply ignore them; we even feel some of their misery. Conversely, when we are unhappy ourselves, the presence of a friend is a comfort and relief. "For grief concealed strangles the soul," wrote Robert Burton, a seventeenth-century minister and scholar, "but when as we shall but impart it to some discreet, trusty, loving friend, it is instantly removed."

These opposites seem to play themselves out every day. Every close relationship is a moving balance between the opposites of individuality and connectedness, personal necessity and friendly concern, privacy and warmth.

Helplessness, Dependency, and Control

Alan Madison: One of the worst thoughts for me is, I don't want people taking care of me. No one wants to give up that control. I come from proud people. I've always felt the need to do it on my own.

123

The balance between dependency and control is most often a problem for people whose HIV infection isn't controlled by drugs and who have intervals of illness during which they depend on others for things they normally provide for themselves.

No One Wants to Give Up Control

Like Alan, all people want to "do it on their own." By that, they usually mean that they do not want to rely on other people; they want to rely on themselves. They take care of their own needs. They want to do their fair share in a relationship, not only taking advice and help, but also giving it. When something goes wrong, they fix it; when they have a problem, they solve it. They can do what they set out to do. In short, they have the sense that they are in control of their own lives.

HIV infection can seriously undermine a person's sense of control. Their dependency ranges from needing someone to shop, clean, and cook for them to needing someone to dress, bathe, and feed them. They dislike this dependency. They say that being dependent is hard on their self-esteem, their sense of self-worth.

Others worry about financial dependency on the welfare system: Helen says, "I'm surely not one for welfare." Both the social service and medical systems require people to give up control, one system over their personal resources, the other over their bodies. The requirements, though necessary, are distressing. People who give over control of their resources and their bodies feel they have little left of their own. They feel powerless, ineffective, and incompetent.

Coming to Terms with Loss of Control

The trick is to balance acceptance of help with preservation of control. First, don't give up independence easily. "I have a friend with AIDS," says Steven, "who sometimes asks me to bring stuff down from his attic or install his screen windows—things I know he can do for himself. I say no. I know, because I have other friends with AIDS, that he has to take some responsibility. Lots of people give up, but mental and physical health go hand in hand." People feel better about accepting help if they think they've done their best to accomplish the task on their own first.

For some people, some help is going to be necessary. Helen, who had worried about depending on her parents or on welfare, made her peace with getting help. "I know I'm not going to be able to count on myself for everything," she finally said. "I'm not going to be afraid of saying I need help. My father and stepmother have been very supportive. My church will always help." Some people feel they need help so badly they have no choice but to accept it. Some people feel they can accept help because they have helped others: what goes around comes around, they say. Some can accept help because they understand that their caregivers need to be involved with them. Some know that if circumstances were reversed and their caregivers were sick, they would help their caregivers. Some feel they have led good enough lives that they are worthy recipients of care.

Control What You Can

Finally, after you accept what you must, control whatever else you can. A friend of Steven's felt he was being a burden to his parents and moved into a private home for people with AIDS; he liked the home particularly because he felt needed by other people there. Edward has had periods of sickness and always recovers but hasn't much energy. He says he needs to balance dependence and independence: "I had to learn to ask for help," he said. "And I had to grow new wings. But I dare not try to be too independent. You never know, you dare not burn bridges. It's a humbling experience. It's really important to maintain supports."

If you cannot control your life in big ways, control it in small ways: you never lose control over everything. Lisa would ask her husband, "Do you want the water glass here or there? Do you want to wear your blue shirt or your white one? Do you want cocoa or coffee?" When Dean went to the hospital, he took along his own lamp and radio. You can always affect the course or quality of your life somehow.

This strategy of controlling what you can extends to the social service and medical systems. For more on dealing with the social services, see chapter 9; for more on dealing with the medical system, see chapter 7.

Control and the Caregiver

For caregivers, problems with control are different. Caregivers need to balance several things at once. They need to deal with their own sense of helplessness, to allow the people they're caring for to maintain a sense of control, and to care for them, all at the same time. Maintaining this balance is tricky and confusing. "My husband is so much in control and I always push that," Lisa said. "But it backfires. When he really needs help, like with getting meals when he's sick, he doesn't ask. Sometimes I help him anyway. I also wish I could help him with the emotional things too, by just sitting and talking. But I'm afraid of smothering him. I just don't know where the line is."

On the whole, caregivers should probably try to let the people they care for determine where the line is. The problems and feelings that people with HIV infection face can be resolved only by them. In fact, for people with HIV infection, being told solutions to problems they know are insoluble, or whose solutions only they can find, is annoying and intrusive. The best help caregivers can give is listening. Caregivers find it hard just to listen; they feel passive and helpless. Nevertheless listening, as Dean said, "really helps."

Listening means being quiet, not interrupting, not judging, not giving advice, not trying to fix what's wrong. It means paying sympathetic attention, drawing the person out. Try saying, "I'm interested in that if you want to tell me." Or, "That sounds hard. How are you handling it?" If the person is crying, don't interrupt or make him or her stop. If you want to know why he or she is crying, wait until the crying is over to ask. Let the person cry it out—some things deserve tears. Listening also means picking up cues: perhaps the person does not want to talk, or wants to talk but is afraid of being a burden, or does not want help, or wants help but does not want to ask. The cues will help the caregiver decide how to act.

Relabel What You Cannot Control

Some people maintain control by what mental health professionals call *reframing* or *relabeling* (see chapter 11). Relabeling means looking at situations in such a way that they seem benign or comforting or controllable. Try paying attention not to where your family or friends fail you, but to where they help. Try calling something a challenge rather than a struggle, a preference rather than a need. If the disadvantages of a situation are undeniable, so are the advantages. It's as though your life were a story and you are writing it. It is your story, your life, and you can say whether it's bad or good. You're in charge of how you see things.

Edward was pleased that doctors caught an infection of cryptococcal meningitis early before he began getting the headaches he'd seen his friends endure. Edward also said that now that his partner has had to take over more of his care, they spend more time together and have become closer: "My being sick has made us closer, made us cherish our time together. It's not depending, it's mutual caring." People with HIV infection who have to quit work say they are happy to have more time to spend on gardening, developing photographs, working on old cars, or anything else they enjoy. They say repeatedly that they are happy to have more time to spend with the people they love.

Relabeling can be done only by the person with the problem, not by anyone else, no matter how well-meaning the other person is. Having your problems relabeled by someone else is usually annoying.

Feelings about Sex

Steven Charles: A lot of stuff about dating gets mixed up when you get a disease from loving someone. Maybe one day. But it would have to be a very special person. I'm happy. I have a lot of friends.

Alan Madison: My partner is negative and I want him to stay that way. We're playing safe, though there's a burnout to playing safe. But I have to use a condom every time I have sex until I die. That's permanent.

People's feelings about sex are varied. At different times and to different people, sex is a joy, a comfort, a distraction, a release, intimacy, reassurance, bonding. To some extent, people's feelings about sex depend on feeling healthy, enjoying life, liking themselves, trusting others, feeling relaxed, having the freedom to be spontaneous. HIV infection changes much of this. Everyone knows these facts: the virus occurs in great numbers in blood and semen, and in smaller numbers in vaginal fluid. So while making love, people with HIV infection can unthinkingly transmit the virus. Even when both partners are infected, they can communicate variants of the virus to each other. To avoid this, people have no alternative but to have no sex at all or to practice safer sex. But both safer sex and the fact that sex can communicate the virus create emotional problems for people.

Problems with Feelings about Sex

Probably the most difficult problem is that some people equate making love with getting infected. They feel guilty having sex. They mourn the loss of the free sexual life they once had. They feel violated by the virus; the virus invaded their bodies when they were doing something enjoyable and natural. And all these feelings come at a time when people intensely need the closeness that sexual intimacy brings. "We've seen couples pull apart," said Dean. "We need closeness a lot more now."

Another problem for some people is that they feel safer sex is no fun. Safer sex seems to detract from spontaneity and a feeling of relaxation. It sometimes seems to add a barrier of constraint or artificiality between partners.

In addition, some people not in long-term sexual relationships fear that if they meet someone they like, they will have to begin the relationship by telling that person something unpleasant to hear. Perhaps that person will respond by rejecting them. Perhaps that person will spread the information about their diagnosis. "I told this guy I was dating I had HIV and he lost interest," said Steven. "I'd figured he'd be ok because he'd been wearing an AIDS memorial T-shirt. I didn't know it was just a fashion statement."

Solving the Problems

Some people react to these feelings, as Steven did for a while, by becoming celibate, not having sex at all. Celibacy is one solution. If you are uncomfortable having sex, or if you feel no desire to, don't bother with it.

But Steven didn't want to live without sex permanently, so he figured out how and when to tell people that he had HIV infection. "People find out I'm positive and still want to get to know me," he said. "I like to have them get to know me first—though not sexually. Then when you move forward in the relationship and sex gets inevitable, I tell them. I was dating one person for a month, and just told him the other day. I just got down to it, didn't beat around the bush. I said, 'I'm really enjoying what's happening and I want to get to know you and honesty is important to me and I need to tell you I'm positive. This is me, it's what I live with and you deserve to know it.' Then I have to deal with their emotions and questions. I tell them anything they might not know. Everyone I've dated is negative, and has remained negative. So always safer sex. I insist on that. The expression and varieties of sex are still there."

After a while, people adjust to safer sex. "The way I've adjusted to safer sex," says Alan, "is by psyching myself into thinking I prefer it. It wasn't easy, but I did it, and now I can't not practice safer sex, even if my partner wants to do it differently. I can't ejaculate inside someone any more."

Lisa and her husband had also worked out a mutually satisfying solution. "The virus was pretty hard on our sexual relationship. Oral sex had been an important part of our lives. I tried oral sex with him while he was wearing a condom, but it tasted too bad. We ended up having sex with him wearing a condom, and with mutual masturbation. It was satisfying enough."

Some people set limits on sex. Edward and his partner had sex less often. That made Edward feel guilty, but his partner said, "I can handle that better than he can." Some couples have sex quickly, and say that is better than nothing. Some couples in which only one person is infected give control to the uninfected person to determine how often they make love and what happens during lovemaking.

One good solution is to accept the necessary changes in sexual practices, and where those changes are less than satisfying find other ways to accomplish the same intimacy, reassurance, comfort, and bonding.

"Sex always created a bonding between my husband and me," Lisa said. "Safer sex could do that too. But I also tried to re-create that bond by doing more things together and having more communication." Dean said the same thing: "We gave up having sex and make love now."

All kinds of physical intimacies that are not sexual can also create bonding: holding hands, touching, sitting close, giving baths, giving massages, combing hair, napping together, taking showers together, playing card games, lying in bed together, sitting together to read the morning paper or to watch TV or listen to music; sitting together and reading aloud to each other. Lisa found that her husband responded as she had hoped: "My husband had always had a fear of intimacy. I saw that dissolve. He told me things he never had before. It took time and love to overcome the fear and guilt."

Relationships with Your Children

Many of the problems people with HIV infection have with their children are, on the surface, the same problems they have with any other relative: how to tell them about the infection, how to deal with their worries. Under the surface, however, the problems are complicated by the uniqueness of the parent-child relationship. Parents and children are not equal partners in a relationship. Parents take care of children, not the reverse. Young children truly are helpless and cannot care for their parents. Older children may be unable emotionally to care for their parents, or the parents may be unable to accept care.

Problems with Telling

In many ways, telling your children about HIV infection is different from telling most other relatives. People feel responsible for their children; they want to protect them against fear and worry and life's hard facts. They think of themselves as their children's safe haven, and they want to avoid bringing uncertainty into their lives. As a result, many people decide to put off telling their children until they have to.

For people who feel and seem healthy, telling their children can be put off indefinitely. Steven has a nice story about a friend, a gay man who in the late 1970s adopted a baby. When the boy was 10, the man became infected with HIV. His doctor at the time told him he might be dead in the next couple of years. So the man decided to put off telling his son and to try to live until his son graduated from middle school. The son graduated. Then the man decided to try to live until his son's high school graduation. The son graduated. Then the man wanted to live for the college graduation. The son graduated. Now the son is several years out of college, is married, has a career, has never needed to know his father has HIV infection, and still doesn't.

People with HIV infection won't tell, they say, unless they start getting sick. "With this virus," said Helen, "you don't know anything definite about the future. I have two kids, aged 16 and 17, who live with their father. They would be anxious, a little for themselves even, though they would believe I wouldn't hurt them." Edward's daughter by his earlier marriage is now 17: "She knows I'm gay and doesn't seem to have a problem with that—she loves my partner," he said. "I told her that I have AIDS only within the last several weeks. I waited that long because I didn't know what to say to a 17-year-old. A lot of it has to do with innocence—you're not supposed to have to deal with the harsh realities as a teenager. She cried at first and was upset, but so far she seems to have dealt with it all right. I worry what effect this is going to have on her. I hope it'll be a good one—that's what you hope, that people will grow from unpleasant experiences. But who's to say?"

Sometimes, people find that they must tell their children sooner than they had planned, because the children, who always see more than they seem to, sense that their parents are preoccupied. The children worry. Sometimes they suspect the truth; sometimes they come to entirely wrong conclusions. One mother had two children she wasn't telling about her diagnosis. The children noticed her medications and frequent doctor appointments, talked to each other about it, and decided she was dying of cancer. The children were upset: one child became a workaholic, going to school and then working into the night until early the next morning; the other got into trouble at school. When their mother finally told them she was infected with HIV and wasn't dying any time soon, they were almost relieved. At the least, they no longer had to deal with uncertainty.

Telling your children you have HIV infection usually also means telling them how you got the virus. People want their children to respect and look up to them. They don't want to look vulnerable or fallible. Most people, however, get infected in ways that society judges harshly: through using drugs by injection or through gay sexual relations. Often people have hidden these behaviors from their children. People worry their children will make the same judgment society makes, and will reject them. Drug users especially worry that they have set a bad example. Helen is proud that her children do not use drugs and have never seen her use drugs: "I'd rather die than lose my kids' respect," she said. One couple with two children told them that the father (who had HIV infection) had cancer. Several years before, the father had experimented with bisexuality and had become infected. Both parents were ashamed of this. The mother said she didn't want them to see her as a secret-keeper, but she couldn't tell them their father was bisexual.

Edward and his 17-year-old daughter managed to resolve the issue of homosexuality by talking openly and lovingly about his life and his daughter's place in it, and her relation to his partner. "Now my daughter just accepts it," Edward said. "She says, 'Dad is gay and has AIDS.' She brings her friends to our house. When the kids are around, my partner and I hold back our normal affections and don't use terms of endearment with each other." Sometimes children have more trouble with the situation than Edward's daughter, and are upset at their father's homosexuality. Sometimes they dislike their father's partner.

In general, people find telling the truth works out best. They naturally feel sadness and guilt and regret about the truth, and those feelings will complicate how they talk to their children. They find that the simplest truth works: the simplest truth does not necessarily go into details of why or how. The parents leave the child with the impression that though they are regretful, they are responsible. They say things like, "You know I used to have a drug problem. At that time, I did things I wasn't proud of, and I got AIDS." Children in their teens understand this sort of information best.

The Children's Worries

Children fear abandonment. Younger children, when faced with a parent's illness, will ask directly, "If you get sick, who is going to take care of me? Who will live with me if you go to the hospital?" Older children, though they are bothered by the same questions, try to tough it out, and often they will not ask.

Some children worry that their parents are not caring for themselves well enough. Helen's son, though he does not know she has HIV infection, sees that she occasionally loses weight and asks her, "You aren't getting high, are you? You're eating, aren't you? You're taking care of yourself, aren't you?" Other children worry not only about their parent's health, but about everything else the parent is normally responsible for: bills, rent, mortgage, car, groceries. These children are beginning to see themselves as their parent's caregivers, and they are trying to take on the role of a responsible adult.

Children often do not express their worries directly. Instead, they act their worries out; their worries are evident only in their behavior. Some children get depressed, some become withdrawn and stop talking, some become unusually aggressive. Parents who see this happening can try to encourage the child to express his or her worries directly. They can also get help from mental health professionals, especially those who deal specifically with families or children.

The Parent's Worries

A parent's worst worry is whether he or she has unknowingly infected a child. Fathers worry that they have infected their children through casual contact; mothers worry that they have infected their children during the birth process. If the child was born before the mother became infected, the child is almost certainly uninfected. If the child was born after the parent became infected, and if the child does not receive treatment, the child has a chance of also having the virus. Parents do not usually know when they were infected, and do not know if they have passed the virus on to their children. The only way to find this out is to have the child tested. To decide whether to do this, ask, What would be gained by testing? What would be lost? Parents often decide to have their children tested, because a child, if infected, critically needs medical care even when he or she appears well. And if the child is not infected, the parent has the relief of knowing it. If you are worried about this, or if you are about to become a parent, get help with this decision from your physician or pediatrician.

Parents with older children are also concerned about their children's worries. People can often accept that a friend or adult relative worries about them, but they are unhappy to think that their children worry about them. The reversal of the normal role of parents and children makes parents uncomfortable; they feel intensely responsible for their children. The children often understand this without being told, and do what they feel they can do. Some children are less worried about this than their parents are. "I've spent more time with my daughter," said Edward. "I'm very close to her. But now I'm worried because I don't want to become a burden on her. When I tell her that, she just says, 'We'll cross that bridge when we come to it.'"

Parents with younger children—or with children of any age—worry that their own health may prevent them from caring for their children, and they feel a moral obligation to provide for that possibility. They are intensely worried, and they are often more distressed about this than about their own health.

Many agencies offer advice on this subject: the state Department of Social Services, social workers, and such private social services as Catholic Charities, Jewish Family and Children's Services, and Lutheran Social Services can help. Community-based AIDS-advocacy agencies might also be good sources of advice; some agencies include the services of a "pro bono" (free) lawyer. In any case, to guard your rights as a parent, make any arrangements only with the advice of a lawyer.

Relationships with Drug Users

Resolving strained relationships between drug users and their caregivers is not always possible. Relationships between drug users and their parents and partners were often difficult even before an HIV diagnosis. Sometimes addiction is a family illness and everyone is participating in the addiction process: parents or partners pay bills, make excuses, solve problems, make problems bearable. Sometimes everyone in the family is a user of some sort and dependent on alcohol or drugs. Sometimes relationships cannot bear the strain of addiction, and families have already drifted apart. Sometimes, as with gayness, families have known all along. A friend of Helen's called a hospital social worker and said, "My brother is in the hospital, probably with AIDS, probably from using drugs. He won't tell me, and I don't want to ask. Can you help me talk to him?" The social worker agreed to say only that the sister had expressed concerns, and set up a visit. When they got together, he told her his life was changing and he was going to need her support. "Finally," said the sister, "we really got together. We had a wonderful time."

Some families simply accept the addiction. Helen's family says, "This is the way Helen is. We do what we can. We just keep going." Other families try to fight the drug problem by withholding care until the user is off drugs. When a friend of Helen's told his mother he became infected with HIV from injecting drugs, his mother took off her shoe, hit him with it, and said she'd take care of his infection but not his drug problem, so if he wanted help he'd better get off drugs. Like Helen's friend's mother, caregivers often insist on detoxification as a condition for care.

The decision of whether to fight the addiction or accept it is extraordinarily painful. Do you insist on detoxification and risk letting people be sick without your care and support? Or do you accept them as they are and risk letting them continue to hurt themselves? Get help with the decision from mental health professionals—psychiatrists, psychologists, social workers—or from professional drug counselors. Professional drug counselors can be found in drug rehabilitation programs and programs in psychiatric hospitals, regular hospitals, Veterans Administration hospitals, or family and children's social service agencies.

Substance abusers, whose main priority is finding alcohol or drugs, often have problems in complying assiduously with the complex regimen necessary to treat HIV infection. Substance abusers also have problems taking the medications if they have periods of intoxication or if they are confined and detoxifying. Still, the medical profession has been notoriously unsuccessful in predicting who will comply with a medication regimen and who won't, especially when it has based its predictions on socioeconomic status. The physician's common assumption is that the person who lives next door is affluent, compliant, and a model patient; while the homeless, jobless addict from the inner city won't follow a complex medical regimen. Such assumptions are often wrong. Everyone needs a chance, and people can usually predict, based on self-knowledge, how likely they are to comply.

The relationships between drug users and their caregivers are not always unstable. If the relationship was stable before HIV infection entered their lives, it will be stable afterward. Caregivers of drug users, however, often need help from mental health professionals.

Chapter 6

The Complications
of HIV Infection
and Their Treatment

- Overview
- What to do when you feel sick
- Lung problems
- Skin problems
- Mouth problems
- Problems of the digestive system
- Gynecological problems
- Eye problems
- Head and nerve problems
- Problems affecting the whole body

The availability of effective drugs to treat HIV (highly active antiretroviral therapy, or HAART) has brought a dramatic decline in HIV-related complications and the number of people whose HIV infection progressed to AIDS. HAART has not been universally successful, however: some people don't adhere to the treatment, some have taken HIV drugs extensively and are now resistant, some cannot tolerate the drugs, and some people simply seem to have bad luck. This chapter deals with the classical complications of HIV infection.

Overview

HIV produces an average of about 10 billion new viruses daily. These new viruses attack and kill CD4 cells, destroying 10 billion CD4 cells each day. The immune system retaliates by replacing the lost CD4 cells. In the long run, however, the virus reproduces more effectively than the immune system retaliates, and over a period of years, the number of CD4 cells gradually declines.

From the point of view of the person with HIV infection, the battle within—the fight between HIV and the CD4 cells—is silent. The person remains asymptomatic until the immune system begins losing the battle. The average person has 1,000 CD4 cells per milliliter of blood—a total of about 100 billion CD4 cells in the body—and does not become vulnerable to complications until the CD4 count falls to 200 cells per milliliter or less. HIV-infected people with CD4 counts above 200 usually deal with the microbial world with aplomb. There are a few exceptions, but not many. Most people actually do well until the CD4 count is substantially lower than 200. The average CD4 count with the first major complication is about 50.

For about 50 percent of people with untreated HIV infection, this first complication occurs within ten years of being infected; this is only an average. A very few people, less than 1 percent, progress rapidly from infection to an AIDS-defining diagnosis within one year. At the other extreme are the people who go for years without any apparent consequences of HIV infection: they have no symptoms, and the number of their CD4 cells is normal. Some of these people go without consequences long enough that they are called "chronic non-progressors." To be chronic non-progressors, people must meet three criteria: they must have had HIV infection for at least eight years; have a normal CD4 cell count (see below); and have received no treatment against HIV. Apparently 2 to 3 percent of people with HIV infection are chronic non-progressors. The reason for non-progression may be that these people have been infected with an especially hapless virus. The reason may also be that many of these people have a robust immune response—a highly effective CD4 response that's specific to HIV. This latter reason is more common.

The reasons that people progress to the first complication vary. Many people never knew they were infected until this first complication prompted them to get their first HIV tests. Other people failed therapy. Some refused therapy. Many were depressed or substance abusers. For those who are newly diagnosed and whose first complication has not left permanent damage, the prognosis is excellent.

The stage at which the first symptoms or conditions of a weakened immune system occur usually happens five to eight years after infection. This stage may or may not mean that the immune system is weakening. The most common early conditions are thrush, oral hairy leukoplakia, shingles, and idiopathic thrombocytopenic purpura. Some of these complaints are experienced by people who do not have HIV; the biggest difference is that in someone with HIV infection, the symptoms tend to be chronic, that is, they persist for several weeks or months. Most people with these early symptoms have a relatively low CD4 cell count, usually less than 300; most people have no symptoms until the CD4 cell count is less than 50.

The late stage of HIV infection, usually eight to ten years after infection, entails severe immunosuppression, that is, severe weakening of the immune defenses of the body. The exact definition of AIDS has historically been a moving target, but in 1993 the definition was set to include anyone with HIV infection and a CD4 count below 200. People with AIDS are susceptible to opportunistic complications caused by microbes to which everyone is exposed on a regular basis but which are usually defeated by a modest effort of the immune system. The most common and important complications are described below. *Pneumocystis jiroveci* pneumonia and Kaposi's sarcoma are the most common of the complications; the others occur less frequently.

This whole process is highly variable. Based on four different studies (done before any effective treatment was available), the time lapse between transmission of HIV and AIDS is as follows: after 1 year, 0 percent of the people with HIV infection were diagnosed with AIDS; after 2 years, 0 percent; after 3 years, 3 percent; after 4 years, 6 percent; after 5 years, 12 percent; after 6 years, 20 percent; after 7 years, 27 percent; after 8 years, 36 percent; after 9 years, 45 percent; after 10 years, 53 percent. Some people with AIDS lived five years or more after their first major complication, without therapy, but they were unusual.

HIV infection, untreated, affects virtually every part of the body. The virus's effect is either indirect—through medical complications—or direct. Moreover, its effects, both direct and indirect, resemble symptoms of other diseases. As a result, people easily become confused and worried: Which symptoms should I see the doctor about? Which should I ignore? Which result from HIV infection and which are the normal flus and headaches everyone has? How are the complications diagnosed? What are the usual treatments? What are the side effects of the treatments?

What to Do When You Feel Sick

This chapter, which discusses the medical complications of HIV infection, is most relevant to people with advanced disease, that is, with a CD4 count of less than 200. Included here are the symptoms for which people should see a physician, the most likely diagnosis of those symptoms, the tests that establish the diagnosis, and the best treatment. The chapter is organized by anatomy: lungs, skin, mouth, digestive system,

Table 5. Prognosis by CD4 Cell Count and Viral Load (without Treatment):
Probability of an AIDS Complication

| | | Probability of AIDS without Treatment in | | |
| | | 3 Years | 6 Years | 9 Years |
CD4 Count	Viral Load	(%)	(%)	(%)
over 500	under 2,000	1	5	11
	2,000–40,000	5	20	41
	40,000–120,000	10	35	60
	over 120,000	33	67	76
350–500	2,000–40,000	6	30	53
	40,000–120,000	15	57	79
	over 120,000	48	78	94
under 350	2,000–40,000	4	30	42
	40,000–120,000	40	73	86
	over 120,000	73	93	96

Source: Adapted from J. Mellors et al., *Annals of Internal Medicine* 126 (1997): 946. To
simplify presentation, numbers have been rounded off and aggregated. Viral load levels
are for the HIV RNA PCR (Roche) assay.

gynecological problems, eyes, and head and nerves, and concludes with
a segment on the constitutional symptoms—like fever and fatigue—that
affect the whole body. So, for example, someone worried about a red
rash would look up skin problems, find the symptom of red rash, and
read which diagnoses are possible.

Our intent is not to provide a substitute for medical care, in part because diagnostic tests and treatments are subject to rapidly changing
guidelines, and some of this information can quickly become antiquated.

HIV, in those who are untreated or who fail therapy, affects the body
in two different ways. The first way it affects the body is directly, causing an early mononucleosis-like disease or a late dementia called HIV-
associated dementia. These are complications caused by the virus directly. The second way HIV affects the body is indirectly, specifically by
reducing the number of CD4 cells (see chapter 3). Most of the symptoms
that people with HIV infection have are a result of complications that
would not happen with the usual number of CD4 cells. As noted previously, the usual CD4 cell count is about 1,000; a person with HIV infection loses, on average, about 30–80 CD4s each year, so that after
seven or eight years the count is down to 200–300. Different people lose

CD4 cells at different rates, but the CD4 count at which complications occur is less than 200, and often substantially lower.

Some complications, however, do not depend quite so much on CD4 cell counts. Those include Kaposi's sarcoma, lymphomas, bacterial pneumonias (but not pneumocystis pneumonia), *Candida* vaginitis, salmonellosis, herpes zoster or shingles, and tuberculosis.

Most of the common and serious complications occur when the CD4 count is below 200 per milliliter, and many people have few medical problems until the CD4 count is consistently below 50. These include pneumocystis pneumonia, disseminated (widespread) cytomegalovirus infection, disseminated (widespread) *Mycobacterium avium* complex infection, cryptosporidiosis, toxoplasmosis, cryptococcal meningitis, and HIV-associated dementia.

We should emphasize that when HAART arrests the growth of HIV, it also halts all HIV-related complications, both direct and indirect. Since 1996, when HAART was introduced, nearly all the complications discussed in this chapter have decreased, most by 50 to 80 percent, and some have nearly disappeared.

Lung Problems

Most infections of the lung, or pneumonias, regardless of their cause, have the same symptoms: cough, shortness of breath, and fever. In some lung infections, the cough is productive—that is, the cough produces sputum; in other lung infections, the cough is dry. Cough and shortness of breath may be accompanied by chest pain. The person with advanced HIV infection should watch out for these symptoms and should seek prompt medical attention for them. They can be symptoms of complications that almost invariably respond to antibiotics if taken early enough.

Cough and shortness of breath are relatively common symptoms of other medical conditions as well. Causes of these symptoms include asthma, influenza, bronchitis, and chronic lung diseases like those brought on by long-term smoking. When these symptoms occur in someone who has not previously had lung problems, when they are more severe than usual, or when they are accompanied by fever, the cause could be pneumonia. People with HIV infection get different kinds of pneumonias, but the most important are pneumocystis pneumonia, tuberculosis, and certain common bacterial pneumonias. The standard diagnostic tests for these symptoms include a blood count, a chest X-ray, and culture of the sputum. Additional diagnostic tests will largely depend on the specific symptoms and on the results of the first set of tests.

Dry Cough, Shortness of Breath, and Fever

Symptoms that include a dry cough, shortness of breath, and fever when the CD4 count is below 200 are most likely to be *Pneumocystis jiroveci* pneumonia (PCP). The most characteristic symptom of PCP, compared to other pneumonias, is a dry cough that does not produce sputum and that begins subtly and progresses slowly. People with PCP first notice shortness of breath only with exercise, then begin to notice it with minimal activity; eventually, they notice it even when they are at rest. Nearly all people with PCP have a temperature of at least 100 degrees F at some point during the day, usually in the late afternoon or the evening. These symptoms of PCP usually come on over a period of many days or several weeks. By contrast, most other forms of pneumonia become serious much more quickly.

PCP is caused by a fungus called *Pneumocystis jiroveci*. PCP is relatively common late in the course of HIV infection: of the first 100,000 people who had AIDS in the United States, 80 percent had PCP sometime during the course of the infection, and 60 percent had PCP as their first major complication. These numbers are now way, way down. The reason the numbers are down by so much is that both HIV treatments and PCP prophylaxis are so effective. Nevertheless, PCP is still the most common important complication of late HIV infection.

PCP in people with AIDS evolves slowly, and most people have had the symptoms for weeks before they seek medical attention. PCP is serious, however, and if left untreated, it is fatal: at first approximately 25 percent of people with HIV died because of PCP. PCP continues to be a major cause of death in people with HIV infection, but primarily in those who do not respond to antiretroviral treatment and don't take the drugs to prevent PCP. This percentage is now decreasing because drugs are given to prevent PCP in people with CD4 counts below 200.

The tests to diagnose PCP can be tedious and unpleasant. People often ask if the testing process can be simplified, and indeed, the person's symptoms and chest X-ray results are occasionally compelling enough to diagnose PCP without looking for the fungus. This approach, though simple and efficient, can occasionally lead to an inaccurate diagnosis; that is, the person is assumed to have PCP, and an alternate and treatable infection may be overlooked. Similarly, a delay in treating PCP may allow it to progress to the point where it is difficult to reverse. For these reasons, most physicians experienced in caring for people with AIDS will treat PCP aggressively when symptoms suggest it. They will also want a proven diagnosis before starting the three-week course of treatment.

A variety of drugs can be used to treat PCP. The most common are antibiotics: trimethoprim-sulfamethoxazole (the trade names are Bactrim and Septra), dapsone plus trimethoprim, clindamycin plus primaquine, atovaquone (Mepron), and pentamidine. Most people respond well to treatment, but recovery is slow. Those who recover are likely to develop PCP again; in fact, the recurrence rate is about 70 percent within one year. Recurrences can be prevented. The drugs that prevent the recurrence of PCP include pentamidine taken by aerosol, trimethoprim-sulfamethoxazole taken by mouth, dapsone taken by mouth, or atovaquone (which is very expensive) taken by mouth. People who are candidates for preventive treatment include not only anyone with HIV infection who has previously had PCP, but also people with HIV infection who have not had PCP but whose CD4 counts are less than 200. The best way to prevent PCP is to increase the CD4 count by treating HIV infection. When the CD4 count has increased to 200 to 250 or more for three months, many studies show you can safely stop treatment, but treatment should resume if the CD4 count decreases to 200 later on. Otherwise, when the CD4 count is below 200, the best treatments are the antibiotics listed above to prevent PCP.

Productive Cough, Shortness of Breath, Fever

Productive cough, shortness of breath, and fever are symptoms of tuberculosis and pneumonia caused by certain types of bacteria; these symptoms may also be caused by PCP, certain viruses, Kaposi's sarcoma in the lung, and several other unusual conditions.

Tuberculosis (TB). The most common symptoms of TB are cough, bloody sputum, shortness of breath, fever, weight loss, chest pain with breathing, and night sweats. As with PCP, the tempo of tuberculosis is generally slow, usually progressing over a period of weeks or months. During this time the person is usually fatigued, has night sweats, and loses weight. The cough usually lasts more than a month and less than a year. TB starts in the lung, but it can spread to almost any part of the body. TB in someone with HIV infection, either in the lung or outside the lung, is now considered an AIDS-defining diagnosis. People with HIV infection often have TB relatively early in the course of the infection, when the CD4 count is fairly high: TB apparently has enough clout that it does not require a severely weakened immune system to cause disease.

Mycobacterium tuberculosis, the only contagious mycobacterial infection, can be transmitted from one person to another by close contact, usually over a period of several months. For this reason, the people most likely to be infected are those who live with the infected person. But an infected person who has been treated with drugs against TB for several days is less likely to transmit the infection to others. This means that once treatment has started, the likelihood that it will be spread to others is reduced or nil. The only way to find out whether a person has dormant or inactive TB is to take the skin test most people are familiar with, done on the forearm. The skin test is a shallow injection of a protein called a purified protein derivative, or PPD, made from *Mycobacterium tuberculosis*. If the area around the injection becomes red and thickened two or three days later, the person's immune system has responded to the bacterium. That means that *Mycobacterium tuberculosis* is in the body and the person has TB, either active or inactive. A positive skin test is followed by sputum tests for TB and X-rays. If the sputum test is also positive, or if the X-ray shows new changes, the person has active TB. Otherwise, the TB is inactive.

It is especially important for people with HIV infection to have a skin test. The risk of developing active TB is 100 times greater with HIV infection than without HIV infection. About 5 percent of all people with HIV infection get active tuberculosis, and about 5 percent of people with tuberculosis have HIV infection. Consequently, everyone with HIV infection should have a tuberculosis skin test, and everyone with tuberculosis should have an HIV blood test. However, TB in people with HIV infection often fails to obey the usual rules: the skin test is often falsely negative and the chest X-ray, though often abnormal, does not show the changes usual in TB. Both of these findings make detecting TB in people with HIV infection more difficult.

Physicians are under appropriate pressure to pursue tuberculosis aggressively and to take precautions to prevent its spread. A patient in a hospital who might have tuberculosis must be in a single room, and anyone entering the room must wear a mask. Visitors are often excluded, and patients are not allowed to leave the room except for medical procedures. The patient feels lonely and bored, but isolation is necessary: hospitals have had big epidemics of TB, and health care workers often get infected by exposure in the workplace. TB is the major microbial cause of death in the world. Virtually everyone is vulnerable, and strict public health measures are an important method of control.

Inactive TB can be treated with a drug, isoniazid (INH), which will prevent active TB. Active TB is treated more aggressively, usually with four drugs. People with tuberculosis must take the full course of the these drugs for at least six months and should do so under direct observation. If they don't take the full course, they cause two problems: the infection recurs, and this time they are likely to have a resistant strain that will be difficult or impossible to treat. Direct observation means going to a clinic to have someone give the medicine.

Bacterial pneumonias. Bacteria have always been a major cause of serious pneumonias. The symptoms of bacterial pneumonias are chills, fever, shortness of breath, and a cough that often produces thick yellow or green sputum. For some people, the major symptom is chest pain, especially when they breathe. Unlike PCP and TB, bacterial pneumonias usually begin rather abruptly, and people see physicians within days rather than weeks or months. Bacterial pneumonias can occur relatively early in the course of HIV infection. Unlike PCP, bacterial pneumonias do not necessarily indicate a severely weakened immune system. One bacterial pneumonia, caused by a microbe called *pneumococcus,* is common in people without HIV infection, though people with HIV infection before the era of HAART had pneumococcal pneumonia 100 times more frequently than people without.

The diagnosis of bacterial pneumonias is usually established with a chest X-ray and sometimes with sputum tests. Treatment with antibiotics is highly effective when begun early in the infection. Trimethoprim-sulfamethoxazole, which prevents PCP, will help prevent pneumococcal pneumonia as well. Pneumococcal vaccine (Pneumovax) may also prevent pneumococcal pneumonia and is advocated for people with HIV infection; it helps best when it is given early in the course of HIV infection. Bacteria other than pneumococcus cause pneumonias as well. *Haemophilus influenzae* is common and easy to treat. *Pseudomonas aeruginosa* occasionally causes pneumonia in the late stage and is hard to treat.

Viral pneumonias. Influenza viruses are like many viruses that attack the respiratory system. They are common in people without HIV infection, and there is no evidence that they are more common or severe in those with HIV infection, even those in advanced stages of HIV infection. Most people with a viral pneumonia have bronchitis—cold symptoms with a cough—but a negative X-ray because the lungs are not infected. Influenza vaccine is advised for people with HIV infection in part because symptoms may cause undue concern about PCP and other lung problems. In addition, we're not sure that influenza is totally safe in people with HIV infection, and the vaccine usually works well. Many other viruses can cause similar symptoms.

Miscellaneous lung conditions. Other causes of lung problems in people with HIV infection are less common than those above. *Mycobacterium avium* complex (MAC), though it usually infects other parts of the body, sometimes infects the lungs. Cytomegalovirus, or CMV, may cause pneumonia in the late stages of HIV infection when the CD4 count is less than 50—though this is unusual. Kaposi's sarcoma may be found in the lungs, where it causes cough and shortness of breath. People with Kaposi's sarcoma in the lungs will probably have changes on a chest X-ray and will also have Kaposi's sarcoma on the skin (see below, "Skin Problems"). Lymphomas are tumors of the lymph system that are common with HIV infection and often cause lung complications. Occasionally, people with HIV infection will have a pneumonia called lymphocytic interstitial pneumonia, which appears to be due to HIV itself and often responds to treatment with corticosteroids.

Skin Problems

The skin is commonly affected in people with HIV infection. The conditions affecting the skin include a diverse array of infections and an unusual tumor called Kaposi's sarcoma. Other skin conditions—seborrhea, molluscum, fungal infections, and allergic rashes—are also common in people without HIV infection, but they are more common and more severe in people with HIV infection. Since most of these conditions are treatable, people should see their physicians, especially if the skin problem is painful, disfiguring, or accompanied by a fever.

As expected, the diagnosis of a skin condition is largely dictated by its appearance. In many cases, a diagnosis can be established simply by observation, but occasionally diagnosis will require a biopsy.

Purple or Black Spots

Purple or black spots on the skin are characteristic of Kaposi's sarcoma (KS), a tumor of the cells of the blood vessels. In most cases, there are several tumors, each approximately a quarter of an inch to an inch in diameter. They can usually be felt as a nodule or a fleshy collection of tissue. They can—but do not usually—cause pain. In light-skinned people, the tumors are usually purple; and in dark-skinned people, they are very dark brown or black. The tumors are not like freckles, either in color or to the touch.

KS tumors can appear any place on the skin, including the face, scalp, back, chest, abdomen, arms, legs, and inside the mouth. They appear most commonly on the tip of the nose, around the eyes, on the ears, behind the ears, and on the arms, the legs, the chest, and the genitals. Usually tumors appear in different places. At times the tumors occur symmetrically, appearing in almost identical places on both arms, on both sides of the face, or on both feet. KS can cause edema (swelling) of the leg or the face. It can also cause disease in such internal organs as the gastrointestinal tract or the lungs.

KS is caused by a virus called Kaposi's sarcoma herpes virus (KSHV), or human herpes virus 8 (because there are seven previously known herpes viruses). KS is not the same as the herpes virus that causes genital infections or cold sores; it is only related to that virus. Among gay men with HIV infection, KS is disappearing, due to changes in behavior, to reduced rates of HIV infection in gay men, and to higher CD4 counts following HAART.

When KS on the skin is suspected, it can be diagnosed with a biopsy of the tumor. The skin biopsy is a simple outpatient procedure; Novocain is injected into the skin to make the procedure painless.

The treatment and prognosis depend on the severity of immune suppression and the number and location of the KS tumors. When KS tumors are few and confined to the skin, the prognosis is good and treatment is usually done for cosmetic reasons or for relief of any unpleasant symptoms: cosmetic problems can often simply be covered with opaque makeup. Skin tumors can also be treated with radiation, freezing, laser treatment, or injection of a drug called vinblastine. When the CD4 count stays below 150, when there are more than twenty-five skin tumors, or when the internal organs are involved, treatment is often cancer chemotherapy. If the tumors are obstructing lymph channels, treatment can be radiation or cancer chemotherapy.

The best advice about treating Kaposi's sarcoma will come from any physician with extensive experience in this area, particularly from an AIDS physician (see chapter 7), from a dermatologist, or from a cancer specialist (an oncologist). Which physician does the treatment will depend on which therapy is used: radiation treatment will require referral to a radiation therapist, cancer chemotherapy might require referral to an oncologist, and drug injections are usually done by a dermatologist or an oncologist.

Red Rash

A rash is usually either diffusely red all over or red only in spots or blotches. It usually appears on the chest, back, arms, face, and legs. Rashes can be accompanied by other symptoms, including fever, swelling of the face, giant welts, or itching.

The most common cause of a red rash covering large areas of the body in people with HIV infection is an adverse reaction to a drug. The most common offending drug is a sulfa drug—especially trimethoprim-sulfamethoxazole (Bactrim, Septra), the drug usually taken for the treatment or prevention of *Pneumocystis jiroveci* pneumonia. Sulfa drugs are also treatments for many other infectious diseases in people with and without AIDS. Rashes that are a reaction to sulfa drugs are especially common in people with HIV infection: 30 percent to 50 percent of people with HIV infection have these rashes. In addition to rashes, many people also have fever, low white blood cell counts, or tests showing hepatitis. All these symptoms disappear when the sulfa drug is stopped. Many people tolerate trimethoprim-sulfamethoxazole if they take it again, especially if they take it in a lower dose.

Rashes are also caused by other drugs, including dapsone, clindamycin, penicillin, amoxicillin, sulfadiazine, voriconazole, atovaquone; and several anti-HIV drugs, including abacavir, efavirenz, fosamprenavir, nevirapine, and atazanavir. Most skin rashes cause no serious problems, even with continued use of the drugs causing them. Rashes often itch, and the itching may be treated with steroid creams or antihistamines like atarax. If the drug causing the rash is stopped, the rash usually improves within 48 hours; if the rash doesn't improve, it is caused by something else. If the drug is really important to treatment, it may be worth "riding it out," because the rash may improve even with continued use of the drug that caused it.

A few conditions or drugs require special attention. Abacavir or nevirapine may cause a rash that indicates a serious problem, especially within the first 8 weeks of starting abacavir and the first 16 weeks of starting nevirapine. These particular rashes are not distinctive, but they are usually accompanied by other symptoms: a fever, gastrointestinal symptoms, or stomach pain. If you're taking abacavir or nevirapine and develop a rash, you must call your doctor.

Other types of skin reactions are serious and require medical attention: skin rashes that involve the mouth or eyes, cause fever, cause blisters, or cause joint pain and weakness.

Itchy Skin

People with HIV infection often have itchy skin. When the itchiness is accompanied by a rash, the cause is usually a reaction to a drug as outlined above. Almost any drug can cause itchiness, but those that do most commonly are the same ones listed above that also cause a rash.

Many people with HIV infection develop bumps, called nodules, that itch so badly that people actually tear the skin with scratching. The condition is called *prurigo nodularis,* which is Latin for "itchy nodules." The cause is unknown. The treatment is to soothe the itching and thereby stop the cycle of scratching–bleeding lesions–scars–more scratching. Applying steroid creams and covering the lesions often helps.

Sometimes the steroid is injected into the nodules. Sometimes the nodules are removed with surgery, either by lasers or with cryotherapy. Sometimes the treatment is antihistamines, taken by mouth, or phototherapy—a light treatment called PUVA.

Itchy skin without bumps or a rash could be scabies, a highly contagious infection whose symptoms are pinhead-sized bumps with ulcers on top of them. They itch more at night. Scabies is treated with a lotion applied over the whole body. People who have been in close contact with the person with scabies should also be treated.

Itchy skin without bumps or a rash could also be a symptom of a serious underlying disease like liver or kidney disease, or lymphoma.

Finally, some people with HIV infection itch but have no bumps or rash, and no underlying disease. They just itch. In this case, the best treatment is oatmeal baths, menthol lotions, anesthetics applied to the skin, or antihistamines or cortisone taken by mouth.

Blisters

Blisters are small, fluid-filled bubbles that often break, becoming open sores filled with clear fluid or pus. Blisters can occur in groups in one specific area of the skin, or they can be distributed all over the skin. Like red rashes, blistering rashes can be caused by adverse reactions to drugs. The most common causes of blistering rash in people with HIV infection, however, are two related viruses, herpes simplex and herpes zoster.

Herpes simplex infection. Infection by the herpes simplex virus is extremely common in healthy people, causing water blisters, pain, and fever. There are actually two different types of herpes simplex viruses: Type 1 and Type 2. Type 1 most frequently causes the infection of the mouth called cold sores (see below, "Mouth Problems"). Type 2 most frequently causes sores on the genitals and the anal region and is regarded as a sexually transmitted disease. When the infection is on the mouth, transmission is usually through oral contact (like kissing) with a person who is infected with the virus and who may or may not have apparent sores on the mouth. When the infection is in the genitals, transmission is usually through sexual contact; the person who is the source of the infection may or may not have sores on the genitals.

After the initial infection clears up, the virus remains in the nerves nearby and is either silent with no symptoms, or it is periodically reactivated. When the virus is reactivated on or in the mouth, it causes what people call cold sores. When the virus is reactivated on the genitals, it causes sores on the genitals or in the anal region. These reactivations are less severe than the initial infection.

Studies of blood tests show that 50 percent of people have had herpes simplex on the mouth and 20 to 30 percent have had herpes simplex on the genitals, even though most do not recall it. Most of these people have either no problems or rare outbreaks; some have attacks more frequently, but these are brief, not severe, and restricted to the lips or genitals. By contrast, people with advanced HIV infection can have herpes simplex infections that cover a larger area of the skin, can be more painful, can last longer, can even affect the internal organs, and are often difficult to treat.

Treatment is generally successful in providing relief from an outbreak of sores, if taken early enough. Acyclovir (Zovirax), famciclovir (Famvir), or valacyclovir (Valtrex) are the usual drugs. They are taken by mouth. Occasionally, people have strains of herpes that are resistant to these drugs and require foscarnet (Foscavir), given by vein. The relief with treatment is usually temporary; treatment does not eliminate the herpes virus and does not cure the infection. When the outbreaks recur frequently enough, treatment is taken continuously.

We now think that herpes on the genitals is important in transmitting HIV infection, probably because the sores are an easy place for HIV to enter. The sores can be obvious blisters, but they can also be tiny and go unnoticed. The drugs used to treat genital herpes—acyclovir, valacyclovir, and famciclovir—all reduce herpes outbreaks, including any tiny sores, and in general reduce the amount of herpes virus that is shed. This means that chronic use of the drugs for genital herpes will reduce not only the outbreaks and transmission of herpes, but also the transmission of HIV.

Herpes zoster, or shingles. Herpes zoster is caused by the same virus that causes chickenpox. Like herpes simplex, the herpes zoster virus stays quiet or dormant in the nerve cells. Every adult who had chickenpox during childhood has the shingles virus living in his or her nerves for life. Usually the virus causes no problems. Sometimes, however, many years or decades after the original bout with chickenpox, it becomes active, causing a disease called shingles. It seems to become active at times of stress or in people with weakened immune systems, but sometimes it becomes active for no apparent reason. The assumption is that the virus is continually present but is held in check by the normal immune defenses. Shingles is common not only in people with HIV infection, but in the elderly and in others as well. Shingles, although it is more common in the late stages of the infection, is one of the few complications of HIV infection that can occur with a high CD4 count.

The symptoms of shingles are blisters that are identical to those seen with chickenpox. The blisters are small and filled with a watery fluid;

later, the blisters break, the fluid becomes pus, scabs form, and the skin heals. Unlike the blisters of chickenpox, however, the blisters of shingles are often extremely painful. In addition, they are not spread all over the body, but instead are distributed in bands or lines on the chest, the abdomen, down the leg, on the arm, or on the face. In most cases, the blisters occur on only one side of the body and stop abruptly at the middle of the body. The blisters follow this pattern because they are following the path of the nerve in which the virus is living, and each nerve serves only one side of the body.

The worst complication of this infection is pain. The pain may come before the blisters appear, or it may accompany the blisters. The pain may also occur months or even years after the blisters are gone and the skin is healed; this pain is called post-herpetic neuralgia. Fortunately, people with HIV infection who get shingles do not often develop post-herpetic neuralgia. This complication is most common in people over 60 years old, with or without HIV infection.

A note about transmission: the blisters contain the virus that causes herpes zoster. Adults who have had chickenpox already have this virus, have antibodies to it, and are not susceptible when exposed to someone with chickenpox or shingles. However, young children and the occasional adult who has escaped chickenpox could become infected with the virus that causes herpes zoster. These people may acquire chickenpox by contact with the blisters or by inhaling the virus. To prevent transmission, people who have not had chickenpox should carefully avoid contact and should even avoid being present in the same room. People who are hospitalized should expect strict isolation precautions—gloves, masks, and gowns—to be taken, to prevent transmission to the health care workers. The so-called varicella vaccine now prevents chickenpox and will protect people who have not had chickenpox. This vaccine should not be taken by people with HIV infection because it is a "live vaccine" that could cause the disease if the immune response is impaired. Chickenpox in people with advanced HIV infection can be severe and can be prevented. Many people who think they never had chickenpox do have antibodies, which indicates that they did in fact have it but didn't know it. For the person with HIV infection who is exposed to chickenpox or to zoster and who has no history or antibody-evidence of prior chickenpox, the recommendation is an expensive immune globulin called VZIG.

Shingles is not life-threatening and inevitably cures itself. But it can be especially severe in people with advanced HIV, or when the eyes are involved. And people are in pain—potentially terrible pain—so treatment is generally recommended. The treatment is with famciclovir or valacyclovir. Treatment makes the blisters clear faster and may reduce the pain, but it needs to be started early. Drugs such as nortriptyline may be taken to control the pain. Famciclovir and valacyclovir may be taken by mouth, but hospitalization for intravenous treatment with acyclovir is sometimes advocated. Foscarnet and cidofovir are usually effective against strains of the virus that are resistant to oral drugs.

Thick, Discolored Nails; Red, Flaking Circles

Thick, discolored toenails or fingernails are usually caused by a fungus. Patches of red, flaking skin, on the feet or in the groin area, are called athlete's foot or jock itch. When the patches of red, flaking skin are in circular patterns on the scalp or the skin, they are called ringworm. Athlete's foot, jock itch, and ringworm are caused by fungi. These fungi cause infections of the skin and nails but are not capable of causing much else. Treatment of ringworm with antibiotic ointments—clotrimazole (commercial name, Lotrimin) or miconazole—applied on top of the involved area is usually effective. Most of these ointments are available without prescription. When the nails are involved, when large areas of the skin are affected, or when ointments do not work, other antibiotics, like itraconazole or griseofulvin, can be taken as pills and are usually effective.

Small, Colorless Bumps

A crop of small, colorless bumps is usually caused by a virus called *Molluscum contagiosum*. Each of the bumps often has a central indentation. The most common location is on the face, especially around the mouth, and in the genital region. *Molluscum contagiosum* seems to be especially common in people with HIV infection. The major problem is cosmetic. No antibiotics are successful, but a dermatologist can remove the bumps by freezing, electrosurgery, curetting, or a topical treatment.

Flaking, Scaling Rash in Patches

Red, scaling patches, most frequently on the scalp, face, ears, chest, and genitals, are symptoms of seborrhea. Some people have the patches symmetrically on both cheeks, in what is called a "butterfly" distribution. Many people simply have seborrhea on the scalp, where it is referred to as dandruff.

Seborrhea appears to be caused by a fungus, generally involves only the skin, and, at least when severe, is usually cared for by dermatologists. Seborrhea occurs in 50 to 80 percent of people with HIV infection. As the infection progresses, seborrhea is more frequent and more severe.

The treatment of seborrhea of the scalp is to use shampoos containing coal tar, available without prescription at drugstores. For best results, apply the shampoo, then leave it on for twenty to thirty minutes before rinsing it off. Seborrhea on the rest of the skin can be treated with ointments containing cortisone or ketoconazole. Cortisone ointments are available without prescription, but severe or persistent cases of seborrhea are best treated with stronger concentrations of cortisone, which require a prescription.

Excessive Bleeding

Excessive bleeding from nosebleeds, cuts, and injuries may be a symptom of idiopathic thrombocytopenic purpura (ITP). The gums may bleed excessively with toothbrushing, or small razor cuts might bleed excessively. Other symptoms are easy bruising and bloody or tarry stools that result from intestinal bleeding. Some people will have many small red dots about the size of a pinhead on the lower legs and feet, called *petechiae*, which are tiny hemorrhages. Others have larger hemorrhages into the skin, called *purpura*. Unlike other red rashes, these hemorrhages do not disappear when pressure is applied to them. In other words, if you push on the red spot, the spot does not clear for several seconds but remains red.

Idiopathic thrombocytopenic purpura means low numbers (penia) of blood platelets (thrombocytes) that promote blood clotting, causing bruises or hemorrhages in the skin (purpura) for reasons that are unexplained (idiopathic). The cause of ITP is unknown: for some reason, either the body produces antibodies that attack blood platelets or the bone marrow stops making platelets. The purpose of the platelets is to help the blood to clot, explaining ITP's excessive bruising and bleeding. ITP can occur in people who do not have HIV infection. It can occur in people with HIV infection either when the CD4 count is high or when it is low, but usually when it is low.

Most people who have ITP are unaware of it; ITP is usually discovered with routine laboratory testing when a complete blood count (CBC) shows that the number of blood platelets is low. The usual count in healthy persons is 150,000 to 300,000 platelets per milliliter of blood. People with HIV infection often have slightly lower counts—80,000 to 120,000 platelets per milliliter—though these counts cause no problem. People with ITP often have counts that are lower yet—5,000 to 30,000 platelets per milliliter.

Treatment of ITP may consist of drugs, like corticosteroids, that suppress the antibodies attacking the platelets, drugs directed against HIV, or gamma globulin given intravenously. The treatment chosen depends on the situation. If bleeding is active and severe, people will need transfusions and injections of platelets. If the platelet count is low and bleeding intermittent, physicians will always treat HIV first. If that fails, the next step is cortisone and sometimes gamma globulin (which is very expensive). If the person has no symptoms, the physician simply advises precautions and follows up with periodic platelet counts. The major worry with ITP is the possibility of internal bleeding, during which large amounts of blood could be lost or vital organs like the gastrointestinal tract, the brain, or the lungs could be damaged. Obviously, the person with extremely low platelet counts should be extremely careful to avoid cuts and injuries. This means using an electric shaver and avoiding anything that would cause cuts or bruises.

Mouth Problems

Many of the complications of HIV infection involve the mouth. Because of this, it is important for all people with HIV infection to inspect their mouths regularly, pay careful attention to oral hygiene, and get regular dental care. Though most complications occur in the later stages of the disease, some occur early.

Pain in the Mouth

The most common causes of pain in the mouth include thrush, oral hairy leukoplakia, herpes simplex, aphthous ulcers, and Kaposi's sarcoma. All of these are described below. Most of them can be diagnosed largely on the basis of their appearance. The biggest problem with pain in the mouth is adequate nutrition. It obviously makes sense to avoid foods that cause pain: foods that are highly seasoned, for instance, or citrus fruits or certain vegetables that are highly acidic. Also avoid foods that are very hot or very cold. Instead, eat bland foods, foods that are soft, and nutritious liquids like milkshakes. Exactly what you eat should suit your own preference, as long as it is nutritious. (See the following section, "Problems of the Digestive System.")

White Patches in the Mouth

White patches in the mouth, sometimes painful, often painless, are most commonly symptoms of thrush, and less commonly symptoms of oral hairy leukoplakia.

Thrush. Thrush is a yeast infection of the mouth caused by the fungus *Candida albicans. Candida albicans* is found in the mouths of most people; thrush occurs only when the fungus begins growing out of control. Since most people have the fungus in their mouths, thrush is not considered contagious. Thrush is commonly viewed more as a nuisance than as a serious problem.

Symptoms include white or grayish-white patches that look a little like cottage cheese along the gums, along the inside of the cheeks, or on the tongue. Thrush can be unnoticeable, or it can cause pain severe enough to interfere with chewing or swallowing. Thrush becomes more serious when it extends to the back of the throat and to the esophagus: the pain from swallowing might cause people to stop eating, and the treatment given may be somewhat different than for thrush that is restricted to the mouth.

Thrush indicates advanced HIV infection but is often the first HIV-related complication. It is more frequent in people taking cortisone and antibiotics. Thrush virtually never occurs without some underlying medical problem. It is also one of the infections people with HIV infection who are not on HAART most frequently develop: about 80 percent of those with HIV infection have thrush at some time. The CD4 count is usually 50 to 250.

What appear to be patches of thrush can also simply be food particles in the mouth. The distinction is easily made by rinsing the mouth to remove food particles. Thrush cannot be removed without direct scraping, and scraping will leave an inflamed spot where the white patch was. Diagnosis of thrush in the mouth can be done by a physician simply inspecting the mouth; microscopic examination of the patch to identify the fungus can be done but is usually not necessary. Diagnosis of thrush in the esophagus is usually presumed if thrush is in the mouth and if people also have trouble swallowing. The distinction is important because thrush in the esophagus is treated differently and because it means that HIV disease is more advanced.

Common treatments for thrush include gargling with and then swallowing nystatin solution, sucking clotrimazole troches, or taking such pills as fluconazole (Diflucan) or itraconazole (Sporanox). All of these are prescription drugs. If any of the drugs fail, another will usually work. Thrush is generally controlled after one or two weeks of treatment. Occasionally people do not do well with any of these treatments, either because the diagnosis was wrong to begin with or because the infection has extended to the esophagus.

In people with HIV infection, thrush tends to recur once treatment is discontinued. As a result, it is common practice to give these drugs for a long time, initially to control the infection and then to prevent its recurrence. Fluconazole (Diflucan) is probably the most effective drug, but prolonged treatment may cause strains of the fungus to become resistant to the drug and the infection to become progressively difficult to treat. The best ploy is to avoid long-term fluconazole, and to try to increase the CD4 count, avoid antibiotics, and when thrush recurs, use the gargles or troches.

Oral hairy leukoplakia (OHL).   White patches on the tongue, along the side of the tongue, and occasionally in adjacent areas in the mouth are symptoms not only of thrush, but also of oral hairy leukoplakia (OHL). Oral hairy leukoplakia is named for its location in the mouth (oral), and its appearance as white patches (leukoplakia) with microscopic hairlike protrusions (hairy) from the tongue's surface. The patches can be a fraction of an inch in diameter or they can coat most of the tongue. Some people with oral hairy leukoplakia have a sore mouth and occasionally have voice changes.

The symptoms of OHL resemble the symptoms of thrush, though OHL is somewhat less common. Sometimes the first clue to a diagnosis of OHL is that the person does not respond to treatment for thrush. The best way to distinguish clearly between thrush and OHL is to look at tissue taken by biopsy under the microscope. Often the patch itself is sufficiently distinctive in appearance to make a biopsy unnecessary. Most people discover the patches themselves, when they examine their mouths.

There is little need for treatment except for pain, for interference with nutrition, or for voice changes. The usual treatment is HAART, but if that doesn't work, you can use acyclovir, taken by mouth. Occasionally other antiviral drugs like ganciclovir are also successful. The patches disappear within two or three weeks when treated, but like thrush, they recur when the medicine is discontinued.

Sores, Blisters, or Ulcers on the Lips or in the Mouth

Sores or blisters on the lips or in the mouth or throat are usually caused by one of two conditions. One is an infection by the virus herpes simplex; the other is a condition called aphthous ulcers, whose cause is unknown.

Herpes simplex.   The sores in the mouth called cold sores or fever blisters can be an infection caused by the herpes simplex virus. The sores usually start as an area of irritation or pain that becomes inflamed, then forms a watery blister that breaks and forms an open sore with pus, and finally scabs over and heals. The sores occur on the lips, in the mouth along the cheeks, on the roof of the mouth or palate, or on the back of the mouth. These sores are usually round or oval, measure about a quarter of an inch or less in diameter, and can have a characteristic red border. The sores of herpes can be very painful and often interfere with chewing; when in the back of the mouth or in the esophagus, the sores can interfere with swallowing.

Herpes simplex remains in the nerves serving the area of the mouth for the remainder of the person's life; it can be reactivated and cause new sores. The interval between outbreaks is unpredictable, but outbreaks are frequently associated with stress, exposure to sunlight, surgery, colds, menstrual periods, fever, and pneumonia. These associations explain the common name of these sores: cold sores or fever blisters.

Infections of the mouth from herpes simplex are extremely common: probably 50 percent of healthy Americans have had this infection at some time. Herpes simplex infections of the mouth are more frequent, more severe, last for longer periods and are harder to treat in people with advanced HIV infection.

The usual treatment is with acyclovir (Zovirax), famciclovir (Famvir), or valacyclovir (Valtrex) taken by mouth, or penciclovir applied to the sores. All treatments work best if taken early; often they're not taken at all because the benefit from them is so modest. If the herpes simplex infection is severe, however, it should be treated. Because herpes simplex infections tend to recur when treatment is discontinued, some people with repeated and severe attacks sometimes take one of the three drugs continuously to prevent recurrence. Like most other HIV complications, herpes simplex is less common and less severe when the CD4 count is high, so the best management is to control HIV.

Aphthous ulcers. Aphthous ulcers are open sores that may look like herpes simplex sores, occurring in the mouth, usually on the inside surface of the cheeks, on the gums, and on the tongue. Aphthous ulcers are usually very painful, especially when touched or when food or liquids pass over them. The pain can severely limit a person's desire to eat. Like thrush and herpes, the ulcers may extend to the esophagus and impair the ability to swallow. The ulcers can occur in people with or without HIV infection, but they are more common and severe in those with HIV infection. They can occur when the CD4 count is high.

Aphthous ulcers are often mistaken for herpes simplex infection, which they resemble. But laboratory tests of aphthous ulcers do not show any specific microbe, and the treatment for herpes simplex infection is unsuccessful in treating aphthous ulcers. The cause of these ulcers is not known. Aphthous ulcers are not transmitted to others. They may recur over a period of many years.

The usual treatment is to rinse the mouth with viscous lidocaine (2% concentration) or to take a combination of viscous lidocaine and benadryl by mouth. Both are available without prescription. Severe ulcers may require prescription drugs such as corticosteroids taken either as a pill or as a gel applied to the surface of the ulcer, or thalidomide in pill form. Aphthous ulcers in the esophagus are usually treated with corticosteroids or thalidomide and usually respond well. Thalidomide is effective but very hard to get because it is a major cause of birth defects in pregnant women.

Bluish or Purplish Bumps in the Mouth

Raised or thickened tissue that is bluish or purplish is a symptom of Kaposi's sarcoma (KS) in the mouth. Most people with KS in the mouth also have KS on the skin (see above, "Skin Problems"), though this is not invariably so. KS can appear anywhere in the mouth but most frequently appears on the roof, or hard palate. The tumors can cover a relatively small area or they can be spread over the entire palate. Common complications of KS in the mouth include pain, bleeding, or intrusion of the tumors onto the teeth causing tooth loss. In many cases, KS in the mouth causes few problems; it either remains stable for prolonged periods or simply grows very slowly.

In the absence of pain, bleeding, or intrusion of KS onto the teeth, there is little reason to treat the tumors. When treatment is appropriate, the KS tumors can be surgically removed if small, or treated with radiation, lasers, or chemotherapy using cancer drugs. Which treatment is used will depend on the location of KS tumors, the severity of the symptoms, and the bias of the physician. The person with KS obviously needs to agree to the treatment the physician recommends; agreement should be based on an explanation of the benefits, the costs, the convenience, and the side effects of various treatments.

Bleeding Gums

Bleeding gums are usually a symptom of gingivitis. *Gingiva* is the medical term for the gums, and *itis* means inflammation. Some people have severe bleeding of the gums, severe pain, and severe gingival disease with rapid tooth loss over a period as short as two or three months. This rapid loss of the structure that supports the teeth is called *periodontitis*.

The cause of gingivitis and periodontitis is not clearly established. Most dentists think the cause is the same bacteria normally present in the mouth, which have, for some reason, gone out of control. Like other conditions, gingivitis is also common in people without HIV infection, but it is more frequent and more severe in those with the infection. Care must be taken to distinguish gum bleeding caused by gingivitis from bleeding caused by the low numbers of blood platelets that are a part of ITP, which is an entirely different complication of HIV infection. The distinction between the two is easily made by a blood test that counts the number of platelets, or by consultation with a dentist, who will identify diseases of the teeth and gums.

For gingivitis and periodontitis, the treatment is usually mouthwashes containing germicides, such as chlorhexidine in a concentration of 0.12 percent (Peridex) or povidone-iodine (Betadine). Both can be purchased in most pharmacies; Peridex requires a prescription, and Betadine does not. For people who have extensive periodontitis, the dental procedure usually recommended is removal of plaque by planing and scaling, a procedure done by dentists. In many cases, antibiotic treatment with metronidazole (Flagyl) is also recommended. These treatments should be accompanied by rigorously doing what your dentist has always told you to do: use dental floss, brush regularly with a soft toothbrush, and see a dentist regularly.

Problems of the Digestive System

The digestive system includes the mouth; the tube through which food passes after being swallowed, called the esophagus; the stomach; the small intestine, where food is broken down and absorbed; the large intestine or colon, where unabsorbed material is stored for elimination; and the anus. The whole system, taken together, is responsible for digestion of food and elimination of waste. This section will discuss all parts of the digestive system except the mouth: the mouth, which is a common site of problems, has its own section, above.

HIV infection can affect any part of the digestive system, and does so commonly in the later stages. The symptoms are often a clue to which part of the digestive system is being affected. Painful or difficult swallowing is usually a symptom of problems with the esophagus. Pain in the abdomen, nausea, and vomiting are usually symptoms of problems with the stomach. Diarrhea, pain, and malnutrition from the failure to absorb nutrients are all symptoms of problems with the small intestine. And pain, diarrhea, or constipation are symptoms of problems with the colon.

Many of the problems in the digestive system also interfere with nutrition. Anything that interferes with nutrition is especially important to someone with HIV infection, because HIV infection itself causes weight loss and nutritional deficiencies. Severe malnutrition also seems to further weaken the immune system. Anyone with HIV infection and such problems with the digestive system should be under the care of a physician.

Loss of Appetite

Loss of appetite has several possible causes. One cause is usually the drugs taken for HIV, or HIV itself, which somehow causes an altered sense of taste: food just doesn't seem to taste good. Other causes are depression, complications, or infections of the mouth. Loss of appetite can substantially reduce the quality of life and, when severe, can cause weight loss and malnutrition.

Treatment depends on the exact cause. When the cause is the drugs taken for HIV, changing the regimen might be necessary. Tell your health care provider. Some drugs—AZT, ddI, and all the PIs—are particularly suspect. Taking AZT with food often helps you tolerate the drug better, but ddI needs to be taken on an empty stomach. Some PIs are better tolerated than others. Ritonavir, however, is a real problem and in fact is used not in full doses but in small doses to boost another PI; and even then, "baby dose ritonavir" can be a problem. When the cause is HIV and an altered sense of taste, the best treatment is to learn your preferences and eat accordingly. A person with an altered sense of taste often has a particular problem with protein-rich foods, particularly with red meat. The solution in that case is to find other sources of protein: poultry, fish, eggs, and cheese are all excellent sources of protein. So are dried beans and rice. A person with an altered sense of taste also seems to have the best appetite in the morning: try to eat large, nutritious breakfasts. If you have a preference for foods at different temperatures, indulge your preference. Try eating foods that smell good: the senses of smell and taste are closely connected. Try adding herbs, bacon, garlic, olives, cheese—anything that livens up the flavor of the food and doesn't disagree with you.

Some HIV-related complications of the mouth (thrush, herpes, aphthous ulcers, and Kaposi's sarcoma), discussed in the preceding section, cause pain with eating. When eating hurts, people often lose their appetites. In this case, avoid foods that cause pain. Stay away from salt and seasoned salts; from hot spices like pepper, chili pepper, and paprika; and from acidic foods like vinegar, citrus fruits and juices, tomatoes, pineapple, and pickles. Try food at moderate or cool temperatures. Try foods that are soft and won't irritate the mouth: mild cheeses, cottage cheese, yogurt, cooked eggs, cream soups, ice cream, puddings, popsicles, ground meats, baked fish, bread, noodles and pastas, and cooked or canned fruits (see also, below, the foods that are least troublesome if you have pain on swallowing).

Another cause of appetite loss is the emotional reaction to having HIV infection. At times, people become anxious or depressed and lose interest in eating. Both anxiety and depression can occur at any stage of this infection. One way to fight this might be to make eating a special event: put on some music, prepare the food so it looks attractive, think of a meal as a break from your worries or a reward for your work, relax, take your time with the meal. Eat your favorite foods unless you are on a special diet. If your HIV medication is a problem, tell your health care provider: there are twenty medications to pick from. Keep snacks around: ice cream, cheese, canned fruit, crackers, peanut butter. Small meals are less filling; try several small meals a day. Eating is often a social event, and many people enjoy food best in someone else's company.

Still another cause of loss of appetite is fatigue: people are simply too tired to eat. Fatigue can also interfere with their ability to prepare a meal if they live alone. If you eat less because you are tired, be careful to eat meals especially high in calories and proteins, so that even if you eat less, you get the same level of nutrition. Try milkshakes, dried fruits, peanut butter, ice cream, cheese, sour cream, hot chocolate, custard, cream soups, scrambled eggs or an omelet with cream cheese, noodles with cheese and cream. Preparing main courses that are high in protein and calories and then freezing them also saves energy: spaghetti sauce, chili, pot roasts, beef or chicken or lamb stews, and soups all taste good made in large amounts, frozen, and reheated; they freeze well. High-protein main courses are also sold prepared and frozen in grocery stores. In either case, frozen food can be reheated on the stove or in a microwave oven. Keep ready-to-eat and nutritious snacks on hand. Many communities also have organizations that will prepare or deliver meals.

In general, the treatment for appetite loss depends on the situation. If you have a sore mouth, get treatment for the sores. If drugs are responsible, you may need to take a "drug holiday," that is, to stop taking drugs for a while. This is safe with some drugs and not safe with others. With anti-HIV drugs, you need the full regimen—usually three or four drugs, all of which are unforgiving; that is, stopping one reduces the potency of the regimen. The best strategy is to substitute one drug to maintain the regimen's potency, or to stop all the drugs, or to try to make the regimen tolerable. Also remember that appetite loss has many causes, and the likelihood that a specific drug is responsible depends on the drug, the dose, and the length of time you've been taking it. It is unlikely that a drug you have taken for a month or more is suddenly causing appetite loss. If the drug is necessary, you might be able to take it instead with meals, or take another drug to reduce nausea. Ask your physician to help you work it out.

When appetite loss is temporary, try to get in as many calories as possible without regard to the nutritional value: you simply are not going to become malnourished in a few days. Try fortifying foods with oil, butter, mayonnaise, a little dried milk, grated cheese, cream. Try making shakes out of combinations of different foods: milk, ice cream, instant breakfast, buttermilk, bananas or strawberries or peaches or apricots or pears, fruit juice, yogurt, honey, cocoa, chocolate syrup, peach or pear or apricot nectars, ginger ale, brown sugar.

Most important is drinking enough fluids: healthy people can survive over one hundred days without food, but no one can survive more than a few days without fluid. Drink fluids that are high in calories and protein—milk, shakes—instead of diet drinks, coffee, or tea. Routinely stir some dried milk into your milk.

If people with HIV infection eat poorly for weeks or months, a physician should be consulted. In some cases, the physician may prescribe an appetite stimulant such as Megace. In extreme cases, the physician may use a feeding tube—a tube placed through the mouth and into the stomach, or through the abdomen and directly into the stomach—so nutrition is maintained despite the inability to eat. An alternative, discussed in a later section on wasting, is to feed people intravenously.

Painful Swallowing

Some people find eating unpleasant and good nutrition difficult because they have pain when they swallow. Sometimes the pain is in the back of the mouth; usually it is in the chest and is a result of esophagitis, an inflammation of the esophagus. The most common cause is infection with *Candida albicans,* the fungus responsible for thrush.

The probability of *Candida albicans* is often so great that physicians treat for *Candida* without testing for it. The treatment is usually fluconazole (Diflucan), taken by mouth. People usually respond well within five days. If *Candida* comes back after treatment is stopped, you may need to take fluconazole until your CD4 count comes back. If the person with esophagitis does not respond at all to this treatment and the cause is therefore obscure, an endoscopy—a special procedure in which a specialist (gastroenterologist) puts a tube into the esophagus and takes a sample of tissue—is often advised. If the cause is a viral infection, like CMV or herpes simplex, esophagitis can be treated with antiviral drugs. All these complications occur only when the CD4 count is low, below 200 and usually below 100. If the cause is aphthous ulcers, the ulcers in the esophagus, like those in the mouth, often respond to corticosteroids.

Anyone with painful swallowing should see a physician. Despite painful swallowing, it is important to maintain nutrition. Eat foods that are soft or liquid: milkshakes, milk, oatmeal, puddings made with milk or cream, custard, jello, ice cream, cottage cheese, cooked and pureed bland vegetables, popsicles, ground meats, baked fish, melons, bananas, scrambled eggs, omelets, French toast, cream soups, noodles, mashed potatoes. Try drinking through a straw. Such a diet, though easy on your throat, can cause loose stools; Metamucil and liquid supplements are sources of soluble fiber that can help prevent loose stools.

Nausea and Vomiting

Nausea and vomiting have a number of causes, the most common being the drugs taken for complications of HIV infection. Drugs whose side effects include nausea and vomiting are amphotericin B, atazanavir (Reyataz), atovaquone (Mepron), azithromycin (Zithromax), ciprofloxacin (Cipro), clarithromycin (Biaxin), trimethoprim-sulfamethoxazole (Bactrim, Septra), dapsone, ddI (Videx), doxycycline, dronabinol (Marinol), ethambutol (Myambutol), fluconazole (Diflucan), fosamprenavir, hydroxyurea (Hydrea), indinavir (Crixivan), inferferon (Roferon, Intron), itraconazole (Sporanox), ketoconazole (Nizoral), lopinavir (Kaletra), metronidazole (Flagyl), oxandrolone (Oxandrin), paromycin (Humatin), pyrazinamide, pyrimethamine (Daraprim), ritonavir (Norvir), saquinavir (Invirase), 3TC (Epivir), zidovudine (AZT, Retrovir).

The probability that a drug is responsible depends on the drug, the dose, and the length of time you've been taking it. If you've been taking a drug for over a month, it would be unusual for it to abruptly cause nausea and vomiting, unless the dose was increased. The treatment depends on the severity of the symptoms, the necessity of the drug, and the possibility of an alternative dosing regimen.

Usually the nausea and vomiting are dose-related, meaning that reducing the dose of the drug will reduce the nausea and vomiting. Or the drug can be taken at times that will not interfere with meals. Or, for many conditions, alternative drugs can be prescribed. Consultation with a physician will usually reveal which drug is likely to be the cause, which is expendable, which can be safely reduced in dose, and which can be safely substituted.

Some of the complicating infections—particularly infections that affect the head or the digestive system—can also cause nausea and vomiting. People who have nausea and vomiting, who are taking no medication, and who have additional symptoms such as fever or diarrhea should see their physicians.

In general, the person who has nausea or vomiting should eat small, frequent meals, and eat slowly. Avoid greasy, high-fat, and spicy foods. When symptoms are not severe, follow a soft and bland diet that is low in fat: rice, noodles, pasta, clear soups, jello, clear fruit juice, ginger ale, crackers, pretzels, tea, dry toast, oatmeal, boiled eggs. For breakfast, eat crackers, dry cereal, or dry toast. Cold meals that have little odor are often easier to eat than hot meals. When symptoms are severe, it is important to replace the liquids and electrolytes lost: try saltines, pretzels, clear fruit juices, ginger ale or colas, caffeine-free Gatorade, clear soups. All liquids should be clear—that is, they should not be thick liquids like vegetable juices, citrus juices, some other fruit juices, or milk. Drink them between meals rather than during meals.

Many drugs reduce nausea and vomiting. Some can be taken by suppository in the event that nothing is retained when taken by mouth. Such drugs should be timed to meals; take them as directed, but try taking the drug after eating meals. Some useful drugs do not require a prescription; these include Dramamine and Pepto-Bismol. Other drugs require a prescription: antihistamines (such as Phenergan or Vistaril) or phenothiazines (such as Compazine), which are drugs that also reduce anxiety. Most of these drugs cause drowsiness.

Diarrhea

Diarrhea is a relatively common complication of HIV infection. It can be acute, meaning that it begins suddenly and lasts for a short time, or it can be chronic, meaning that it persists for several weeks or months. Diarrhea has a number of causes. Many people have diarrhea simply as a result of anxiety. Some people have recurrent bouts of stomach pain and diarrhea, called *irritable bowel syndrome,* that go on for years without any identifiable cause and without complications or progression. Some people have diarrhea because of HIV itself. Some people have diarrhea because they do not have the enzyme called *lactase* that is necessary to digest a milk sugar called *lactose.* Some people with HIV infection who were once able to tolerate lactose become unable to tolerate it. In lactose intolerance, the diarrhea occurs after people eat food containing lactose, including milk, ice cream, cheese, instant coffee, chocolate, cream, cocoa, and cream fillings. Yogurt, however, is tolerated by some people who are otherwise lactose intolerant, and is worth trying because it is a good source of protein and calcium. Other symptoms of lactose intolerance are cramping and gas.

Another cause of diarrhea is the drugs commonly used by people with HIV infection. Among anti-HIV drugs, Kaletra and nelfinavir commonly cause a diarrhea that is usually controlled with loperamide (Imodium). Antibiotics often cause what is called nuisance diarrhea: a few loose stools most days, though they can also cause severe diarrhea accompanied by fever and cramps. The antibiotics that most commonly cause severe diarrhea are clindamycin, ampicillin, amoxicillin, amoxicillin-clavulanate (Augmentin), a group of drugs called cephalosporins, and another group called fluoroquinalones. Drugs that less commonly cause diarrhea are trimethoprim-sulfamethoxazole, erythromycin, penicillin, and the fluoroquinalones (ciprofloxacin, levofloxacin, gatifloxacin, and moxifloxacin). Any person who has severe diarrhea or diarrhea with fever while taking such drugs should discontinue the drug immediately and notify the physician. Less serious forms of diarrhea are often dose-related, that is, diarrhea can be reduced simply by reducing the amount of the antibiotic. Or the person can be prescribed another drug. Some drugs taken for HIV cause diarrhea, especially ddI, nelfinavir (Viracept) and lopinavir (Kaletra). In this case, diarrhea can often be managed by over-the-counter drugs like Imodium or calcium.

Diarrhea in people with HIV infection is also caused by infections of the digestive system, primarily infections of the small bowel and the colon. Infections are especially likely if the diarrhea is accompanied by a fever. Acute diarrhea can be caused by a number of microbes that are either easily treated with antibiotics, or that go away without treatment, or that progress to chronic diarrhea. Acute diarrhea is often due to food poisoning, viral infection, or anxiety, which are occasional problems for everyone, with or without HIV infection.

Infection is another common cause of diarrhea. Infection often causes a brief bout of gastroenteritis—or "food poisoning," or "travelers' diarrhea." Most of these cases of diarrhea come and go in a few days with so-called supportive care: bland food, plenty of water, and a drug like Imodium. In general, people with HIV infection get the same bouts of gastroenteritis as anyone else, and with the few exceptions noted below, no worse than anyone else. You should obtain medical attention promptly if you have severe diarrhea of such large volumes that you get dehydrated, if the stool has blood in it, or if you have severe abdominal pain. The possibility of an HIV-related complication increases when the CD4 count is below 200.

Perhaps the most common cause of chronic and often severe diarrhea in people with AIDS is *Cryptosporidium,* a parasite that is easily detected in a lab test of the stool. Infection occurs when *Cryptosporidium* is ingested, by contact with animals or with infected people, or most commonly by drinking contaminated water.

Anyone can get cryptosporidiosis diarrhea, but people with HIV infection seem unusually susceptible. For a person with a CD4 count of less than 50, the diarrhea can be devastating, with ten to twenty watery stools each day for months. Cryptosporidiosis in healthy people and in those with HIV and good CD4 counts will usually stop after one to two weeks. Cryptosporidiosis has no good treatment, except Imodium or even narcotics to control the diarrhea, fluids to maintain hydration, and nutritional support. Some people try paramomycin, a drug for cryptosporidiosis, but it doesn't work very well. The real key is the CD4 count: if the count is low, raising it even a small amount will often get the cryptosporidia under control.

Other common infectious causes of chronic diarrhea are a tiny parasite called *Microsporidium,* a virus called cytomegalovirus, and a bacterium called *Mycobacterium avium* complex (MAC). These latter microbes cause a diarrhea that persists for months and occurs only with late-stage AIDS, that is, a CD4 count of less than 50. Cytomegalovirus causes cramps and fever; the only treatment is intravenous ganciclovir or foscarnet, and it doesn't work well. MAC causes diarrhea and fever; it responds to clarithromycin plus ethambutol, though the response takes a long time. Microsporidiosis is caused by two types of parasites; one responds to albendazole and the other to fumagillin, but the best treatment is to boost the CD4 count. A substantial portion of the people with HIV infection have a chronic diarrhea for which their physicians can establish no clear cause.

Call your physician if the diarrhea is severe, or if it is accompanied by severe pains in the abdomen or by fever, or if it persists. Chronic diarrhea is more common late in the course of the infection when the CD4 cell count is low, and is often accompanied by severe weight loss and malnutrition, sometimes referred to as "wasting syndrome."

The first consideration is to see if diarrhea is being caused by drugs. If drugs are not the cause, the first test to diagnose other causes of severe or chronic diarrhea should be an analysis of the stool for infectious microbes. If no microbes are found, and if the symptoms are severe, it is often recommended that the digestive system be examined directly with an instrument called an endoscope. An endoscope is a long tube that can be passed through the mouth to look at the top part of the gastrointestinal tract—the esophagus, the stomach, and the small intestine —or passed through the rectum to look at the colon. The physician who performs the test is a gastroenterologist, a specialist in digestive diseases. Endoscopy permits not only a direct view of the wall of the intestine, but also removal of a small piece of tissue (a biopsy) of any area that appears abnormal. The tissue can then be examined under the microscope to identify the nature of the problem. A number of X-ray procedures also allow a look at the intestine. The person should be forewarned that these types of specialized tests tend to be unpleasant and expensive.

The treatment of diarrhea depends largely on the severity and cause. When drugs are responsible, a physician will reduce the dose or—if the drug is not critical or if a substitute is easily available—will discontinue the drug. Regardless of the cause, it is important, first, to drink enough fluids and, second, to eat enough food. The usual recommendation is to eat small, frequent meals and to drink fluids between meals. Avoid insoluble fiber: seeds, brans, nuts, whole wheat bread, the skins of fruits and vegetables. Avoid anything that causes gas: carbonated drinks, beans, cabbage, spicy foods, gum. Avoid fats, milk, cheese, ice cream. Since caffeine is a bowel stimulant, avoid coffee, tea, colas and some sodas, hot chocolate, and chocolate.

Soluble fiber, like pectin, counters diarrhea: oatmeal, jello, apples, bananas, mangoes, melons, fruit nectars, and cooked and skinned fruits and vegetables are sources of soluble fiber. Try white bread, white rice, noodles, and pastas. Drink plenty of liquids: water, clear fruit juices, clear soups, broth, ginger ale and caffeine-free colas (stir out the bubbles). Dietitians call such a diet a BRATT diet: bananas, rice, applesauce, tea (caffeine-free), and toast. The BRATT diet, though helpful in controlling acute diarrhea, lacks many nutrients and should not be continued for more than a week. In addition, avoid drinking fluids during meals; fluids should be taken between meals. As with nausea and vomiting, it is important to replace lost electrolytes: try saltines, pretzels, clear fruit juices, Gatorade, ginger ale or caffeine-free colas, potatoes, bananas, clear soups. When diarrhea is unrelated to eating, there may be an advantage to adding foods containing soluble fiber—as listed above—in an effort to add bulk to the diet.

With severe diarrhea, when malnutrition becomes a worry, supplement the diet with special high-nutrient fluids such as Ensure, Ensure Plus, Jevity, Peptamen, or Perative. High-nutrient fluids, which can be obtained in grocery stores and pharmacies, provide a rich source of calories and protein. These supplements are commonly recommended for wasting, but some—Ensure Plus and Peptamen—actually cause diarrhea and should be diluted before using. All of these dietary decisions are best made with the advice of a physician and a dietitian.

Drugs may also be used to reduce diarrhea. Some treatments that reduce diarrhea are available without prescription: Donnagel, Kaopectate, Lactinex, Pepto-Bismol, loperamide (Imodium), oat bran, psyllium, calcium, SP-303, and the like. All of these seem to work some of the time, and most cost less than $10 a month. If the diarrhea is caused by a microbe, your physician will prescribe drugs to eradicate the microbe, if it can be treated; the specific treatment will depend on the microbe found. As noted, however, many microbes do not respond to antibiotics, and sometimes no microbial cause is found. In these cases, diarrhea is often treated with prescription drugs—including diphenoxylate (Lomotil), tincture of opium, and paregoric—that quiet the motion of the muscles of the intestines. Diarrhea due to nelfinavir (Viracept) or lopinavir (Kaletra) is so common that it is expected. Most cases are not severe enough to require discontinuing the drug, and reducing the dose is unacceptable.

Most cases can be controlled by over-the-counter drugs, like those listed above.

Gynecological Problems

The gynecological problems that women with HIV infection get are the same that all women get. But certain problems are more common or more severe in women with HIV infection: vaginal yeast infections, genital herpes (discussed above), and cervical cancer.

Cervical Cancer

Cervical cancer, which has no symptoms in the early stages, is a concern in women with HIV infection, although the risk is increased only slightly over those without HIV. Cervical cancer is associated with infection by a virus called the human papillomavirus, or HPV. HPV also causes warts in the genital region. But the HPV that causes genital warts—easily seen as fleshy growths—and the HPV that is associated with cervical cancer are different strains of HPV; the HPV that causes visible warts does not cause cancer, and vice versa. Cervical cancer is detected by Pap smears. Pap smears turn out to have abnormal results more frequently in women with HIV infection than in those without. As a result, it is now recommended that women with HIV infection have Pap smears at their initial medical evaluation, then six months later, then every year thereafter. Those with abnormal Pap smears should have a referral to a gynecologist.

Vaginal Discharge, Severe Genital Itching

A discharge that often resembles cottage cheese and severe genital itching are symptoms of vaginal yeast infections. A yeast infection is a complication caused by the same fungus, *Candida albicans,* that causes thrush.

Vaginal yeast infections are common in all women: 50 percent of all women without HIV infection have vaginal yeast infections at some time. In women with HIV infection, vaginal yeast infections are more frequent, more severe, and less likely to clear up with treatment. Yeast infections occur at a relatively early stage of HIV infection, often when the CD4 cell count is over 500; but they become more severe and harder to treat when the CD4 count is low. In addition, women with low CD4 counts often need to take antibiotics, like Bactrim, for other complications, but these antibiotics make vaginal yeast infections more common and more severe. Women therefore need to make a trade-off: antibiotics versus a high rate of yeast infections, including both thrush and vaginitis.

The usual treatment is a cream applied locally to the vagina, like Gyne-Lotrimin. These creams are available at drugstores without prescription. Women with more advanced stages of HIV infection are likely to find that local creams do not work very well, or that the yeast infection may recur rapidly when treatments are discontinued. Management of this problem will often require consulting a gynecologist who might prescribe such drugs as fluconazole or itraconazole by mouth.

Vaginal Discharge, Pelvic Pain, Painful Sexual Intercourse

Vaginal discharge, pelvic pain, and painful sexual intercourse are symptoms of pelvic inflammatory disease, or PID. PID is an infection of the upper part of the genital tract: the uterus, fallopian tubes, and ovaries. The usual causes are sexually transmitted microbes like gonococcus and chlamydia. In its later stages, PID can lead to infertility, high rates of ectopic pregnancies, and chronic abdominal pain. PID may occur in women who do not have HIV infection as well as in those who do, but women with HIV infection appear to have PID more frequently, and in them it is more difficult to treat successfully. The diagnosis and treatment require evaluation by a physician, including a pelvic examination and prescription drugs. The standard drugs, antibiotics, are highly effective in the short run but may not prevent the infertility and pain of the later stages of PID. Because of this, many physicians recommend that women with HIV infection and PID be hospitalized for treatment of PID.

Eye Problems

People with HIV infection do not usually have problems with their eyes, and when they do, the problems are often the usual ones that accompany the aging process. But there are some eye problems that indicate serious complications, and a physician must be notified. The most common and serious is cytomegalovirus retinitis.

Blurred Vision

Blurred vision, along with several other symptoms and a low CD4 cell count, may indicate an infection of the eye called *cytomegalovirus (CMV) retinitis*. In addition to blurred vision, symptoms of CMV retinitis can include a blind spot, pain in the eye, and "floaters." Floaters are spots that float across the line of vision as a result of inflamed cells in the middle of the eye. In many instances the person with CMV retinitis notices no symptoms at all.

In this case, CMV has infected the retina, the layer of cells in the back of the eye that, like the film of a camera, is responsible for recording images. The specific symptoms a person has will depend on which area of the retina is affected. CMV retinitis used to occur in 20 to 30 percent of people with HIV infection, but with HAART, the number of cases has decreased by 80 percent. CMV retinitis is now quite infrequent; it virtually never occurs when the CD4 cell count is over 100 and usually occurs when it is less than 50. For people with CD4 counts below 50, many physicians recommend a routine ophthalmologic examination at six-month intervals.

CMV retinitis can occur in one eye or in both eyes. If the infection in one eye is left untreated, it will often affect the other eye as well. If both eyes are infected and left untreated, the usual result is blindness. Loss of sight caused by cytomegalovirus cannot be corrected with glasses.

With early treatment, vision can usually be saved before blindness occurs. Options for treatment are now extensive. They include a drug, ganciclovir, which can be taken by mouth (Valcyte), by vein (Cytovene), or by a device (Vitrasert) that is implanted in the eye by an ophthalmologist and that slowly releases ganciclovir for six months. All options will temporarily stop or slow the progression of the retinitis; that is, the retinitis will get no worse. None, however, will reverse the damage already done.

Treatment is continued until people take HAART and have a rebound in their CD4 cell counts; the reconstituted immune system protects against progression of CMV retinitis. But treatment will need to start again if the CD4 count goes below 100.

CMV retinitis is now a disappearing disease. Essentially all of the infectious disease–complications of HIV are decreasing in frequency because of HAART, but CMV retinitis has decreased more than any of the others.

Head and Nerve Problems

The nervous system has two parts: the central nervous system and the peripheral nervous system. The central nervous system is made up of the brain, where thinking takes place, and the spinal cord, which is a bundle of nerves that carries directions from and to the brain. The peripheral nervous system is composed of the nerves throughout the body that bring sensory messages to the brain and deliver commands to the muscles. About half of all people with HIV infection develop problems with the nervous system, either the central nervous system or the peripheral nervous system.

The central nervous system—primarily the brain—is somewhat more likely to be affected than the peripheral nervous system, either by HIV itself or by a medical complication. The most common symptoms of central nervous system involvement are (1) mental slowing, with memory loss, personality changes, and impaired concentration; (2) seizures; (3) weakness or paralysis; (4) poor coordination; and (5) headache that is often severe or different from the usual headache. All of these symptoms suggest infection in the brain or meninges (the membrane surrounding the brain) and require medical treatment. In many instances, the person with these symptoms will be referred to a neurologist, a specialist in diseases of the nervous system.

The most frequent and serious diseases of the central nervous system in the era of HAART are complications associated with a weakened immune system, and an infection caused by HIV itself, called HIV-associated dementia. The most common of the complications are toxoplasma encephalitis and cryptococcal meningitis; less common are lymphomas of the brain, Kaposi's sarcoma, cytomegalovirus, progressive multifocal leukoencephalopathy, *Mycobacterium avium* complex, tuberculosis, and the herpes viruses.

All these diseases cause similar symptoms and most occur when the CD4 cell count is less than 200. Diagnosis, therefore, requires special tests. The tests usually done begin with a neurologic examination that includes a physical examination of the nervous system to determine coordination, strength, sensations, reflexes, and mental functioning. An important laboratory test is a lumbar puncture, also called a spinal tap. The lumbar puncture is done to obtain a sample of the cerebrospinal fluid that surrounds the spinal cord and brain; the fluid is then examined for any inflammatory cells or microbes that will provide clues to the diagnosis.

Other major laboratory tests are computerized tomography (CT scan) and magnetic resonance imaging (MRI) of the brain. Both tests are methods of viewing the brain in three dimensions to look for specific changes. These changes indicate the location of the problem and its probable cause. Diagnosis of central nervous system problems, then, is based on the symptoms, the results of a neurologic examination, the results of examination of the cerebrospinal fluid, and any changes in the images of the brain.

Many diseases of the central nervous system can be treated successfully, especially early in the course of the disease. Many of the symptoms suggesting central nervous system infections, however, occur even when there is no problem in the central nervous system at all. Weakness, seizures, and mental changes, for instance, can be caused by medications, changes in the balance of electrolytes in the blood, and fever caused by some other infection. Particularly difficult to sort out are headaches: 90 percent of all people, with or without HIV infection, have periodic headaches.

The final part of this section on head and nerve problems will discuss the problems HIV infection causes with the peripheral nervous system.

Headaches

Headaches are extremely common. In most cases, headaches bother the person who has them far more than they bother the physician who treats them. This is because headaches rarely indicate severe or progressive disease. Most headaches occur when the muscles that cover the top of the skull contract; these headaches are called tension headaches. A less common but more painful type of headache, called a migraine or a cluster headache, results when the arteries of the scalp contract. Another common cause of headaches is a generalized illness such as influenza or infections in the sinuses or ears. Sinus headaches are somewhat more common in people with HIV infection, who frequently have sinusitis.

Certain headaches, however, require a doctor's attention. Like other focal neurologic symptoms and like fever and stiff neck (see below), headaches can be a symptom of an infection of the brain or the meninges. Headaches associated with infections of the brain or meninges have one or more of the following characteristics:

1. They are unusually severe or last unusually long.

2. Either the character of the pain or the location of pain makes the headache different from headaches the person usually has.

3. They occur along with problems with vision.

4. They occur along with weakness of an arm or leg, with dizziness, or with impaired coordination.

5. They occur along with stiff neck, nausea and vomiting, or extreme lethargy or sleepiness.

6. They are severe and occur along with an unexplained fever.

The major infections that cause such headaches in people with advanced HIV infection are toxoplasma encephalitis and cryptococcal meningitis. Both of these infections, as well as a multitude of other infections of the brain and meninges, occur only in the late stages of HIV infection and are relatively easy to diagnose. They are also treatable. A less common cause of headaches in people with HIV infection is lymphoma.

Toxoplasma encephalitis. The symptoms of toxoplasma encephalitis include headache, fever, confusion, personality changes, and what physicians call focal neurologic symptoms that occur generally with a problem in a specific part of the brain: paralysis or weakness on one side of the body, loss of speech, loss of coordination, and certain kinds of seizures.

Toxoplasma encephalitis is caused by a parasite, *Toxoplasma gondii,* which is commonly found in cat stool and in inadequately cooked meat. After infection, the parasite remains—generally dormant—in the human body for life. In fact, 10 to 30 percent of all adults in the United States have blood tests positive for antibodies to *Toxoplasma gondii.* The parasite causes severe disease primarily in people with a CD4 count less than 100.

Toxoplasma encephalitis can be diagnosed with a blood test that detects antibodies to *Toxoplasma gondii,* combined with a CT scan or MRI scan for imaging the brain. Either scan will show a characteristic pattern of inflammation in the brain.

The standard treatment for toxoplasma encephalitis is an antibiotic, pyrimethamine, taken in combination with other antibiotics, either sulfonamides or clindamycin. These drugs are given initially by vein and then by mouth in relatively high doses. Most people improve within one week; brain scans two weeks after treatment generally show reduction in the size of the area of inflammation. People usually respond to treatment impressively, but toxoplasmosis is likely to recur when treatment is discontinued, so treatment is continued until the CD4 count comes back up.

To prevent toxoplasma encephalitis in people whose CD4 counts are below 100, the common recommendations are to take Bactrim, or a combination of dapsone and pyrimethamine, to prevent toxoplasmosis.

Lymphoma. Another common cause of focal neurologic problems in people with HIV infection is lymphoma, a tumor of lymph cells. Almost any part of the body can be affected by lymphoma, but the brain is one of the parts most commonly affected. Lymphoma is often suspected if treatment for suspected toxoplasma encephalitis is ineffective. Treatment is with radiation and the chemotherapy drugs used to treat cancers. Most people improve, but the improvement is temporary. (See also below, under "Problems Affecting the Whole Body.")

Cryptococcal meningitis. Meningitis means inflammation (itis) of the meninges, the fibrous membrane that surrounds the brain and spinal cord. The symptoms of meningitis are usually severe headache, fever, and stiff neck; other symptoms can include seizures and double vision.

Cryptococcal meningitis is caused by a fungus called *Cryptococcus neoformans,* which is found throughout the world and is transmitted when the fungus is inhaled. The infection itself cannot be transmitted from one person to another.

Cryptococcus usually causes either a trivial disease or no disease at all until the CD4 cell count is less than 100 and the immune system is weakened. *Cryptococcus neoformans* is the most common cause of meningitis in people with AIDS. The infection may develop in several different places in the body; it is most damaging and most common in the brain. Cryptococcal meningitis is both serious and treatable, so it is important to make the diagnosis. The test for cryptococcal meningitis is a blood test and a spinal tap. A spinal tap is done so that a sample of the cerebrospinal fluid can be examined for evidence of inflammation and for *Cryptococcus.* For people with a severe headache, a spinal tap will often reduce the pressure and immediately relieve the pain. This is one of the rare cases in which people will beg for a spinal tap.

Treatment usually consists of the antibiotic amphotericin B (given by vein), followed by fluconazole (given by mouth). Treatment is usually successful, but the infection tends to recur when treatment is discontinued. Fluconazole by mouth is continued until the CD4 count rebounds from HAART.

Slowed Mental Processes or Dementia

Slowed mental processes, including forgetfulness, loss of recent memory (that is, the person can remember childhood experiences, but not the morning's events), and difficulty concentrating, can be symptoms of HIV-associated dementia (HAD). HAD, which used to be called AIDS dementia complex, is a mental deterioration that accompanies HIV infection. Other symptoms are irritability, social withdrawal, and apathy. Occasional symptoms are weakness in the legs or arms, tremor, poor coordination, incontinence, and loss of balance. The onset of these symptoms can be either gradual or abrupt.

The progress of HAD often follows a certain pattern. At first, mental slowing is noticed, either by caregivers or people with HIV infection themselves: a comment might be that they are less sharp, or they are not as quick, or their thinking is cloudier. They take longer to organize their thoughts, to respond to questions. This doesn't happen all at once: some days they are slower, and other days they're clear and sharp. Later, mental slowing progresses and can be accompanied by apathy and withdrawal. Most people with HAD eventually have problems controlling their muscles. They walk unsteadily, and they trip or fall easily; their legs are often weak. Their coordination is reduced, and they have problems with eating and writing. Eventually, they may become totally withdrawn. HAD is different for different people. Some people with dementia experience a mild mental slowing that never becomes more serious; for these people, dementia has only a small impact on their lives. For others, dementia progresses rapidly and mental impairment is severe.

During the pre-HAART era, HAD occurred in 20 to 30 percent of people with HIV infection. With HAART, that percentage is lower, though it hasn't decreased as much as the other HIV-related complications have. The reason for this difference is not clear, but it could possibly be that to HIV, the brain and the rest of the body are two separate things. That is, in the body apart from the brain, HAART kills off HIV and reconstitutes the immune system; but in the brain, HAART has less effect on HIV and immune function. Part of the problem in sorting this puzzle out is that no one understands the cause of HAD. Evidence suggests that the cause might be HIV in the brain: the cerebrospinal fluid that bathes the brain often shows evidence of HIV early in the course of the infection, before the person shows any symptoms.

A person with the symptoms of HAD should be examined and tested to exclude the possibility that the symptoms are caused by depression or by an infection of the central nervous system. Diagnosis of dementia will often be made by specialists: neurologists or AIDS physicians. The tests for dementia include a series of tests of mental abilities, a neurological examination, a spinal tap, and a brain scan. The purpose of the tests is to find out what the person can and cannot do mentally, to determine the severity of the dementia, and to exclude other causes—like cryptococcal meningitis, toxoplasmosis, or lymphoma of the brain—that could be causing the same symptoms.

So far, we have little in the way of treatment for HAD. Some medical researchers think what's most important is a drug's ability to get into the brain: drugs often cannot get into the brain, and the brain may serve as a sort of isolated harbor for HIV. In any case, the most important part of treating HAD is to select the HAART drugs that get into the brain especially well. AZT, abacavir (Ziagen), indinavir (Crixivan), nevirapine (Viramune), and efavirenz (Sustiva) get into the brain better than most other drugs.

A note of caution: For reasons medical scientists do not yet understand, most drugs that act on the central nervous system, including drugs for sleep, antidepressant drugs, and anti-anxiety drugs, have a greater-than-usual effect on people with dementia. These include alcohol and all benzodiazepines: Valium, Librium, Xanax, and Ativan. Physicians must be made aware of the diagnosis of HAD so they can prescribe and monitor drugs carefully.

People with a confirmed diagnosis of HAD need appropriate medical care for this and other aspects of HIV infection, need support in their living arrangements, and need to do some long-term planning. They need to start considering some difficult decisions. Some of these decisions include signing a durable power of attorney, writing a will, and writing a living will and a medical order not to resuscitate (see chapter 9). Another decision is when to stop driving a car. Clues that it may be time to stop include these: they feel that their motor abilities or reaction times are impaired, they notice people blowing horns, they start getting traffic tickets, they sometimes forget where they are, or they are worried about hurting others when they're behind the wheel. They must also decide when to stop work, especially if they think they are doing sloppy work or can't work as well as they used to or can't remember what they need to. Quitting work or not driving does not automatically mean that a person is dependent and useless, or that life can't be enjoyable.

One of the biggest questions that people with HIV infection and their caregivers need to answer is how long HAART will be useful. HAART can clearly delay or prevent the onset of HAD, and the drugs can sometimes reverse the changes, especially when the regimen is started in the early stages of HAD. But when HAD becomes advanced and the person is no longer responding, then it is appropriate to consider discontinuing HAART, which is, after all, difficult to administer and substantially toxic. In this case, HAART may reduce the quality of life without providing any perceived benefit. The decision to stop HAART in such cases is complex.

Numbness, Tingling, or Pain in the Feet

The symptoms listed so far in this section on head and nerve problems have dealt with problems in the central nervous system. People with HIV infection also have symptoms of problems in the peripheral nervous system, the network of nerves throughout the body that bring sensory messages to the brain and deliver commands to the muscles. The most common symptoms are numbness, tingling, or pain in the feet. The symptoms may worsen to the point where wearing shoes becomes intolerable and walking becomes impossible.

These symptoms are called *painful sensory neuropathy*, that is, painful sensations due to damaged nerves (neuropathy). Painful sensory neuropathy in people with HIV infection is usually caused either by HIV itself or by one of two anti-HIV drugs, ddI (didanosine, Videx) or d4T (stavudine, Zerit). These drugs must be stopped promptly when these symptoms occur, since continued use will cause progression of the symptoms to the point of irreversibility. Report the symptoms of painful sensory neuropathy to your physician to determine the cause and to begin treatment. Other drugs that produce the same or similar symptoms are metronidazole (Flagyl), cisplatin, disulfiram, INH, phenytoin (Dilantin), and vincristine. The symptoms can also be caused by diabetes and alcoholism.

Treatment is mainly to relieve pain. If the symptoms are severe, you may have to stop wearing shoes or wear only soft slippers. If blankets and sheets cause pain, build a sort of bridge at the foot of the bed that lifts up the blankets and sheets. Nonprescription drugs that may help include aspirin, acetaminophen, and ibuprofen. In some cases, a physician will prescribe narcotics or drugs called *tricyclic antidepressants*, such as amitriptyline (Elavil) or nortriptyline (Pamelor). Side effects of the drugs include drowsiness, so these drugs are best taken at night. Some creams, like HEET or those like Zostrix that contain capsaicin, also relieve the symptoms, though some people complain that they also cause burning pain. HEET requires no prescription.

Problems Affecting the Whole Body

Symptoms that affect the whole body, or constitution, are called *constitutional symptoms*. Constitutional symptoms are the vague, general symptoms that often accompany chronic illnesses. Included are weight loss, chronic weakness, diarrhea, night sweats, fever, lethargy, malaise, and fatigue. All these symptoms are relatively common both in the general population and in people with HIV infection. Some of these symptoms—fatigue, lethargy, malaise—are subjective and difficult to measure. Others—fever, severe weight loss (wasting)—are more objective. These symptoms can be considered the constitutional symptoms of HIV infection only when they have been present for at least one month.

People with HIV infection tend not to have constitutional symptoms until the CD4 count is below 200, unless they are also depressed or have some unrelated medical problem like influenza. In people with HIV infection, the distinguishing feature of all of these constitutional symptoms is that they are chronic; that is, they don't go away. Any of these symptoms may also be caused by certain complications. Because some of these complications are treatable, when these symptoms develop, see a physician.

Three of these constitutional symptoms—fatigue, fever, and wasting—deserve additional discussion.

Fatigue

Fatigue is an especially common constitutional symptom. Its severity is often profound and its causes are diverse. Likely explanations are infections, depression, anemia (low red blood cell count), and HIV-associated dementia. Many cases of fatigue, however, have no clear cause and can be blamed on HIV infection itself. This is true only when the CD4 cell count is low. Fatigue from HIV infection is uncommon and not severe when the CD4 count is over 200; it is common and rarely severe when the CD4 count is between 50 and 200; and it is common and often severe when the CD4 count is below 50.

HIV infection causes fatigue partly because it deprives the body of some of its sources of energy. People with HIV infection often have anemia, or lower numbers of red blood cells. Red blood cells, among other things, carry oxygen; oxygen supplies the muscles with energy. People with fewer red blood cells therefore have less energy and tire easily, though the anemia must be severe before people notice symptoms.

In addition, people with HIV infection and fatigue sometimes experience severe weight loss, referred to as "wasting," because they're not taking in enough calories. Some of the weight loss of wasting may result from the loss of muscle protein, called protein-calorie malnutrition, and some wasting may be the result of the direct action of cytokines, proteins that regulate the immune system (see below, "Weight Loss or Wasting"). For some people, fatigue is caused by chronic serious infections like MAC or CMV.

Medications can also cause fatigue or sleepiness, which is often interpreted as fatigue. These medications include, among others, narcotics, antihistamines, and antidepressants. AZT may cause fatigue. Fatigue accompanied by nausea, vomiting, and stomach pain may come from lactic acidosis, a potentially serious side effect of the nucleoside drugs like AZT, ddI, and d4T. This can occur after months or years of taking these drugs, and the CD4 count may be high or low.

Fatigue is also an indirect result of HIV infection. In this case, it may be accompanied by weight loss, fever, and night sweats. These symptoms are most likely to occur relatively late in the course of the infection when the CD4 count is low in people who either do not take HAART, or who take it and don't respond.

A medical evaluation can help sort out the cause of fatigue. A simple blood count will show if the cause is anemia. Blood tests will indicate if the cause is lactic acidosis due to AZT, ddI, or d4T; lactic acidosis is extremely important to recognize because it can be lethal. Such symptoms as fever, cough, and diarrhea often accompany HIV infection's complications. Most causes are treatable.

For more on dealing with fatigue, see chapter 4, "HIV Infection and Its Effects on the Emotions," under "Fatigue and Accommodation."

Fever

Fever, like other constitutional symptoms, is common; it can be caused by a complication of HIV infection, or it can simply be due to HIV.

Most people with fever are aware of it. Rapid rises in body temperature are commonly preceded by chills. Chills are an indication of the body's attempt to retain heat by constricting the blood vessels of the skin where heat is given off. People with fever cannot tolerate the usual range of heat and cold that most people consider normal room temperature. Along with fever, some people also have "night sweats," sweating at night that can be severe enough to require changes in bed clothing. In people with HIV infection, fevers often begin gradually, occurring off and on for extended periods of weeks or months.

Temperature is measured on two scales: the Fahrenheit, or F scale, commonly used in the United States, and the centigrade, or C scale, used in the rest of the world and in some hospitals in the United States. A temperature of 98.6 degrees F corresponds to 37 degrees C; 99.6 degrees F corresponds to 37.5 degrees C.

The average temperature is 97 degrees F at 3:00 A.M. and 99.3 degrees F at 5:00 P.M. In general, temperatures are about two degrees higher (on the Fahrenheit scale) in the late afternoon than they are in the morning. This daily fluctuation in temperature is exaggerated during fever. For this reason, people with HIV infection who think they have fever should take their temperatures several times during the day, when they feel feverish, and in the late afternoon.

Physicians always want to know when a person with HIV infection has a fever: fever is an objective indication of a problem that is not just a day-to-day variation in health status. Prolonged fever accompanied by chills in people with low CD4 counts indicate the presence of some infection other than HIV. If you have such a fever, see a physician; at least 80 percent of fevers in people with HIV infection occur with an infection that can be diagnosed and treated. Fever with a low white blood count (neutropenia) or a line inserted in a vein for receiving intravenous antibiotics can indicate a serious bacterial infection that requires immediate medical attention.

In people in the late stages of HIV infection, the conditions that are most likely to cause persistent fever are tuberculosis, *Mycobacterium avium* complex infection, cytomegalovirus infection, fungal infection, pneumocystis pneumonia, toxoplasmosis, cryptococcosis, and pneumonia. In people with CD4 counts over 200, the common causes of fever are the same conditions that cause fever in anyone—flu, pneumonia, or gastroenteritis. Drugs may also cause fever. Nearly all drugs may do this, but those that do it most commonly are sulfa drugs like trimethoprim-sulfamethoxazole (Bactrim or Septra) and dapsone. Other drugs that can cause fever include amphotericin B, phenytoin (Dilantin), barbiturates, thalidomide, pentamidine, clindamycin, and penicillin. One drug, aba-cavir (Ziagen) may cause fever that is especially important to recognize because it may be a particularly serious side effect requiring discontinu-ance and careful avoidance in the future. When a drug causes fever, the fever is almost always accompanied by a rash: exceptions are ampho-tericin B and pentamidine. The best way to tell if the drug is the cause is to stop suspected drugs and see if the fever disappears, which usually oc-curs within 24 to 48 hours.

Fever is basically treated by treating whatever is causing it. Treating fever itself is a little controversial. Fever actually has advantages: the im-mune system works better at higher temperatures, and fever is an im-portant indicator of the course of the disease and of the effectiveness of treatment. But fever is also unpleasant for the person who has it and in-creases the metabolic rate, burning more calories and making good nutrition more difficult. Otherwise, there is little evidence that fever is harmful.

When the decision is made to reduce fever, the usual drugs are as-pirin, acetaminophen, or ibuprofen. Acetaminophen carries on the label a warning that it causes liver or kidney damage; although the probabil-ity of this is low, it might be best to limit the amount of acetaminophen you take. The maximum adult dose is 0.6 to 0.9 mg (usually two or three pills) taken every four to six hours. The fever decreases or disappears when people take one of these drugs, but returns when the effect of the drug wears off. For people with persistent fever, these fluctuations in temperature can be more unpleasant than a steady, if high, temperature. For this reason, people with persistent fevers are often advised to take these drugs regularly, every four to six hours, without waiting for the fever to recur.

Weight Loss or Wasting

Wasting is the somewhat unfortunate term given to unintentional loss of 10 percent of the body weight, with no explanation other than HIV in-fection. Wasting once accounted for 20 percent of AIDS diagnoses, but now in the HAART era, it is rare. In general, wasting is seen only in the late stages of HIV infection, in people whose CD4 counts are less than 100 and whose response to HAART is poor. The exceptions to this are wasting due to depression, medications, health conditions unrelated to HIV infection, or early complications of HIV infection like TB or lymphoma. Wasting accompanied by a 25 to 30 percent loss of body weight is considered a medical emergency requiring immediate evaluation and treatment.

Wasting results from one of two problems: inadequate nutrition or metabolic changes. Inadequate nutrition simply means starvation: the body does not get enough nutrients because the person is not eating enough nutrients or is losing too many nutrients. The cause might be loss of appetite, depression, sores in the mouth or esophagus, loss of the sense of taste, or the side effects of drugs. Some people lose weight because of vomiting or severe diarrhea: the food goes through the digestive system without being absorbed.

Metabolic changes can be caused by fever, by an imbalance in hormones called *cytokines,* by any active complication, and by HIV infection itself. All increase the body's metabolic rate: the motor runs more quickly and calories are burned at a faster clip. For instance, fever increases the rate at which the body metabolizes food by 7 percent for each degree F. So a person with a temperature of 103 degrees F through the day will increase the calories needed by 30 percent. People with increased metabolic rates may eat voraciously and still lose weight. The average 160-pound man requires 1,700 to 2,100 kilocalories to maintain basal metabolism, but a person with untreated HIV infection requires 2,700 to 3,600. People with HIV infection consequently need to eat more.

Many men with HIV infection, especially in the late stages, produce low amounts of testosterone, which can cause fatigue, loss of libido, and wasting. The test is a measurement of the level of testosterone in the blood. The treatment is the hormone, given as an injection, a skin patch, a pill, or an ointment.

The weight loss associated with wasting is different from the weight loss that accompanies dieting. People who are dieting lose fat but preserve muscle and protein. People who have wasting lose muscle protein—a condition known in medicine as protein-calorie malnutrition. For many people, the weight loss is a stair-step phenomenon—an infection with weight lost, then control of the infection with weight stabilized at a lower level, then another infection with weight lost, and the same process over again.

People with uncontrolled HIV infection often worry about wasting, and want advice on preventing it. The best ways are to control HIV with antiretroviral therapy, use the appropriate preventive antibiotics when the CD4 cell count is low, and take in enough calories. Beyond that, we don't know how to prevent wasting. The usual advice is to do what is most logical to preserve muscle protein: eat a balanced diet with adequate amounts of protein, and exercise moderately to maintain or build muscles. Foods that contain protein include meat, fish, poultry, eggs, nuts, and peanut butter. The preferred exercises are activities that both build endurance and maintain muscle: walking, jogging, swimming, or bicycling. Strenuous exercise, like Olympic-type training or marathons, is unnecessary and may even harm the immune defenses. Resistance exercise—weight-lifting exercises that require you to resist the pull of gravity—for 20 minutes three or four times a week will maintain strength and preserve or increase weight.

Otherwise, the treatment of wasting depends on the cause: no single treatment is universally effective. Loss of appetite may be treated with drugs like Megace or Marinol; much of the weight added with these drugs, however, is simply fat, and not protein. Cytokine imbalance requires drugs like growth hormone or thalidomide; growth hormone costs over $200 a day and thalidomide is hard to get. Depression requires antidepressive drugs, which are usually effective. Men with wasting often have low testosterone levels and benefit from treatment with testosterone or anabolic steroids; some women do also.

Sores in the mouth or esophagus—like thrush, oral hairy leukoplakia, or herpes—should be treated with antibiotics, and the person should eat foods that are soft, easy to swallow, and bland. Diarrhea requires drugs like Lomotil, loperamide, or paregoric to slow the intestine, antibiotics to treat infections, or dietary modification. Nausea and vomiting require small frequent meals of food that is not aromatic and is easily digested; nausea and vomiting can also be treated with drugs. Fever requires aspirin, acetaminophen, or ibuprofen and drugs to eliminate the cause of the fever. Rapid weight loss during late-stage AIDS often indicates a chronic infection, like CMV, herpes simplex, tuberculosis, or *Mycobacterium avium*. In these cases, the most important treatment is to control the underlying infection.

Many people have difficulty maintaining nutrition because of the demands of the drugs of HAART and their side effects. For instance, indinavir (Crixivan) and ddI both must be taken on an empty stomach, but they can't be taken together, so deciding when to eat can be a problem. Some of these drugs cause nausea, which also confounds nutrition. The key is to discuss these issues with your physician, since an alternative schedule or an alternative regimen may be possible. For more about all these treatments for wasting, see above, "Problems of the Digestive System."

In general, cater to individual tastes, eat small and frequent meals, and eat foods that contain a lot of calories and protein. For the short term, anyway, don't worry too much about a balanced diet and eat snack foods that carry large numbers of calories: peanuts, peanut butter, nuts, raisins, sunflower seeds, M&Ms, Oreo cookies, pizza, milkshakes, potato chips, Fritos, macaroni and cheese, Big Macs, most candy bars, fudge sundaes, marshmallows, and many others. Try asking a licensed dietitian. Also ask about exercise training. Men should ask about testosterone.

When people cannot eat enough to compensate for losses, supplements will help. Supplements like Ensure, Ensure Plus, Jevity, Criticare, Peptamen, or Perative, which can be obtained in grocery stores and pharmacies, provide a rich source of calories and protein. The various supplements are similar in nutritional value. These supplements are commonly recommended for wasting, but some—Ensure Plus, Criticare, and Peptamen—actually cause diarrhea and should be diluted before using. If the supplements are taken in addition to meals, the person will need a few cans a day. If the supplements are the only nutrition the person is getting, the person will need about ten cans a day. Most people don't try to get all of their nutritional needs with these supplements, but they use them to supplement a diet of foods that are more pleasurable and diverse.

When people have problems that prevent the small intestine from absorbing food, different supplements, which are predigested and ready to absorb, will help. Supplements like Vivonex T.E.N. cost about $6 to $8 per can. If these supplements are taken in addition to meals, people will use three to six cans a day; if the supplement is the only source of nutrition, the person will need six to nine cans a day.

All nutritional supplements are available without prescription. But if a prescription is written nevertheless, Medicaid and some insurance plans will cover the supplement's cost.

On the rare occasions when the intestines quit digesting and absorbing food, nutrients might need to be provided by vein—a procedure called parenteral (meaning by vein) hyperalimentation. This is expensive—in fact, extraordinarily expensive—and costs over $10,000 per month. Most physicians prefer to use parenteral hyperalimentation for only a week or two to get past a temporary problem, though occasionally they use it for longer periods for uncontrollable diarrhea caused by cryptosporidiosis.

Causes of Constitutional Symptoms

The causes of constitutional symptoms are diverse. Sometimes the cause is anxiety and depression (see chapter 4). Sometimes it's the medicines. Sometimes it's the common aches and pains—colds, influenza, gastroenteritis, nervous stomach, headaches—that affect everyone.

Sometimes the cause is one of the medical complications. When

Table 6. Nonmedicinal Treatment of Wasting

Cause	Do's	Don't's
Mouth sores	Treat the cause—usually thrush, OHL, esophagitis, herpes, aphthous ulcers	Food that is hot, spicy, sour, or sticky
Loss of taste	Eat the foods you like; use herbs, spices, and additives as desired	Food you don't like
Nausea	Eat small portions; eat saltines, pretzels, toast; drink liquids and eat food separately	Food that is fatty, spicy, or has strong aromas; drugs that cause nausea—use substitutes
Depression	Ask the assistance of a mental health professional	
Dementia	Encouragement by caregiver; may require feeding	
Diarrhea	Small, frequent meals; eat food high in soluble fiber, like oatmeal, pears, bananas, peaches	Caffeine, milk and milk products, fruit juices, fatty food, alcohol; food high in insoluble fiber like whole grain breads and cereals

constitutional symptoms are accompanied by cough and shortness of breath, the cause may be pneumocystis pneumonia. When constitutional symptoms are accompanied by headache or other symptoms of central nervous system infection (see above, "Head and Nerve Problems"), the cause is probably toxoplasma encephalitis or cryptococcal meningitis. When constitutional symptoms last for weeks or months, the cause is probably pneumocystis pneumonia, tuberculosis, *Mycobacterium avium* complex, cytomegalovirus, lymphoma, fungal infections, drugs, or HIV itself.

Tuberculosis. Tuberculosis (TB) is an infection of the lungs by a bacterium called *Mycobacterium tuberculosis.* (See "Tuberculosis," under "Productive Cough, Shortness of Breath, Fever," in this chapter.)

Mycobacterium avium complex (MAC). Mycobacteria are special types of bacteria; the best known, *Mycobacterium tuberculosis,* causes tuber-

Table 7. Drugs Used to Treat or Prevent Wasting

Drug	Cost/Week*	Comment
Megesterol (Megace)	$70–140	Most of the weight gain is fat. Side effects: impotence, reduced testosterone levels, high blood sugar.
Dronabinol (Marinol)	$140–210	Most of the weight gain is fat. Psychoactive component of marijuana, so may cause "high."
Serostim (growth hormone)	$1,750–2,300	Most of weight gain is lean body mass. Requires injection daily.
Testosterone injection	$10	Causes muscle building and masculinizing effects; used by men only. Injected every two weeks.
Testosterone patch	$35	Same as testosterone injection, but applied as a patch to skin daily. Men only.
Oxandrolone	$250	Causes muscle building with fewer masculinizing effects. May be used in low dose by women.
Nandrolone	$15	As above
Testosterone plus Megace	around $30	Popular combinations

*Cost based on average wholesale price.

culosis (TB). TB is the most common complication of HIV infection in developing countries. But in Europe and North America, the most common mycobacterial infection in HIV infection is *Mycobacterium avium* complex, or MAC. In people with HIV infection, MAC is usually widespread and can be cultured in the blood. People who do not have HIV infection also get infections with MAC, but only in the lungs. Before HAART, 30 to 50 percent of people with advanced HIV infection and a CD4 cell count of less than 50 developed MAC infection. MAC is now relatively unusual but still occurs in those with low CD4 counts who don't take drugs to prevent MAC.

MAC may spread widely throughout the body. In the liver, MAC can cause hepatitis; in the lung, pneumonia; in the bone marrow, it can cause a lowered blood count (further lowered from the effect of HIV); in the lymph glands, it can cause enlargements; in the intestines, stomach pain and diarrhea. Accompanying all of these infections are constitutional symptoms; the most common are chronic fever, weight loss, abdominal pain, and diarrhea.

MAC is easy to diagnose because it can be detected in the blood, but labs take at least a week to grow and identify it. MAC is somewhat difficult to treat, however, since many standard drugs don't work well and since, during the course of therapy, MAC often becomes resistant. Physicians have two approaches to this infection. To prevent MAC, the recommendation is to take clarithromycin (Biaxin) once a day, or azithromycin once a week. Preventive treatment is begun when the CD4 count is below 50, and can be discontinued when the CD4 count is above 100. To eliminate or reduce the numbers of mycobacteria, the standard treatment is to give two or more drugs. The most important are clarithromycin (Biaxin) and ethambutol given together. Sometimes these two are combined with a third drug: ciprofloxacin (Cipro), rifabutin (Mycobutin), azithromycin (Zithromax), or amikacin (Amikin). Most people respond to the drugs, though the response is slow, often requiring weeks for fever, fatigue, and positive blood cultures to resolve. In addition, many people have trouble tolerating the drugs, and some develop resistance to the drugs, after which the infection breaks through. Most important is to raise CD4 cell counts, which will help control MAC, prevent resistance, and simplify treatment.

Successful treatment of MAC has one curious and common complication, called "immune reconstitution syndrome," or IRS. IRS is described below but is emphasized here because it seems to complicate treatment of mycobacterial infection far more than treatment of other infectious disease complications. In Africa, the most common form of IRS is immune reconstitution TB; in the United States and Europe, it is immune reconstitution MAC. To understand the mechanism of this reaction, see "Immune reconstitution syndrome," below.

People with MAC usually take two antibiotics for MAC and three to four drugs for HIV infection. The MAC infection does improve somewhat, and the CD4 cell count rises as the HIV viral load falls. The newly reconstituted immune system recognizes MAC and attacks it aggressively. As a result of the attack, the person may have fever, fatigue, sweats, and local symptoms like enlarged, tender lymph nodes, stomach pain, or back pain, depending on the site of the attack.

It is important to note that MAC is transmitted very differently from the mycobacterium that causes tuberculosis. MAC is in soil and often in water supplies, which are presumably the sources of infection. Unlike tuberculosis, MAC is not transmitted from one person to another, and special precautions to prevent its spread are not necessary.

Cytomegalovirus (CMV). CMV infection, like herpes simplex infection, occurs early in life and remains dormant until a weakened immune system allows it to flourish. About 60 to 90 percent of adults have antibodies to CMV in their blood, meaning they have been infected and continue to harbor the virus. The initial infection is usually associated with either trivial symptoms or no symptoms at all. For most people the presence of the virus in the body continues to cause no symptoms until the immune defenses are lowered. About 30 percent of people with AIDS who are not taking treatment develop CMV disease when their CD4 counts are less than 50.

Like MAC, CMV infections are spread throughout the body. In the liver, CMV causes hepatitis; in the intestines, diarrhea; in the brain, encephalitis; in the nerves, a condition called radiculopathy; in the esophagus, difficulty swallowing; in the lung, pneumonia; on the skin, herpeslike sores; in the eye, retinitis. In many people, CMV infection only causes constitutional symptoms, including fever, fatigue, and wasting. The most common and serious of these infections is CMV retinitis. The diagnosis is made by an ophthalmologist. Treatment is important: it prevents loss of sight that could end up in blindness (see above, under "Eye Problems").

CMV is transmitted the way HIV is, through sexual contact or contact with blood. CMV is not transmitted from one person to another by casual contact.

CMV infection is difficult to treat although antibiotics like ganciclovir (given intravenously), cidofovir, and foscarnet are at least partially effective against some forms of the disease. CMV retinitis responds well to many different kinds of treatment, but the problem is relapse: that is, symptoms recur, and eye examinations show progressive changes. CMV at other places in the body responds less predictably. The problem with all the treatments is that they work temporarily, then fail. Depending on the type of treatment, the average time to failure is two to twelve months. Then a new treatment is tried.

For people with a low CD4 count, the best treatment is to start CMV therapy and HAART both. HAART increases a low CD4 count and permits the immune system to control CMV. When the CD4 count is over 100, it is possible to stop treatment for CMV.

Lymphoma. Lymphomas are tumors of the lymph glands that can occur in anyone but are more common and more severe in people with HIV infection. Lymphomas can occur relatively early in HIV infection when the CD4 count is above 200; lymphoma is one complication of HIV infection that has not decreased dramatically with HAART, presumably because lymphomas do not require a major decrease in the CD4 cell count.

In some people, the only symptoms of lymphoma are the constitutional symptoms. In other people, the symptoms of lymphoma are very large lymph glands in the neck, under the arms, or in the groin. In some people, the symptoms of lymphoma differ according to where in the body lymphoma occurs: lymphoma in the intestines causes pain and diarrhea; in the brain, focal neurologic problems (see above, "Head and Nerve Problems"); in the lung, pneumonia. The most common symptoms are fever, weight loss, fatigue, and abdominal pain. A CT scan of the chest and abdomen helps find the lesions if they are not obvious.

In people with HIV infection, lymphomas occur more often and progress more rapidly than they do in other people. Treatment is with radiation and with chemotherapy using the same drugs used for other types of tumors. The treatment is given by specialists, either radiation therapists or oncologists. The success of the treatment is variable; some people do extremely well. Curing lymphoma is increasingly likely, so talk to your physician about the side effects and potential benefits of each treatment.

Fungal infections. Constitutional symptoms can also be caused by fungal infections, including *Cryptococcus neoformans, Histoplasma capsulatum,* and *Coccidioides immitis.*

Cryptococcus neoformans usually causes pneumonia, then spreads to other areas of the body. It spreads most commonly to the meninges, where it causes meningitis (see above, under "Head and Nerve Problems"). It can also cause only constitutional symptoms.

Histoplasma capsulatum is found primarily in the central and eastern parts of the United States, especially in the Mississippi, Ohio, and St. Lawrence River valleys. Most people with histoplasmosis have been in the areas where it is common, but they may have been in those areas years earlier. In most people, it causes infections of the lungs. In people with HIV infection, it causes infections spread throughout the body.

Coccidioides immitis is found in the southwestern United States (California, Arizona, New Mexico, and Texas), where it causes a lung infection called valley fever. As with histoplasmosis, HIV-infected people with coccidioidomycosis have usually visited or lived in the areas where the fungus grows. In people with HIV infection, *Coccidioides,* like *Histoplasma,* tends to spread throughout the body.

All three fungal infections are diagnosed by detecting the fungus.

They are usually treated with amphotericin B, given intravenously, or with the azoles—fluconazole (Diflucan) or itraconazole (Sporanox)—both taken by mouth.

Drugs. Constitutional symptoms can also be caused by drugs. People with HIV infection take many drugs either to treat or to prevent infections, and to treat anxiety, depression, fever, aches, and problems with sleep and appetite. Many of these drugs have side effects, ranging in seriousness from drowsiness to kidney damage and anemia. The only side effects of many drugs, however, are constitutional symptoms, particularly fever and rash. Drugs can also commonly cause hepatitis, low counts of white blood cells, nausea, vomiting, diarrhea, and abdominal pain. AZT, d4T, and/or ddI can cause lactic acidosis, which in turn can cause weight loss and weakening; lactic acidosis is important to recognize because it's progressive and ultimately serious.

For reasons that are unclear, many of these side effects are more common in people with HIV infection. For instance, trimethoprim-sulfamethoxazole (Bactrim or Septra) causes side effects in 10 percent of the people without HIV infection and over 50 percent of those with HIV infection.

Finding out which drugs are causing side effects and stopping the side effects requires the advice of a physician. This advice will depend on the probability for each drug and the necessity of the drug. The physician will either advise what is called a drug holiday—discontinuation of all drugs—or will stop drugs one at a time.

HIV Infection. Some people have constitutional symptoms that cannot be attributed to a medical complication, or to the side effects of drugs. In such cases, HIV itself might be responsible.

Constitutional symptoms with no causes other than HIV usually occur late in the course of the infection. The treatment is drugs directed at HIV—like HAART—or drugs that simply relieve the constitutional symptoms—aspirin, acetaminophen, ibuprofen, or similar drugs. Sometimes prednisone helps. These drugs are often given on a trial basis, in varying combinations and increasing doses.

Immune Reconstitution Syndrome (IRS). The HAART era brings with it an unexpected development. A rapid decrease in HIV viral load is usually accompanied by a rapid increase in CD4 cells, which means the immune system is being rebuilt, reconstituted—exactly what we want. But when people taking HAART also have complications like CMV or MAC or PCP or cryptococcal meningitis, their newly reconstituted immune systems kick in, recognize those microbes, and aggressively attack. The

Table 8. Stages of Untreated HIV Infection and Commonly Associated Complications

Condition	Symptoms	Comments
Asymptomatic infection	None (*asymptomatic* means *without symptoms*)	May have abnormal laboratory tests often indicating suppressed immunity (low CD4 count or normal CD4 count).
Persistent generalized lymphadenopathy	Nodules like marbles under the skin, in the neck, armpits, and groin	Swollen lymph nodes do not represent progressive disease but are sites of virus growth; about 10 to 15% of people will complain of tender swellings in the neck or in the armpits. This symptom occurs early in the course of HIV infection and is not seen as a serious complication.
Early symptomatic HIV infection (Note: All conditions listed as occurring in early stage disease when the CD4 count is above 200 are more common and more severe when the CD4 count is below 200)		These include complications that may occur when the CD4 count is relatively high. Most are more frequent and more severe in the late stages.
Thrush	White patches in the mouth	80 to 90% of people with AIDS have had or will have thrush; more common when taking antibiotics; frequency has become much less, due to HAART.
Vaginitis	Vaginal discharge, often white, cottage-cheese-like, with itching	Common in all women, including those with high CD4 cell counts and without HIV infection.
Oral hairy leukoplakia	White patches usually along sides of tongue	15 to 25% of people with AIDS have had or will have OHL. There are usually no symptoms and no need to treat.

Herpes zoster	Painful blisters, usually on specific part of the skin, making a line or crop of blisters on one side	Caused by same virus that causes chickenpox.
Idiopathic thrombocytopenia	Bleeding, especially from gums, rectum, urine, into the skin, & with minor cuts	May occur relatively early in HIV infection.
Pneumonia	Cough, fever, and sputum	One of the relatively few serious complications that occurs with a CD4 count above 300; most commonly caused by a bacterium called pneumococcus. Treatment with common antibiotics is usually successful.
Tuberculosis (TB)	Cough, blood in sputum, shortness of breath, fever, weight loss	TB rates are high in urban areas and among immigrants, blacks, Hispanics, and injection drug users; CD4 count may be high and averages 200 to 300. This is a contagious disease, so household contacts need to be evaluated.
Lymphoma	Fever, weight loss, lethargy, abdominal pain	5 to 10% of all people with AIDS develop lymphoma; may be difficult to diagnose; becoming more common in the era of HAART, presumably because other complications are less common and HIV infected persons now live longer.
Late symptomatic HIV infection, or AIDS		This includes AIDS-defining diagnoses. The CD4 cell count is below 200 in 90% of people with an AIDS-defining diagnosis.

(continued)

Table 8. (*Continued*)

Condition	Symptoms	Comments
Pneumocystis pneumonia (PCP)	Dry cough, shortness of breath, fever	Most common first serious AIDS-defining diagnosis; 80% of people with AIDS eventually develop PCP unless the CD4 count is kept high or preventive medicine is taken. CD4 count is below 200 in 90% of the people; average CD4 count is 100 without prophylaxis and 30 in people who take prophylaxis. This complication is much less common in the era of HAART.
Constitutional symptoms	Chronic diarrhea, weight loss, night sweats, fever, fatigue	There are a variety of causes in people with HIV infection, and finding the cause is the key to treatment.
Kaposi's sarcoma	Purplish or black nodules on skin	Frequency is decreasing; it now accounts for about 6% of initial AIDS diagnoses. It is one of the few AIDS-defining diagnoses that commonly occurs with CD4 counts above 200.
Candidal esophagitis	Difficult or painful swallowing; usually have thrush	20 to 30% of people with AIDS get candidal esophagitis; most common with thrush; same symptoms may be caused by cytomegalovirus, herpes simplex, or aphthous ulcers; average CD4 count is 50.
Cryptococcal meningitis	Severe headache & fever; may have double vision or stiff neck	8 to 10% of people with AIDS eventually get cryptococcal meningitis; the average CD4 count is 50.

190

Cryptosporidial diarrhea	Diarrhea for over one month	3 to 4% of people with AIDS eventually get cryptosporidial diarrhea; CD4 count may be high or low, but persistent diarrhea over a month occurs only when the CD4 count is below 200.
Cytomegalovirus (CMV) infection spread throughout the body	Symptoms depend on location of the infection. Fever is common. Intestine: abdominal pain & diarrhea Eye: abnormal vision or "floaters" Brain: headache, lethargy, disorientation	20 to 40% of people with AIDS eventually develop CMV disease. An eye infection, "retinitis," accounts for 60 to 70% of CMV disease in people with AIDS. The CD4 count is usually below 50 and averages 20. This complication is uncommon in the era of HAART.
Mycobacterium avium complex infection throughout body	Symptoms depend on location of the infection. Fever usually present. Intestine: abdominal pain & diarrhea Liver: hepatitis & stomach pain Lungs: pneumonia	30 to 50% of people with AIDS eventually develop this complication if the CD4 count decreases below 50 and there is no prophylaxis. Most common symptoms are chronic fever, abdominal pain, weight loss, and anemia. This complication is uncommon in the era of HAART.
Toxoplasma encephalitis	Headache, seizure, fever, lethargy, weakness on one side	3 to 10% of people with AIDS eventually get toxoplasma encephalitis, in the absence of preventive treatment; CD4 count is below 100 and averages 50; this complication is uncommon in the era of HAART.

(continued)

Table 8. (*Continued*)

Condition	Symptoms	Comments
Herpes simplex	Blisters on skin lasting over 1 month, especially around anus, genitals, or mouth	10 to 25% of people with AIDS develop serious herpes simplex infections. Both the mouth and genital forms occur at all stages, but they persist over a month or spread to other parts of the body only when the CD4 count is below 200.
Wasting syndrome	Over 10% weight loss that is unexplained and often accompanied by diarrhea or fever lasting over 1 month	This complication is uncommon in the era of HAART. It is always important to look for a treatable cause and to get the CD4 count up.
HIV-associated dementia (HAD)	Memory loss, apathy, inability to concentrate, inability to control arms or legs	20 to 30% of people with AIDS develop HAD, nearly always when the CD4 count is below 200; this complication is decreasing in frequency in the era of HAART, but the decrease is less impressive than are decreases in other HIV-related complications.
Lymphoma of brain	Headache, behavioral change, seizure, impaired function of arm, leg, speech, etc. No fever.	Lymphoma in the brain occurs in late disease when the CD4 count is below 100.
Peripheral neuropathy	Pain or tingling sensation in feet	Usually occurs in late disease, but occasionally occurs when CD4 count is over 200. Identical symptoms may be caused by drugs like ddI, ddC, or d4T regardless of the CD4 count.

immune attack causes general symptoms of fever and fatigue, along with specific symptoms that reveal the site of the attack: a swollen lymph node in the neck for MAC, a sudden worsening of vision for CMV, or a sudden severe headache for cryptococcal meningitis. The health care provider has to decide: Is this a relapse of the infection? Is it a new reaction to one of the many drugs? Is it a new HIV-related complication? It is none of these; it is an immune system now doing its job. The resulting syndrome is called immune reconstitution syndrome or IRS.

IRS usually occurs after HAART is started, when the CD4 cell count is still low (usually less than 100) and the response to HAART is good (the viral load is falling and the CD4 cell count is rising). The new immune response is to an infection, usually one that is newly treated, but sometimes one not known to have existed. Though the symptoms can be pretty awful, the syndrome is a good sign: the immune system is working. IRS is managed by continuing HAART, treating the complicating infection, and quieting down the immune system with ibuprofen or cortisone.

Consider the case of a 42-year-old man who sees a physician because he has fever and weight loss. The physician runs tests and learns that the man has HIV infection, a CD4 count of 50, and a blood culture positive for MAC. The physician treats the man with HAART and for MAC. The man slowly responds, and after four months, his CD4 cell count has increased to 96 and his viral load has decreased from 56,000 to 450. He then develops fever and a large, tender swelling in his neck. This is MAC IRS: his HIV is under control; his CD4 count is on a roll; and his MAC, which used to be disseminated throughout his body, is now isolated in one lymph node, where the immune system is doing its job. The physician doesn't want to stop treating either HIV or MAC, so to make the man feel better, the physician prescribes corticosteroids to cool down the overactive immune system.

Chapter 7

Options for Medical Care: Medical Personnel and Procedures

- Medical care systems
- Limits on your options for medical care
- Physicians
- Comprehensive care programs
- Case management
- Hospital care
- Hospital people and practices
- Patients' rights in hospitals
- What matters

A person with HIV infection is confronted with questions about medical care that are as confusing as they are important. What kind of physicians treat HIV infection? What kind of medical care is available? What kind of hospital provides the best care? This chapter outlines the options for medical care available to a person with HIV infection and provides some general guidelines for people considering those options. The chapter also provides a general guide to hospitals and describes the rights people have when they are patients in a hospital. And finally, the chapter outlines the alternatives to hospitalization.

Medical Care Systems

Medical care comes in two general types: managed care and fee-for-service. In managed care, an organization takes financial and medical responsibility for your care. There are several types of managed care organizations; the most common among people with HIV infection are health maintenance organizations, or HMOs. In fee-for-service, the patient or the patient's insurance company pays the bills for medical services. In the past, most health care in the United States was fee-for-service. In the past several years, however, more and more people have come under managed care organizations or HMOs. Policies for coverage in either managed care organizations (like Kaiser) or fee-for-service plans (like Blue Cross–Blue Shield) may be purchased as an individual or as part of a group. An individual must qualify; a group plan is usually available through employment.

With managed care organizations, the good news is that the organization will provide all the medical care services without a charge beyond the monthly fee. The bad news is that most organizations have their own networks of health care providers and facilities, so that options for selecting health care providers or for choosing hospitals are limited. This means that patients cannot pick their own doctors, or that they may not continue to see a doctor they had picked previously unless they pay for the service.

The driving force in these organizations is cost saving. Savings are often accomplished with three general tactics: (1) limitations on the availability of services, (2) reduced or capitated reimbursement for services, or (3) substitutions. The organization assigns a fee per patient per month. The fee may be a full cap, which covers everything; or a partial cap, which covers some services but not all; or subcapitation, which covers some services done elsewhere. Substitution means an aide does the work usually assigned to a nurse, or a physician's assistant does the work usually assigned to a physician, or a general practitioner does the work of a specialist.

In the battle to reduce cost, the highest priority is allocated to eliminating hospital care, which is by far the most expensive component of the U.S. health care bill. Another tactic to reduce cost, called "cherry picking," is for the managed care organization or HMO to enroll patients who are unlikely to need medical services. Quality is neither recognized nor rewarded. In fact, many HMOs provide financial incentives to physicians to avoid consultations, expensive tests, or expensive treatments.

People with HIV infection frequently need medical services and are seen by managed care organizations or HMOs as high risks. Many people with HIV infection will find themselves victims of cherry picking; if they succeed in enrolling in an organization, their access to services and to medical expertise may be limited. They may have particular difficulty finding experts in HIV infection, in part because no managed care organization or HMO wants to be the selective referral source for patients who might be expensive to treat. Mental health services are especially difficult to find in these organizations.

Fee-for-service might also impose sharp limitations on medical care for people with HIV infection. There are three types of limitations: access to insurance, denial of payment for preexisting conditions, and limited coverage for a diverse range of services. Most insurance companies limit the access of individual applicants who are considered high risks; acceptance in group policies through employment plans is much more readily available. Services covered are specific to the plan. All plans cover the high-priced item—hospitalization—but may have a cap, a co-pay, or a restriction on services. Coverage of other medical care services—including outpatient visits, pharmacies, home care services, and nursing home services—is quite variable. The most important plan for people with HIV infection is the pharmacy plan. HIV drugs now account for half the total HIV medical bill: the average HAART regimen costs $10,000 to $15,000 per year. Most insurance companies will not cover preexisting conditions in individual applicants (see chapter 9).

Medical care is provided by different kinds of people offering different services in different settings. The providers of medical care are professionals: they are physicians, physician's assistants, and nurse practitioners. The setting in which care is provided can generally be divided into two components: *outpatient facilities* and *inpatient facilities*. Outpatient facilities are individual physicians' offices, clinics staffed by physicians who practice as a group, managed care organizations or HMOs, and public health department clinics. Inpatient facilities, which are primarily hospitals and nursing homes, are generally used by people who need more intensive care.

In recent years, because hospital care in the United States is now enormously expensive, there has been a growing demand for alternatives to hospitals. These alternatives now include chronic care facilities (like nursing homes), home care programs, day care centers, infusion centers, hospice care facilities and programs, and outpatient clinics. Some of the alternatives provide the services—including transfusions and other infusion services and same-day surgery—previously provided only in hospitals. Hospitalization in acute care hospitals accounts for about 15 to 20 percent of the total cost of HIV care. So for managed care organizations or HMOs, these less expensive alternatives to hospitals are a high priority.

Financing for this complex network of resources varies: the principal modes of funding are Blue Cross–Blue Shield and other insurance companies, managed care organizations or HMOs, self-pay, and the government programs for assistance with medical bills (Medicaid and Medicare). Chapter 9 will discuss how to finance medical care—since financing is obviously a major factor in deciding which option to choose.

Regardless of which option for medical care you choose, it is important to have

—a physician who has extensive experience with HIV infection;

—a close physician-patient relationship;

—the services of medical specialists as they are needed;

—the services of psychiatrists, psychologists, or support groups as they are needed;

—emergency medical services;

—a hospital with appropriate resources;

—such alternatives to hospital care as home therapy, chronic care facilities, and hospice care.

It is particularly important to have access to a physician or hospital or clinic that will provide the special medical resources and skills needed to treat people with HIV infection. The treatment of HIV infection is a fast-moving field: medical therapy now makes a substantial difference in the progress of the disease, and new treatments are continually being developed. HIV care is now a specialty with its own research agenda, journals, care programs, conferences, and experts. It is important for a person with HIV infection to have care from someone included in this HIV care network.

Limits on Your Options for Medical Care

Your options for medical care will depend on where you live. The kind of care specific to HIV infection is likely to be better in a big city: most big cities offer many options for treatment of HIV infection. Smaller cities and rural areas are likely to offer fewer options, and the physicians in these areas are less likely to be familiar with HIV infection. This is because most of the people who became infected in the early stages of this epidemic lived primarily in large cities like New York, San Francisco, Los Angeles, Miami, and Washington, D.C.; disproportionately fewer people living in smaller cities and rural areas were infected. As a result, physicians who trained or who practice in small cities or rural areas often lack experience in treating HIV infection.

As a consequence, when people with HIV infection who live in small cities and rural areas want medical treatment or periodic consultation about medical treatment, they often travel to the nearest physician or clinic specializing in HIV infection (see below, under "Choosing a Physician"). Some people also travel to more distant clinics or physicians to get the anonymity they cannot get locally.

The options for medical care may be substantially fewer for people who are in managed care organizations or HMOs, for people receiving Medicaid, and for people who have limited financial resources and no health insurance. Managed care organizations or HMOs and city health clinics offer medical services that vary in quality, some very good and some not so good. Large urban areas have federal funds from the Ryan White Act to provide medical care and support services for people with HIV infection. The range of services offered and the quality of those services are both variable. Most people served under this act are uninsured or underinsured and have limited financial resources.

Managed care organizations or HMOs are networks of service providers that contract for all the health care of their subscribers. These organizations provide comprehensive services—but to be profitable and competitive, they prefer to have healthy subscribers who don't need health care. Conditions like HIV infection that are chronic and expensive to treat are avoided when possible, and quality services tailored to the specific needs of people with HIV are rare. These organizations may also limit access to any component of health care that is expensive: hospitalization, laboratory tests, radiology procedures, or consultations with specialists. Some organizations are exceptions to these rules, so the person with HIV infection may be lucky, or may need to search them out. Some organizations do not allow patients to see physicians other than those physicians who participate in that organization, or do so only on a case-by-case basis. People enrolled in those organizations therefore have no choice in what specialists they see. The organization can also limit the hospitals people may be admitted to.

The process of selecting among medical options begins with finding out what your finances allow and what publicly funded resources are available. This disease is expensive, and managed care organizations or HMOs, insurance plans, and Medicaid will each pay for some things and not for others. Many insurance plans especially restrict the outpatient services they cover. Medicaid covers a broad range of services but reimburses physicians at so low a rate that most physicians refuse to accept patients paying through Medicaid. Many employers offer a choice between joining a managed care organization or HMO or being reimbursed by the insurance company, and you may be able to switch back and forth as your needs dictate. In any case, you need to know your options. You can begin by finding out what your organization, insurance company, or government medical assistance will allow (see chapter 9), and then discussing these issues candidly with your physician or with a social worker.

Physicians

Most people receive medical care for HIV infection from one or more kinds of physicians: primary care physicians, AIDS physicians, and specialists.

Primary Care Physicians

The medical management of HIV infection has not only become increasingly complicated but also changes with extraordinary frequency. Most medical authorities, including the U.S. Public Health Service, conclude that HIV care should be managed by an expert, that is, a physician who has a specific interest in HIV infection, who attends the professional meetings, follows the HIV Web sites, and cares for many patients. The need for an expert to do HIV care is now well accepted in medicine, and most metropolitan areas have many HIV experts. In fact, most nonspecialists consider HIV care too complicated and will not provide it at all. So the challenge to the person with HIV infection is to find the right HIV physician in the right plan that provides the right services.

Some primary care physicians in private practice work in groups of between three and ten. Physicians in such groups usually have different areas of expertise: some treat stomach problems, for example, and some treat lung problems. The person with HIV infection will usually see the same physician for general health care, but will see other physicians for specific problems. The advantage of group practice is that these physicians are all under the same roof, and communication between physicians with specializations is good.

AIDS Physicians

AIDS physicians are physicians who devote most of their time to caring for people with HIV infection. By strict definition of the word *specialist,* there is no such person as an "AIDS specialist": rather, some physicians simply adopt the treatment of AIDS and HIV infection as a special interest, and are called, informally, AIDS physicians.

A little background on what makes a specialist:

Physicians practice in a variety of specialties, including family practice, pediatrics, internal medicine, surgery, and obstetrics and gynecology. Becoming a physician requires graduating from medical school, doing postgraduate training as a resident, passing standard tests, and getting a license through the state licensing board. By law, a physician requires a license to practice medicine. The type of postgraduate training determines the specialty.

Becoming a certified specialist requires certification by a professional specialty board within the American Board of Medical Specialties. Certification requires postgraduate training for a specified number of years in an approved training program, followed by passing an examination in the specialty called a *board examination*. To be certified as a cardiologist, for example, the physician must take three years of postgraduate training in internal medicine, then pass the board examinations to be certified as a specialist in internal medicine, then take three additional years of postgraduate training in cardiology, and then pass the board examinations in cardiology. Any physician can claim to be a cardiologist, but only those who satisfy these requirements can call themselves board-certified cardiologists.

There are no recognized accredited training programs for specializing in HIV infection and no board examinations to certify competence in treatment of HIV infection. This means there is no official medical specialty in HIV infection. In the absence of a certification process, however, many groups are now defining criteria for the HIV specialist based on experience and continuing education. The criterion of experience is usually based on the number of patients cared for: the usual requirement is that the physician cares for at least 25 to 50 patients with HIV. The criterion of continuing education means that the HIV specialist must have at least 5 to 10 hours of HIV-related postgraduate instruction each year. The group defining the criteria decides the actual numbers of patients and hours of education.

In this era of HAART, there is grand testimony about the need for experience in HIV care. First, the medical issues have become incredibly complicated—so complicated that most physicians don't feel competent to provide medical care. Second, medical care changes fast. In no other facet of medicine are new drugs, new treatment strategies, and new medical issues introduced with such speed. In fact, 60 medical journals (including one or two that are good) are now devoted to HIV infection, and five to ten major national or international HIV conferences take place each year. Third, and most important, the HIV care specialist makes a big difference. Research studies have shown that care by a physician with HIV experience means patients live longer, have lower costs, and require fewer and shorter hospitalizations. In short, although HIV infection is a specialty without official recognition by the usual accrediting group, a working definition of "specialist" based on experience is becoming generally accepted because it is so well justified.

The official, accredited specialty that has provided most of the AIDS physicians is infectious diseases, which, like cardiology, is a subspecialty of internal medicine. Specialists in infectious diseases become AIDS physicians because HIV infection is an infectious disease, and because most of HIV infection's complications are those commonly encountered during infectious disease training. Specialists in infectious diseases primarily treat about 40 to 50 percent of all people with HIV infection who are getting care in the United States.

Other medical specialties also supply AIDS physicians. Some specialists treat AIDS because of the nature of their specialties: oncology, pulmonary medicine, dermatology. Others, like gay physicians, treat AIDS for more personal reasons. Many AIDS physicians are primary care physicians who specialize in HIV infection.

AIDS physicians keep current with this fast-moving field by attending medical meetings dealing with HIV infection, by following the Web sites with HIV-related news, and by subscribing to the better medical journals devoted to HIV infection. Their practices may be limited almost exclusively to people with HIV infection, and they are themselves often community leaders in the social, medical, and political issues related to HIV infection.

Other Specialists

HIV infection directly or indirectly affects virtually every organ of the body, and no physician, regardless of training, can alone treat all the conditions associated with HIV infection. As a result, people with HIV infection, especially people with AIDS, are likely to be referred to such specialists as neurologists, psychiatrists, oncologists, gastroenterologists, ophthalmologists, dermatologists, and pulmonary specialists. Referrals to such specialists almost always come from the primary care physician or the AIDS physician. These physicians will select specialists based on the reputation of the specialist within the medical community, on their own previous interactions with the specialist, and on the specialist's specific interest or expertise in AIDS.

Choosing a Physician

What is the best way for someone with HIV infection to go about selecting a physician? First, remember that this may be one of the most important decisions you will make. HIV care is now extremely complicated, so having a physician with substantial experience with the disease, the drugs, and the side effects is critical.

Begin by asking your primary care physician if he or she feels comfortable caring for a person with HIV infection. You may appropriately ask about his or her experience; since about 90 percent of HIV care in this country is provided by about 5 percent of physicians, the answers you will probably hear are "no" and "none." If so, then ask for an appropriate referral: the medical community has an effective communication network, and your physician will either know or can easily find out who has a good reputation within the profession for the care of people with HIV infection. Group practices and managed care organizations or HMOs will often have one or more physicians who specialize in care of people with HIV infection. Physicians are the best source of advice about other physicians.

If you do not already have a primary care physician, another source of information is by word of mouth from other people with HIV infection, although some caution is called for here: watch out for people who confuse medical competence with a good bedside manner. What impresses patients and what impresses physicians are often quite different, and your highest priority is competent and comprehensive care.

Other sources are AIDS hotlines, community organizations devoted to AIDS, nurses, and the centers that run tests for antibodies to HIV. The yellow pages may have listings for physicians with a special interest in AIDS, but the relevant listings are more likely to be of physicians specializing in infectious diseases. You can then contact the infectious disease specialists directly and ask for either an appointment or a referral; they will know well the available local resources for treating HIV infection. City, county, and state medical societies often have lists of physicians with specialized interests; however, these lists may reflect those who have paid their dues and need the patients, rather than those who offer high-quality services. Also, if you are thinking of contacting a physician whom you know of only through an advertisement, be aware that physicians who advertise often do so because other physicians no longer refer patients to them.

In general, to choose a physician, ask another physician, check certification, be cautious about a physician who advertises medical services, ask about a physician's reputation among his or her peers, and look for a physician who has privileges to admit patients to a good hospital. Hospitals review physicians carefully before allowing them the privilege of admitting patients, and hospitals of good quality will accept only reputable physicians.

Many people with HIV infection select an AIDS physician for conditions related to HIV infection, and continue to see their primary care physicians for all other conditions. To repeat, the best physician to manage HIV infection is someone who specializes in the field; the field has simply become too complicated for the generalist. Research shows that doctors with extensive AIDS experience have patients who live longer, go to the hospital fewer times, and stay in the hospital for less time; these doctors also answer their patients' questions better. If HIV expertise is not available, you need to find an AIDS physician and periodically consult with him or her or ask your own physician to consult with an AIDS physician by phone.

Regardless of what kind of physician you see or where you live, if you have questions about your medical care, you can ask for a second opinion or get a consultation with another physician. That is, you can go to another physician or clinic that specializes in the treatment of AIDS and ask to have the program of your medical care reviewed. If you belong to a managed care organization or HMO, you may have to pay for this, but a second-party review is often worthwhile. The need for a second-party review will be driven to a large extent by your own perception of your care—that is, whether your viral load has lowered, whether the side effects of the drugs are being managed, and whether the treatment regimen is acceptable. To have the program reviewed thoroughly, you need to bring (or send) copies of all your hospital records and your physician's office records. These records will most importantly include your treatment regimen, your viral load results, and your CD4 test results. Other information of interest includes the results of the CBC, the lipid test, X-rays, scans, biopsies, and any other tests, plus the diagnoses of HIV-related complications. Remember that these records are yours, and the office or hospital that has them is obliged to give them to you if you sign a request. These records not only simplify the consultation but also prevent unnecessary duplication of visits or tests.

You need not worry that you will offend your own physician by asking for such a consultation. In normal medical practice, second opinions are often encouraged and, for many procedures, are sometimes required. Moreover, given the seriousness of HIV infection and the speed with which recommendations for treatment change, second opinions are simply considered a very good idea.

Comprehensive Care Programs

Some hospitals, clinics, and managed care organizations or HMOs, especially those in large urban areas, have comprehensive programs of care tailored to the specific needs of people with HIV infection. The goal of comprehensive care programs is to provide all the care needed by a person with HIV infection in one setting and under one roof. These "HIV centers" have become the accepted standard of care in most of Europe and in Brazil, Australia, and Canada. The HIV centers provide a diverse array of HIV-related services and health care providers who share a career commitment to HIV. Such centers are also available in the United

States, often at major academic institutions. The centers' advantages are that they have extensive resources specific to HIV, they have access to the latest drugs, and they are usually on the cutting edge in the management of a disease where recommendations change with unparalleled frequency.

In the United States, the type and extent of services provided, and the type of specialists available, vary from one program to another and from one HIV center to another. The people and programs in comprehensive care programs can include HIV counselors, medical specialists, support groups, home therapy programs, dietitians, psychologists and psychiatrists, social workers, case managers, hospice care programs, drug rehabilitation programs, and dental care. Most comprehensive care programs will have some but not all of these services.

HIV counselors are specifically trained to provide information about HIV infection, especially information about the progress of the disease, the meaning of a positive blood test, and preventing transmission. These counselors also give advice on where, in a local community, to go for legal advice, for financial advice, and for personal planning services.

Medical specialists associated with a comprehensive care program are the same experts a primary care physician or AIDS physician is likely to consult about some of the complications of HIV infection that require specialized knowledge or a specialized procedure. The specialists most likely to be consulted are neurologists (brain and nerves), ophthalmologists (eyes), gastroenterologists (intestines), dermatologists (skin), oncologists (tumors), psychiatrists (mind), obstetricians (pregnancy), gynecologists (women's health), and pulmonary physicians (lungs). The specialist in a comprehensive care program may deal primarily with the specialty as it applies to HIV infection. That is, instead of a gastroenterologist who deals with all problems of the digestive system, you may find one who has a special interest in the gastroenterological problems of people with HIV infection.

Support groups offer a person with HIV infection emotional support and help with adherence to the drug regimens in the company of people facing similar problems (see chapter 11). The support groups are ideally made up of no more than five to eight people affected by HIV infection who have common interests and concerns. The groups are often led by a mental health professional. The benefit of a support group is sharing experiences and problems—medical and nonmedical—that are not easily shared with others.

Home therapy programs extend comprehensive services to the person's home. These services are most useful to the person whose physical condition is stable and who may be staying in the hospital only to receive certain types of treatment, like intravenous drugs. Nurses working in home therapy programs can give intravenous drug treatments, draw blood for necessary laboratory tests, and do general nursing care—all at home, and all much less expensively than in the hospital. In most instances, the person with HIV infection or the caregiver is taught how to administer the drugs intravenously by himself or herself, so that visits by a trained professional are few. This style of giving intravenous drugs may sound somewhat risky, but it has now become commonplace in medical practice.

A dietitian's job is to help people with HIV infection solve the eating problems that can interfere with proper nourishment and complicate the proper use of HAART. Eating problems may result from depression, altered taste, medical complications in the mouth or esophagus, side effects from medications, dental problems, severe diarrhea, or HIV itself. Food helps the absorption of some drugs and interferes with the absorption of others. Some drugs, like indinavir, can be taken with a light snack, but not everybody knows the definition of a light snack. Dietitians teach people with eating problems how to deal more effectively with nutritional needs depending on the cause of the problem.

Psychologists and psychiatrists treat the array of emotional difficulties that face people with HIV infection. Some of these difficulties are serious, some short-lived; some are treatable with medications, some are best treated by talking them out. Psychological social workers, mental health nurses, psychologists, and psychiatrists—four kinds of mental health professionals who provide somewhat different services—can determine the severity of the emotional difficulty and can decide on the best course of treatment (see chapter 11, under "Mental Health Professionals").

Social workers and case managers help sort out many of the nonmedical problems people with HIV infection face: dealing with hospitals and insurance companies, keeping finances straight, sorting out living arrangements, and much more (see the sections in this chapter on case management and on social workers).

The services offered in comprehensive care programs are more likely to be extensive in metropolitan areas and in hospitals or clinics that serve large numbers of people with HIV infection. Some people, especially those in the early stages of the infection, have no need for such a complex network of services. Some AIDS physicians work in private offices but have established a network of referrals that is comparable to a comprehensive care program. Some people with HIV infection prefer the simplicity of a single physician; others prefer the availability of many specialized services. The people who most benefit from the advantages of a comprehensive care program are either those who need more complicated and specialized care or those whose primary care physicians are uncomfortable treating many of the complications of HIV infection.

Case Management

Case managers are usually social workers or public health nurses who help coordinate the lives of people with HIV infection. People with HIV infection are in extraordinary need of help with work, home life, medical care, medical insurance, legal issues, finances, and psychological problems. Furthermore, people with HIV infection are subject to so many sudden changes in health that planning becomes difficult. Fortunately, the complexity of their needs has been recognized, and increasing numbers of organizations, programs, and other resources now satisfy these needs. The quality and quantity of these resources vary. Case management is a way of linking the people with HIV infection to the resources in their own communities.

Working together with medical care providers, case managers commonly make two plans for each person with HIV infection: a medical care plan and a social work plan. The medical care plan includes plans for a range of continuing medical services, including home care; care in a clinic, hospital, nursing home, or hospice; and, when necessary, care in an addiction program or a mental health program. The social work plan includes financial plans, insurance benefits, benefits from publicly funded programs, resources for drugs, housing plans, and employment plans. The social work plan also links the person with HIV infection to community organizations that provide such services as support groups, home health care, companionship, meals in the home, and the like.

The primary goal of the case manager is to be an advocate for the person with HIV infection. This means obtaining for him or her all the services that are available and appropriate. A second goal is to obtain the best services at the lowest price. In short, a case manager knows the system, and his or her job is to make the best use of it.

Case management services are sometimes funded by state health departments, by other sources of public funds, or by foundations. Insurance companies will sometimes pay for case management services. You can find out how to arrange funding for case management services by talking to the case manager or to a social worker.

Both the availability and the quality of case management services vary widely in different communities. Some are not run as well as others. Some may not be networked into both the agencies that provide social services and the agencies that provide health care services for people with HIV infection. And even those that seem to be well run and well networked are difficult to evaluate. Case management has been used to care for the elderly, for the mentally ill, and for crippled children; evaluations of the usefulness of these programs have been quite variable. As for HIV infection, there is probably no other disease in medicine where the fundamental philosophy of case management is more sound, at least in theory. In practice, it is not clear that case management has successfully achieved any of its major goals: improved quality of life, prolonged survival, or reduced cost of care.

Case managers can increasingly be found not only in comprehensive care programs but also in hospitals, clinics, state or city health departments, and community organizations dedicated to HIV infection. To find a case manager, ask if your hospital employs a case manager, and if not, if it will refer you to one. AIDS physicians and social workers will also know the names of the good case managers.

Hospital Care

Many people with HIV infection are admitted to a hospital at some time during the course of the infection. But since 1996, when HAART was introduced, people's need for hospital care has changed greatly. Over the following three years, the number of hospitalizations for complications of HIV infection decreased between 60 and 80 percent.

Nevertheless, hospitals remain an important part of HIV care. Patients may or may not have a choice of what hospitals they are admitted to. As discussed in a later section, the choice is largely dictated by the type of insurance they have and the hospitals for which their physicians have admitting privileges.

People are often frightened about going to a hospital—to be sure, hospitals are confusing places. This section discusses hospitals, and their people and practices, in an attempt to lessen the fear and confusion.

Teaching and Community Hospitals

Hospitals differ in the services provided and the style of care. One of the biggest differences is between teaching hospitals and community hospitals. Teaching hospitals are generally larger hospitals that provide on-the-job training for medical residents and often for medical students as well. Teaching hospitals are often affiliated with medical schools, the physicians are often on the medical school faculty, and physicians may be responsible both for patient care and for research programs.

The advantage of teaching hospitals is that their resources for testing and treatment are both extensive and up-to-date. This is important in a field that changes as rapidly as research in the treatment of HIV infection. Teaching hospitals are also more likely to have comprehensive programs for the care of people with HIV infection. This access to comprehensive services is very important to some people with HIV infection and less important to others. Some people need a good AIDS physician who knows the disease well and can give guidance for most of its issues. Other people's cases are more complex, with needs that range from social support, to mental health consultation, to availability of cosmetic surgeons. These latter people might do better in an HIV center, which provides extensive services (see above).

Community hospitals tend to be smaller hospitals with fewer resources and whose staff physicians often have less experience with HIV infection. Nevertheless, many community hospitals have devoted physicians who provide excellent care in an environment less overwhelming than that of a large teaching hospital.

Experience counts, however. Surveys of hospitals caring for people with HIV show that survival is better and the length of stay is shorter in hospitals that treat many people with HIV, compared to hospitals that treat few people with HIV infection. Still, there is no doubt that many of the common complications of HIV infection can be easily managed in a community hospital.

Choosing a Hospital or Care System

For many people with HIV infection, choice of a hospital or care system is limited. Participants in managed care organizations or HMOs are required to use specific hospitals. People from small cities or from rural areas often have only one hospital near enough to choose. In medical emergencies, a public ambulance is required to take the patient to the nearest hospital, leaving the family and the patient little say in the matter, unless they hire a private ambulance.

In most instances, the physician responsible for the care of the person with HIV infection will make a recommendation depending on which hospital has the resources necessary for that person, and in which hospital the physician has admitting privileges (meaning the physician is allowed to admit and treat patients).

A large teaching hospital might best be chosen by a person who has unusual complications that require specialized services. If you have a strong wish to go to a certain hospital, you should tell your physician. In the event that your physician is not on the admitting staff of that hospital, he or she can transfer your medical care to another physician.

Hospital People and Practices

Both teaching and community hospitals present the patient with a bewildering array of people with different titles offering different services. Hospitals also follow certain practices that may likewise be confusing. To help eliminate some of this confusion, the following are the people and practices a person in a hospital can expect to see.

Physician-of-Record

Your physician-of-record is the physician medically and legally responsible for your care—that is, for all medical recommendations, including decisions about diagnostic tests and about your treatment. Your physician-of-record is most often your primary care physician, but sometimes it is the physician assigned from the hospital staff. Even though you might see nurses and residents more often, the physician-of-record has ultimate responsibility for your medical care. Every person in a hospital has a physician-of-record.

Primary Care Physician

A primary care physician is a general practitioner, a family physician, or an internist. That is, primary care physicians are usually generalists who deal with a lot of different medical problems—high blood pressure, diabetes, wax in the ear, and sinusitis. Primary care physicians are the backbone of managed care organizations or HMOs, and subscribers are invariably assigned to one. Whether in private practice or employed by a managed care organization, primary care physicians may or may not be HIV-savvy.

Residents, Fellows, and Interns

Residents and fellows are physicians who have recently graduated from medical school but who are not yet practicing medicine on their own. Residents are still in residency, that is, they are still in training to obtain their credentials in a specialty, usually in family practice or internal medicine. Most residents receive three years of training. What used to be called "interns" are now called "first-year residents." Fellows are physicians who have finished their residency training and are now training in a subspecialty—for example, infectious diseases. Residents and fellows are found in teaching hospitals that have the credentials for training specialists.

If you are in a teaching hospital, the physicians you are likely to see most often are residents in internal medicine or family practice, and fellows in infectious diseases or some other subspecialty. Their autonomy in making decisions about your medical care varies, depending on their training, the rules of the hospital, and the idiosyncrasies of the physician-of-record.

Specialists

In addition to the physician-of-record, the residents, and the fellows, the other physicians you will see in a hospital are the specialist physicians. Because AIDS affects so many different parts of the body, and because it takes so many forms in so many different people, no single physician can treat all aspects of the disease. Specialists (technically, these are subspecialists) that are most likely to be consulted in HIV infection are neurologists, ophthalmologists, gastroenterologists, obstetricians, dermatologists, psychiatrists, and pulmonary specialists. Each has a specific area of expertise that may be sought by the physician-of-record. In most instances these specialists make recommendations or provide special procedures. The person ultimately responsible for carrying out their recommendations and approving their procedures is the physician-of-record.

Physician's Assistants and Nurse Practitioners

Physician's assistants and nurse practitioners are midlevel practitioners, meaning that their responsibilities lie somewhere between those of a nurse and those of a physician. Midlevel practitioners assess medical problems, order tests, and recommend treatments. They work with varying degrees of independence, depending on state laws, the medical problems they care for, and their relationship with the other health care providers.

Midlevel practitioners often have specialized training in one area of medical care, including care of people with HIV infection. They are especially valuable in highly specialized areas of medical care because they have often acquired, through training and experience, an expertise not usually found among physicians who care for people with many different diseases. Many comprehensive care programs for people with HIV infection rely heavily on midlevel practitioners.

Physician's assistants have two years of specialized training, must pass a board exam every six years, are required to have at least one hundred hours of postgraduate education every two years, and are licensed.

Physician's assistants must practice under the supervision of a physician. They may prescribe drugs in some states but not in others.

Nurse practitioners are registered nurses who have nine additional months of advanced training or have received a master's degree in nursing. Nurse practitioners do much of what physician's assistants do, but they are not required to serve under the direct supervision of a licensed physician.

Nurses

Registered nurses make certain kinds of medical assessments, including assessments of patients' medical conditions, their ability to provide self-care, their psychiatric needs, and their nutrition. Registered nurses also provide psychological support, are responsible for certain types of treatments, and administer medications. Nurses can also be valuable sources of information about your care: ask them questions.

All hospitals are required to have a registered nurse on each unit of the hospital twenty-four hours a day. Each patient in the hospital is assigned a nurse for every eight-hour shift.

Nursing support technicians, licensed practical nurses (LPNs), and nursing aides are paramedical personnel who are less extensively trained than registered nurses and do many of the jobs that were previously done by nurses: these include taking pulses and temperatures, measuring blood pressure, handing out medications, bathing the patient, changing beds, handling bedpans, and dressing wounds.

Gatekeeper

"Gatekeeper" is a new term in health care. Gatekeepers are a common feature of managed care organizations or HMOs. They make decisions about access to such specialized and often expensive services as specialty consultations, lab or radiology tests, and, most importantly, hospitalization. Hospital care is by far the most expensive part of health care, so care in alternative settings is a major objective. Gatekeepers are often primary care physicians, but might also be other health care professionals like physician's assistants or nurses.

Social Workers

A social worker is a college graduate either with a degree in social work or with two years of postgraduate training and a Master's of Social Work. Most states require these credentials for a license to practice social work. The actual graduate training is primarily devoted to counseling. In a hospital, a social worker's primary role is to help people plan what to do when they leave the hospital. These plans, called discharge plans, include making decisions and arrangements for nursing home placement, home care, or outpatient care.

Good social workers also get involved with much more. They arrange for such special services as rehabilitation from injection drug use, treatment of alcoholism, psychiatric care, physical rehabilitation, and contact with community organizations. The job of the social worker usually ends when the person is discharged from the hospital.

Social workers can be found not only in hospitals but also in clinics, in private practice, in community organizations devoted to HIV infection, and working as case managers assigned to an individual person. All U.S. hospitals that receive federal funds must have social workers; this means essentially that all hospitals have social workers, since Medicare and Medicaid fund so much of this country's health care in hospitals.

Information about social workers or case managers may be obtained through the hospital social worker, by referral from physicians, through contact with the local health department, or through the yellow pages of the telephone directory (listed under social workers, therapists, or counseling).

Patient Representatives

Many hospitals have a public relations office with patient representatives who serve as links between the hospital and the patients. Patient representatives have varied jobs: for example, they answer questions about bills, provide translators for persons who speak foreign languages, and provide clothing for those in need. Patient representatives also serve as a complaint department. People with complaints document their concerns in writing, and the patient representative tries to deal with these concerns to the satisfaction of all parties.

Rounds

Rounds is a well-established ritual in medicine in which physicians, nurses, and often other members of the care team go "around" to see the patients every day. At the beginning of the twentieth century, rounds were very formal: a professor at a teaching hospital led a parade of residents, medical students, and nurses through the wards of the hospital, reviewing each patient, writing down the findings, discussing the patient's condition, and making plans. At present, rounds are much more informal. In teaching hospitals, the rounding team usually consists of residents, medical students, and nurses, with or without the physician-of-record. In community hospitals, rounds are simpler and usually involve the physician-of-record and sometimes a nurse. Rounds are traditionally held every morning, although many private physicians find it more convenient to round in the afternoon when test results are in hand and consultants are more likely to be available. Most agencies that fund medical care require that the physician see every patient under his or her care nearly every day of hospitalization.

For the person in the hospital, rounds are an opportunity to ask brief questions about progress and plans. Long discussions with more detailed questions are probably best asked in the more private company of the resident or the physician-of-record.

Universal Precautions

Universal precautions are a set of rules to protect health care workers from certain infectious diseases. Included among those diseases are HIV infection, hepatitis, and any other infectious disease transmitted through body fluids (blood, saliva, urine). All hospitals in the United States are required to practice universal precautions.

Though the rules of universal precaution apply to all body fluids, the major concern is for blood and bloody fluids. The rules require a barrier between the health care worker and the fluid. The barrier rule means that gloves are to be worn when dressing wounds and the like.

It should be emphasized that universal precautions are universal. They apply to all people participating in the care of any patient in the hospital. There are *no* precautions that are special to people with HIV infection. Exceptions are the complications of HIV infection—like salmonellosis, tuberculosis, and shingles—that pose a threat to health care workers. But these infections require the same precautions regardless of HIV status.

The Hospital Bill

The anticipated charge for the average private or semiprivate room in a private hospital is $500 to $1,000 a day (in 2005 dollars), but it can be over $2,100 in such large metropolitan areas as New York City. Intensive care units are usually $2,000 to $2,500 a day. Additional charges include medications, laboratory tests, physicians' fees, and specialized procedures like bronchoscopy or operations. The hospital bill is likely to be long and full of medical jargon with lists of numerical codes for every pill, syringe, gauze pad, and procedure. Physicians' fees are billed separately from the hospital bill, except for Medicaid patients. Insurance companies determine the customary and reasonable charges for both the hospital and the physician and, on that basis, make their payments. Questions about the hospital charges should be directed to the hospital billing office or to the patient representative. Questions about a physician's charges should be directed to the physician. If finances are going to be a problem, the person should inquire about charges for various tests and their alternatives before the tests are done.

Patients' Rights in Hospitals

The medical care system is large, complicated, overwhelming, and bewildering. Everyone who is a patient in the system has a right to have questions answered. Questions about medical care are best addressed to the medical care providers—the nurse or midlevel practitioner or physician. Questions about the medical system itself are best addressed to a patient representative (see above), a patient advocate now in most hospitals and in many of the larger clinics.

People who become patients in the medical care system have specific rights they should be aware of. The following is an adaptation and amplification of the "Patient's Bill of Rights" offered at the Johns Hopkins Hospital in Baltimore, Maryland.

1. The person should expect medical care regardless of race, color, religion, national origin, source of pay, or medical condition. Specifically, no one can be denied care because of HIV infection. Early in the AIDS epidemic, some hospitals and clinics avoided providing AIDS care, on the grounds that treating people with AIDS might deter other people from using that hospital or clinic. Much of this image problem is now in the past, but people with HIV infection should nonetheless be aware of their right to medical care in hospitals.

2. The person should expect to be treated with respect. He or she should be addressed by proper names and not be treated with undue familiarity. He or she has the right to an appropriate response to questions.

3. People should expect privacy and confidentiality in all aspects of their care. This is an especially sensitive issue for people with HIV infection. Privacy and confidentiality have some limits, however. Important diagnoses such as HIV infection or the complications of

HIV infection cannot be excluded from the medical record. Moreover, these medical records are available to those who have a justified need to see them, including physicians involved in the person's care, insurance companies, Medicaid/Medicare, managed care organizations or HMOs, and public health officials. Furthermore, all cases of AIDS are reported, by law, to the Centers for Disease Control and Prevention; and many states require that blood tests that are positive for HIV also be reported to state health departments. Although this is a sensitive issue, we are not aware of a breach of confidentiality that has ever occurred as a result of such reports. And hospitals take seriously their responsibility to protect medical records from people who have no need to see them (see chapter 9 and Appendix B, "Understanding Tests for HIV"). Insurance companies have a justified right to this information and may use it to deny subsequent policies.

4. People should know the physician who is responsible for their care. They have the right to participate in decisions involving their medical care. These decisions should be based on a clear explanation of the medical condition, the proposed procedures, the proposed treatments, and the risks involved.

5. People should expect efficient and courteous attention from all hospital personnel. They should also respect the possibility that other patients' needs might be more urgent.

6. People have the right to be interviewed and examined in surroundings that assure privacy. They also have the right to know the role of any observer and to ask observers to leave. People also have the right to restrict visitors and can do this simply by notifying the nurse or physician responsible for their care.

7. Mentally competent people have the right to reject any form of proposed treatment or diagnostic test. In particular, many people have profound feelings about resuscitation and life support measures like breathing machines or artificial kidney machines. Uncomfortable as this subject is, decisions about life support measures should not be left until the person is too ill to participate in a rational discussion. Preferences about such issues should be discussed candidly, at the appropriate time, and should be documented in the medical record, in a living will, and by assigning a durable power of attorney for health care. This empowerment for life decisions is now mandated by the Patient Self-Determination Act (see chapter 9). In the event that there are no such provisions, and the person is not ca-

pable of making medical decisions, this role is entrusted to a hierarchy of others, starting with a court-appointed legal guardian, then spouse, child over eighteen years, parent, or sibling (brother or sister), in that order (see chapter 9).

8. People may be asked to participate in research projects called clinical trials (see chapter 8, under "Experimental Drugs and Clinical Trials"). Clinical trials can involve people only with their written consent and with the approval of the person's physician. Furthermore, once involved in a clinical trial, the person has the right to discontinue participation at any time.

9. People have the right to unrestricted communication with anyone. This includes physicians, lawyers, clergy, and representatives of AIDS-advocacy groups.

10. People may leave the hospital against the advice of their doctors at any time. They will usually need to sign a form entitled "Discharge against Medical Advice." The implication of the form is that the physician will not be responsible for any harm that results from this action. In addition, the refusal of care by the person or the person's legally authorized representative may, upon appropriate notice, result in termination of the patient-physician relationship. The exception to the discharging-against-advice right is that some states have laws requiring people with certain contagious diseases who are considered potentially harmful to others to remain in the hospital. This may occur with tuberculosis, which is often difficult to control in patients with HIV infection and which is a public health risk. It is conceivable that this ruling could also be applied to people with HIV infection who are known to behave irresponsibly. We are not aware that this ruling has ever been applied in this way.

11. People may not be transferred from one facility to another unless they receive a complete explanation of the need for the transfer and the alternatives to the transfer, and unless the receiving facility accepts the transfer. People who desire transfer to another hospital should notify their physicians, who will make the arrangements. Almost all transfers between hospitals are based on discussions between physicians, usually the physicians-of-record of the two facilities. The admitting office of the receiving hospital must also be involved to assure that the source of medical insurance complies with their requirements.

12. People who are discharged from the hospital have a right to information regarding continuing health care requirements, including

recommendations for medications, nutrition, activity, return to work, and follow-up medical evaluations.

13. The person has the right to inquire about any charges by the hospital, the clinic, or a physician, and to be presented with various options for payment.

What Matters

What matters most for HIV care in the HAART era is to have a physician who is skilled in this disease. In the early 1990s, HIV care was a "primary care disease"; that is, most of the care was done by generalists like family physicians and internists. Medical science frankly had little to offer its patients, so HIV care was adopted as a condition that every doctor should be prepared to treat. In 1996 and 1997, HAART was introduced, and with it came some complex care issues, including a heavy menu of drugs, complex side effects, sophisticated laboratory monitoring, and resistance tests. HIV care was now complicated, the field moved rapidly, and new findings and new strategies for treatment made HIV care a specialty. In fact, it is now estimated that of the 600,000 physicians in the United States, only 3,000 care for 80 percent of the people with HIV infection. These specializing physicians go to the meetings, read the HIV medical journals, and talk to each other. In a sense, HIV care is a little like oncology: the disease is serious, and we have many tools, but their use requires skill and devotion. These are the characteristics that you want your care providers to have.

You also want an insurance plan that covers most of the outpatient pharmacy costs. These costs have now become the largest component of the bill for HIV care—a bill that totals $10,000 to $15,000 per year for most people with HIV infection. The coverage of outpatient medications varies greatly, but it's critical in HIV care. Many people are covered by Medicaid or the Ryan White Care Act Title II funds, though even these have income thresholds. To date, the somewhat fractured U.S. health care system has been generous to people with HIV infection through a number of these entitlement programs. But we are increasingly concerned that this generosity won't be sustained, and in particular, that outpatient benefits might be in jeopardy. In any case, you need to address these coverage issues as early as possible, perhaps with the help of an HIV-savvy social worker.

Chapter 8

Traditional Medicine

- Traditional medicine
- Experimental drugs and clinical trials

In the early years of the AIDS epidemic, medical treatments could do little except relieve unpleasant symptoms. As researchers understood more about HIV—how it infects, how it multiplies—they began to find drugs that slow the infection, and even to understand how to custom-build drugs to attack HIV. The result of their understanding was and continues to be a rapid succession of new drugs to treat HIV itself.

We now know that certain drugs reduce the numbers of HIV the way antibiotics reduce other microbes that cause infections. We know that when the numbers of HIV go down, the immune system comes back. We know that certain vaccines and antibiotics will delay or even prevent the medical complications that accompany AIDS. These drugs and vaccines are part of traditional medicine.

The medical care of people with HIV infection can be divided into traditional medicine and alternative medicine. Traditional medicine is traditional to us in the West—in the United States and the Western world—and is based on specific scientific standards. Alternative medicine has diverse forms: some borrow heavily from Eastern (Chinese, Japanese, or Indian) philosophy; some use methods based on the mind-body interaction; and some are based on nonapproved drugs or diets or other treatments that, measured by the yardstick of the science of medicine, have no established merit.

Most people with HIV infection receive traditional medical care. As many as a third of the people with HIV infection in some large urban areas receive some form of alternative treatment as well. Both traditional and alternative medicine make the same claims: the treatments kill HIV or prevent HIV from reproducing, or strengthen the immune system, or relieve symptoms. People with HIV infection hearing these conflicting claims are understandably confused. The confusion was great in the first ten years after 1986 when AZT was introduced, because it was never clear whether AZT did much to combat the infection. In retrospect, this skepticism may have been justified. The drugs that were related to AZT (ddI, d4T, 3TC, and ddC) seemed to improve people's health when used in combination, but the advantage wasn't great. In 1996, however, the benefit claimed for new protease inhibitors was powerful, convincing, and indisputable. Some people continued using alternative medications, some used a combination of alternative and traditional medicine, and many were simply confused. In the late 1990s, in studies of health, in clinical trials, and in the personal experiences reported in clinics, the benefit of HAART became obvious.

The purpose of this chapter is to discuss the drugs of traditional medicine and their side effects, and—another source of concern for people with HIV infection—how to pay for them. It also explains how drugs are tested to find out whether they are useful and how best to use them.

Traditional Medicine

Traditional medicine is a tightly controlled system of regulations, accreditation, approval, and licenses. Providers of health care—physicians, midlevel practitioners, nurses—must be licensed, and their licenses depend on training, postgraduate education, and certifying examinations. The settings in which health care is provided—hospitals, chronic care facilities, and home care programs—must be accredited by the Joint Commission on Accreditation of Healthcare Organizations (JCAHO). The drugs must be approved by the Food and Drug Administration (FDA), the federal agency responsible for judging the safety and effectiveness of new drugs. The organizations that finance health care (private insurers, Medicaid, Medicare, Blue Cross/Blue Shield) are regulated by agencies of the federal and state governments. (In a way, the financers of health care largely drive the system: they will not reimburse for care by unlicensed care providers, for stays in nonaccredited facilities, or for treatment with unapproved drugs.)

This system of controls is set up to safeguard the public. The controls are meant to stop people or programs or institutions from claiming to offer services or cures that are in fact unnecessary, useless, or unproven.

The health care providers and the health care facilities of traditional medicine are discussed in chapter 7, and financing health care is discussed in chapter 9.

Traditional Medicine's Drugs

Most of the drugs offered by traditional medicine have been tested by a scientific method that starts with studying the drug in a test tube and ends an average of twelve years later after studying the drug in thousands of people (see below, "Experimental Drugs and Clinical Trials"). The results of those tests are analyzed statistically, to see if some apparent benefit is actually due either to simple chance or to "outliers," those rare and exceptional cases that lie far outside the average case. Such analysis is especially important in a disease like HIV infection, because people vary so enormously in the rate at which the disease progresses and in the types of complications they get. Once the test is completed, the results are written up in a manuscript and submitted to medical journals. The medical journals send the submitted manuscripts to experts in the field for "peer review," meaning that two or three HIV experts analyze the study to determine whether it can be accepted for publication as is, needs to be altered to become acceptable, or should be rejected outright. Some prestigious journals, like the *New England Journal of Medicine,* reject 95 percent of the manuscripts submitted.

The important part of this process is the rules by which the study was done in the first place. Certain protocols are now standardized for HIV treatment. The number of participants, or sample size, needs to be adequately large. The participants need to be randomized, that is, assigned randomly to either the new drug regimen or the standard drug regimen for comparison. The study must be long enough, usually 24 to 48 weeks. The study's end point—usually measurements of the viral load, the CD4 cell count, and/or the presence of HIV-related complications—needs to be clearly defined. Information about the drugs' safety also needs to be clearly defined.

If the results survive the peer review process, they are published in medical journals and presented at meetings, especially the HIV/AIDS medical meetings attended by 3,000 to 6,000 people whose careers are committed to HIV. This entire process ensures that physicians learn about new treatments and reassess old ones. The process by now has a twenty-year history and has become thoroughly standardized.

A second way that drugs get reviewed is the FDA's regulatory process. The FDA licenses new drugs for sale in the United States. Other countries have similar agencies. The FDA's purpose is to assure the safety and efficacy of new drugs; to let doctors and patients know that drugs sold in the United States are safe, within reasonable and well-defined limits; and to make sure drugs work for selected and well-defined conditions. Safety is always qualitative, since no drug is completely free of side effects. Efficacy must be proved by certain specific outcomes within specific amounts of time.

FDA reviews are tedious, expensive, and time-consuming, but the need to assure safety and efficacy is an incredible demand. For the average drug, the total cost of development is around $1 billion; three thousand patients need to be studied; and the review takes six to twelve months. The length, extent, and cost of this process may be appropriate and necessary for new drugs for non-life-threatening conditions like sinusitis, headache, and joint pain. But it may be unnecessarily rigid and slow for serious conditions that kill people, like AIDS and cancer. Because of this argument, the FDA has developed a fast-track review of drugs for critical medical conditions, including AIDS. By the start of 2006, 21 of 22 drugs submitted in the past twenty years by pharmaceutical companies for the treatment of HIV were approved. The time required for review after submission was generally three to six months, and the sample size required was substantially lower than for other drugs. This fast review process has helped create a rich pipeline of new drugs, thereby drastically improving HIV care. The process remains rigorous, using the same protocols for clinical trial design to establish safety and efficacy.

Approved Drugs

The drugs used in traditional medicine can be classified into *approved* and *unapproved* drugs. An approved drug is a drug that is approved by the FDA and that can be sold to the public (see below, under "Experimental Drugs and Clinical Trials"). Approved drugs are further divided into nonprescription drugs, prescription drugs, and controlled drugs. Nonprescription drugs, like aspirin and cold remedies, can be bought by anyone—that is, they are "over the counter" drugs. Prescription drugs can be bought only with a prescription or with a licensed physician's telephone call to a pharmacy. Controlled drugs, like narcotics and sleeping pills, can be physically addictive and are often subject to abuse. Controlled drugs can be bought only with a special prescription signed by a physician with a special license for prescribing controlled drugs.

Most approved drugs have two names: a generic name, which is usually also the medical name (like pentamidine), and a trade name, which is usually selected by the drug's manufacturer (like Pentam). Drugs that have been patented by a single manufacturer have only one trade name. Once that manufacturer's patent runs out, many manufacturers can make the drug, and each manufacturer now puts a different trade name on the drug. As a result, there can be several trade names for a single generic drug (trimethoprim-sulfamethoxazole is called both Bactrim and Septra).

Unapproved drugs, often called underground drugs, are drugs that are neither approved by the FDA nor in the process of being approved. They are widely taken without prescription by people with HIV infection. They are discussed further below, under "Alternative Medicine."

Types of Drugs Used for HIV Infection

People with HIV infection take three kinds of drugs: drugs against the virus, drugs and vaccines to prevent the complications of HIV infection, and drugs to relieve unpleasant symptoms.

Drugs directed against HIV are called *antiviral* or *antiretroviral* drugs. Antiretroviral drugs come in three groups, defined by how they act against HIV. See also chapter 3.

Nucleoside analogs ("nukes"). This group of drugs attacks HIV by interfering with one of HIV's enzymes, called reverse transcriptase. HIV uses reverse transcriptase to change its RNA to RNA's mirror image, DNA. The viral DNA then becomes part of the DNA of an infected cell like the CD4 cell. So when the CD4 cell reproduces, it produces more HIVs and is itself eventually destroyed. When the nukes interfere with reverse transcriptase, they therefore interfere with HIV's takeover of the CD4 cell's DNA. The first nuke was AZT; it was first tested in 1986 and was approved for use in 1987. Since then, five other nukes have been introduced. They all work the same way, by interfering with reverse transcriptase. The drugs have a letter name, a chemical name, and a trade name (see table 4).

Protease inhibitors (PIs). These were introduced in late 1995. PIs attack HIV at a different place in its reproductive cycle. Once HIV is inside the cell and has taken over the cell's DNA, it uses the enzyme called protease to help make the complete virus. So by inhibiting protease, the PIs inhibit HIV from ever completing the virus's life cycle. The PIs are more potent than the nukes, both in the test tube and in the body (see table 4).

Nonnucleoside reverse transcriptase inhibitors (NNRTIs). As the name implies, these drugs, like the nukes, inhibit reverse transcriptase, but they are not chemically or biologically like nucleosides (see table 4).

Entry inhibitors. A fourth class of anti-HIV drugs, the entry inhibitors, block HIV's entry into the CD4 cell. The first entry inhibitor was enfuvirtide (T20, Fuzeon), approved by the FDA in 2003. Enfuvirtide needs to be injected twice daily. Several more entry inhibitors, to be taken by mouth, are being developed. Many experts feel that this new class of drugs will have an important impact on HIV infection and its management.

Aside from all the antiretroviral drugs, another category of drug taken by people with HIV infection prevents complications. A multitude of drugs prevent the most frequent and serious of the complications, pneumocystis pneumonia. Other drugs prevent other frequent complications such as tuberculosis, toxoplasmosis, and *Mycobacterium avium* complex (MAC). Vaccines prevent influenza and pneumococcal pneumonia. We know that these prevention strategies work, because proper clinical trials have shown that they do. For these complications, we know ways to detect who is most susceptible: for pneumocystis pneumonia, a CD4 count under 200; for toxoplasmosis, a CD4 count under 100 coupled with a positive blood test; for MAC, a CD4 count less than 50; and for tuberculosis, a positive skin test. For these complications, we know which drugs work best. For other complications the picture is cloudier. That is, the evidence that prevention works is less impressive; or the preventive measure has consequences—unpleasant side effects, likelihood of drug resistance, or high cost—that outweigh the benefits.

The third type of drug taken by people with HIV infection provides relief from unpleasant symptoms, including insomnia, anxiety, depression, fever, aches, problems with sleep and appetite, nausea, diarrhea, and pain. These drugs don't cure the problem causing the symptoms, but they do reduce the person's suffering. Relieving symptoms is the strategy used for most noninfectious diseases.

A fourth type of drug is used to treat the side effects of the drugs listed above. For example, the high levels of blood cholesterol that many antiviral drugs cause can be treated with statins. Diarrhea can be treated with loperamide. Sometimes the best treatment is simply to switch drugs, but if the side effect is not serious, if the goals of treatments are achieved, and if the alternative options are limited, our tendency is to press on and continue treatment aimed just at the symptoms of the side effect.

Side Effects of the Drugs

Many of these drugs have side effects, referred to by physicians as *adverse drug reactions, ADRs* for short. The ADRs of most drugs are well known and well defined, based on the experience of thousands of people who took the drug during its clinical trials, and on the experience of everyone who took the drug once it was on the market. Although anyone can develop ADRs, for some reason ADRs are more common in people with HIV infection. For instance, trimethoprim-sulfamethoxazole (Bactrim or Septra) causes ADRs in 10 percent of the people without HIV infection and 50 percent of those with HIV infection.

ADRs are classified as either *allergic* or *toxic*. Allergic reactions mean that the cells of the immune system have recognized the drug as foreign and have responded by causing a rash, a fever, or both—like the rashes that penicillin causes in some people. In allergic reactions, the dose of the drug is unimportant: the immune system will respond similarly regardless of the dose. Serious allergic reactions often imply that neither that drug nor any related drugs should be taken again.

Toxic reactions are caused not by the immune system but directly by the drug itself. An example is the drowsiness caused by Dramamine or other antihistamines or the kidney damage and anemia caused by amphotericin B. Toxic reactions are usually dose-related; lowering the dose will relieve the symptoms.

People usually develop ADRs after they have been taking the drug for one or two weeks. Some people, however, will have a serious ADR after one dose; others will have no ADRs until after they have taken the drug for months or years; some develop ADRs after repeated courses of the same drug. Therefore, ADRs are unpredictable: because a drug was taken once and tolerated does not mean that it can be taken later and cause no ADR.

Sorting out and controlling ADRs will be done by a physician. The physician will either give the person with a suspected ADR what is called a drug holiday—discontinuation of all drugs—or will stop drugs one at a time, starting with those that are most likely to cause ADRs and those that are most dispensable.

Table 9 lists the prescription drugs commonly taken by people with HIV infection, their generic and trade names, their doses, the conditions they treat, and their side effects.

Costs of the Drugs

The costs of the drugs differ, depending on the pharmacy and whether they are generic or trade-name drugs. Nearly all people with HIV infection taking HIV drugs get those drugs from a prescription plan through an HMO, a commercial insurance company, Medicaid, Medicare, or the Ryan White Care Act funds. Few people can afford the full price of these drugs, so some prescription plan is nearly always necessary. Some people prefer mail order pharmacy services for convenience, cost savings, and anonymity. Ask your physician to write prescriptions, when appropriate, for drugs under their generic rather than their trade names. Many drugs required by people with HIV infection still have a patent; these tend to be expensive, usually $2,000 to $10,000 yearly if continuous use is required. The patent protects the exclusive right of the drug company that discovered the drug to sell it. This protection means that the company can charge what the market will bear—even if the drug is easy to make— and is the reason that drugs are so expensive. The situation angers consumers and insurance companies. Nevertheless, patent protection is the reason we have such progress in drug development in this field, the reason people with HIV infection now live fifteen years longer, and the

Table 9. Drugs Commonly Taken by People with HIV Infection

Drug (trade name or abbreviation)	Dose (adult)	Cost/Week or Cost/Dose* (dollars)	Conditions Treated	Side Effects (less frequent side effects in parentheses)
Acyclovir (Zovirax)	Mouth: 200–800 mg 2–5 times/day	25–120	Herpes simplex Shingles	(Rare—kidney damage, headache, rash, nausea, diarrhea, liver disease)
Amphotericin B	Vein: 30–50 mg/day	115	Fungal infections: *Candida, Cryptococcus,* histoplasmosis	Kidney damage, anemia, nausea, vomiting, chills, fever, electrolyte disturbances, metallic taste—sometimes called "amphoterrible" because of the side effects
Ampicillin or Amoxicillin	Mouth: 250–500 mg 3–4 times/day	4	Bacterial infections: sinusitis, pneumonia	Rash, diarrhea
Ativan (Lorazepam)	Mouth: 1 mg 2 times/day	10	Anxiety	Sedation, memory loss, dizziness, incoordination, fatigue, confusion, dependency with long-term use; avoid alcohol and other mind-altering drugs
Atorvastatin (Lipitor)	10 mg/day; increase by 10 mg at 2–4-week intervals	2.50/10 mg dose	Increased cholesterol	Liver disease, muscle disease with leg pains
Atovaquone (Mepron)	Mouth: 750 mg 2 times/day	160	Pneumocystis pneumonia	Bad taste, rash, nausea, diarrhea

(continued)

225

Table 9. (*Continued*)

Drug (trade name or abbreviation)	Dose (adult)	Cost/Week or Cost/Dose* (dollars)	Conditions Treated	Side Effects (less frequent side effects in parentheses)
Azithromycin (Zithromax)	Mouth: 250 mg/day or 1,200 mg/week	30–40	*Mycobacterium avium* complex Toxoplasmosis Cryptosporidiosis	Nausea, vomiting
Benadryl	Mouth: 25 mg/day	2	Insomnia Allergies	Sedation
Bupropion (Wellbutrin)	Depression: 150 mg/day; increase to 300 mg/day Smoking: 150–300 mg/day for 7–12 weeks	1.00/75 or 100 mg dose	Depression; smoking cessation	Agitation, insomnia, anxiety, nausea, weight loss, seizures
Buspirone (Buspar)	Mouth: 5–10 mg 3 times/day	20–40	Anxiety	Insomnia, nervousness, headache, diarrhea, nausea; fewer problems with dependency and other complications compared to benzodiazepines like Valium, Xanax, Ativan, Halcion, etc.
Ciprofloxacin (Cipro)	Mouth: 500–750 mg 2 times/day	50–70	Tuberculosis *Mycobacterium avium* complex	(Rare—nausea, vomiting, headache, malaise, dizziness)

			Common infections: pneumonia, infectious diarrhea	
Clarithromycin (Biaxin)	Mouth: 250–500 mg 2 times/day	50	Myobacterium avium complex; Common infections: sinusitis, pneumonia	Nausea, vomiting
Clindamycin (Cleocin)	Mouth: 300–450 mg 3 times/day; Vein: 600–900 mg 3 times/day	50–70; 300	Pneumocystis pneumonia; Toxoplasmosis; Bacterial infections	Diarrhea (rash, nausea)
Clotrimazole (Lotrimin, Mycelex)	Mouth: 10 mg troche 4–5 times/day	25	Thrush	(Rare—nausea, vomiting, liver damage)
Dapsone	Mouth: 100 mg/day	1	Pneumocystis pneumonia	Fever, rash, nausea, low white blood cell count, anemia that may be severe
Dronabinol (Marinol)	Mouth: 2.5 mg 2 times/day	40	Wasting	Euphoric "high," paranoia, sleepiness, mood changes, dizziness, nausea
Erythromycin	Mouth: 250–500 mg 4 times/day	4	Bacterial infections: pneumonia, sore throat, sinusitis; Anemia	Nausea, vomiting

(continued)

Table 9. (*Continued*)

Drug (trade name or abbreviation)	Dose (adult)	Cost/Week or Cost/Dose* (dollars)	Conditions Treated	Side Effects (less frequent side effects in parentheses)
Erythropoietin (EPO)	Injected under skin: 6,000 units 3 times/week	220	Anemia	(Rare)
Ethambutol (Myambutol)	Mouth: 400 mg 3 times/day	20	*Mycobacterium avium* complex Tuberculosis	Eye problems in 1%—report changes in vision and color immediately
Feeding supplements	Mouth: 4 cans/day	50	Malnutrition	(Rare—diarrhea, supplements taste bad)
Finofibrate (Tricor)	54 mg/day with increase to 160 mg/day if necessary	1.00/54 mg tablet dose	Increased triglycerides	Liver disease, flu-like symptoms, muscle pain
Fluconazole (Diflucan)	Mouth: 50–200 mg/day	30–100	Cryptococcal meningitis Candidal infections	(Rare—rash, nausea, vomiting, liver damage)
Fluoxetine (Prozac)	10–40 mg/day	2.60/10 mg dose	Depression; obsessive-compulsive disorder	Nausea, anxiety, dysfunctional sex, dry mouth
Foscarnet (Foscavir)	Vein: 90–120 mg/day	500	Cytomegalovirus infections	Kidney damage, electrolyte problems with tremors, tingling, seizures (Rare—ulcers on penis)

Drug	Dose/Route		Indication	Side effects
G–CSF (Neupogen)	Injected under skin: 1–50 mcg/day	130–170	Low white cells	(Bone pain)
Ganciclovir (Cytovene)	Vein: 350–700 mg/day Mouth: 1 g 3 times/day	160–210 300	Cytomegalovirus infections: retina, lungs, intestine	Reduced white blood cells predisposing to infections, headache, low platelets predisposing to bleeding (Rare—liver damage, mental changes, seizures)
Gemfibrozil (Lopid)	600 mg 2 times/day	1.25/600 mg dose	Elevated blood lipids	Gallstones, gallbladder disease, stomach intolerance
Growth hormone (Serostim)	Injected: 6 mg/day	1,200–1,600	Wasting	Joint pain, low blood sugar
Halcion (Triazolam)	Mouth: 0.25 mg/day	5	Insomnia	Sedation, along with memory loss, fatigue, confusion; dependency with long-term use
Haloperidol (Haldol)	Mouth: 2 mg 2 times/day	2	Delirium	Lethargy, drooling, involuntary movements, lack of coordination
Interferon (Roferon A, Intron A)	Vein: 10–20 mil units/day or 3–10 mil units 3 times/wk (hepatitis)	90–1,000	Kaposi's sarcoma Hepatitis B Hepatitis C	Flulike illness, fever, fatigue, headache, muscle aches, depression, confusion, nausea, vomiting, abdominal pain, low white blood cell count, low platelets, rash, hair loss: all are dose-related

(continued)

Table 9. (*Continued*)

Drug (trade name or abbreviation)	Dose (adult)	Cost/Week or Cost/Dose* (dollars)	Conditions Treated	Side Effects (less frequent side effects in parentheses)
Isoniazid (INH)	Mouth: 300 mg/day	0.15	Tuberculosis	Nausea, vomiting, liver damage (headache, rash, dizziness)
Itraconazole (Sporanox)	Mouth: 100–200 mg 1–2 times/day (liquid or tablets)	30–120	Fungal infections: *Candida*, histoplasmosis, cryptococcosis	Nausea, vomiting (Rare—hepatitis, rash)
Ketoconazole (Nizoral)	Mouth: 200–400 mg/day	15–30	Candidal infections, esp. thrush	Nausea, vomiting (liver damage, reduced libido, menstrual problems, headache, dizziness, itching, rash)
Levofloxacin (Levaquin)	Mouth: 500 mg/day	50	Pneumonia, sinusitis	(Nausea, vomiting, diarrhea)
Lomotil	Mouth: 5 mg 4 times/day	25	Diarrhea	(Rare)
Megace (Megestrol)	Mouth: 80 mg 4 times/day	60	Wasting	(Rare)
Metronidazole (Flagyl)	Mouth: 750–2000 mg/day	1	Gingivitis Other infections	Nausea, vomiting, metallic taste, headache (painful feet and legs with prolonged use, reaction with alcohol withdrawal)
Nortriptyline (Aventyl, Pamelor)	Mouth: 25–75 mg/day	6–16	Peripheral neuropathy Depression	Dry mouth, blurred vision, sedation, fatigue, anxiety, decreased libido, dizziness, involuntary movements

Nystatin (Mycostatin)	Mouth: gargle 500,000 units 4 times/day	10	Thrush	(Rare—nausea, vomiting, diarrhea)
Oxandrolone (Oxandrin)	Mouth: 2.5 mg 2–4 times/day	10–200	Wasting	Masculinizing of women; liver toxicity
Pegylated interferon (Pegasys, Peg Intron)	180 mg/day (Pegasys); 1.5 mg/kg of person's weight (Peg Intron)	364/180 mg dose	Hepatitis B or C	See Interferon
Pentamidine (Pentam)	Aerosol: 300 mg/month	25	Pneumocystis pneumonia prevention	Aerosol: Cough (Rare—asthma reaction)
	Vein: 200–300 mg/day	500–700	Pneumocystis pneumonia treatment	Vein: Kidney damage, nausea, vomiting, low blood sugar, low blood pressure with fainting, rash, anemia, low white cell count predisposing to infection
Pravastatin (Pravachol)	40 mg/day; may be increased to 80 mg/day	2.80/10 mg dose	Elevated blood lipids	Muscle pains, liver toxicity, nausea, heartburn
Prednisone, Cortisone	Mouth: 20–80 mg/day	1–3	Severe pneumocystis pneumonia / Aphthous ulcers / ITP / Kidney failure	Side effects are dose- and duration-related: infections due to same organisms found in late stage HIV infection, euphoria or depression, skin bruises, round face

(continued)

Table 9. (*Continued*)

Drug (trade name or abbreviation)	Dose (adult)	Cost/Week or Cost/Dose* (dollars)	Conditions Treated	Side Effects (less frequent side effects in parentheses)
Prozac	Mouth: 20 mg/day	15	Allergic reactions Depression	Nervousness, dry mouth, insomnia, nausea, constipation
Pyrazinamide	Mouth: 1,000–2,000 mg/day	30	Tuberculosis	(Rare—liver damage, joint pain, nausea, vomiting, increased uric acid: gout)
Pyrimethamine (Daraprim)	Mouth: 25–100 mg/day	3–7	Toxoplasmosis	Must take folinic acid (Leukovorin) to prevent anemia (Rare—anemia, low platelets, low white blood cells predisposing to infection)
Ribavirin (Rebetol, Rebetron)	800–1,200 mg/day	10/200 mg dose	Hepatitis C	Anemia, cough, stomach problems
Rifabutin (Mycobutin)	Mouth: 300 mg/day	50	*Mycobacterium avium* complex prevention; prevention of tuberculosis	Same as rifampin (see below); with high doses, eye inflammation
Rifampin (Rifadin)	Mouth: 600 mg/day	30	Tuberculosis	Orange discoloration of tears, urine, sweat (Rare—liver damage, rash); causes liver to eliminate some drugs faster, so doses of those drugs must increase; one of these drugs is methadone—and consequence can be

232

		withdrawal symptoms—and another is birth control pills

Drug	Dose	Cost	Indication	Side effects
Sulfonamides	Mouth: 2–8 mg/day	1	Toxoplasmosis / Nocardia	Rash, fever, liver damage, low white blood cell count, nausea, vomiting
Testosterone	Injection: 200 mg every 2 weeks / Patch: 4–6 mg/day	8	Wasting	Acne, enlarged breasts, skin flushing, increased libido
Thalidomide	Mouth: 100–300 mg/day	40	Wasting / Aphthous ulcers	Severe congenital abnormalities when given to pregnant women
Trimethoprim	Mouth: 750–1,400 mg/day	1	Pneumocystis pneumonia	Nausea, vomiting, rash (Rare—anemia, low white blood cell count)
Trimethoprim-sulfamethoxazole (Bactrim, Septra)	Mouth: 1 DS/day	1	Pneumocystis pneumonia prevention	Nausea, vomiting, fever, rash, low white blood cell count, liver damage: all are dose-related
	Mouth: 6 DS/day	3	Pneumocystis pneumonia treatment	
Xanax (Alprazolam)	Mouth: 0.25 mg 2 times/day	7	Anxiety	Sedation, lack of coordination, memory loss, fatigue, confusion, dependency with long-term use

*The cost figure is the approximate wholesale price of the indicated drug for 2005; the cost to the consumer will usually be higher.

reason they're likely to live even longer in the future. Once the drug goes off patent, the price drops precipitously. AZT, for instance, went from $12 per day to $.50 per day in one month. The cost of the standard therapy, Highly Active Antiretroviral Treatment (HAART), is $10,000 to $15,000 yearly. Many people question our ability as a society to pay this high price, especially with 800,000 candidates for the therapy. One method to evaluate price is by cost-effective analysis—a method by which we can compute the amount of money required to preserve life for one year. Computing the cost of a year of life preserved balances all costs of tests, treatment, hospitalization, medication, and physicians' fees. For treatment in the HAART era, the cost is $15,000 to $20,000 per year of life preserved. By comparison, the cost of a year of life preserved for mammography is $40,000, and for coronary bypass, it is $113,000 per year of life preserved. The point is that on the basis of other well-accepted, standard treatments, the cost of HAART seems justified.

Paying for the Drugs

The question of who pays for drugs is complicated and controversial. All insurers, public or private, differ in whether they pay for drugs, how much they pay, and which drugs they pay for. Medicaid and the Veterans Administration both provide coverage for prescription drugs; Medicare, through its prescription drug plans, covers only some drugs. Commercial insurance companies' plans and Blue Cross/Blue Shield's plans vary in their coverage. Medicaid is a state-based program, so that coverage depends to some extent on where you live. In New York and Maryland, coverage is generous; in most southeastern states, coverage is frugal. The Ryan White Care Act (Title II) funding for medications is also state-based, and again, availability and the extent of coverage depend on where you live. Title II has three criteria for access: limited income and assets, lack of an alternative source of payments, and a formulary that includes the requested drugs.

In general, where Medicaid has frugal coverage, the Title II funds will be not be extensive because a frugal Medicaid plan places demands on the Title II funding. The frugal states have people waiting for access to Title II support, and drug availability is limited.

The companies and plans that do cover drugs sometimes put limits on their coverage. They will pay only for FDA-approved drugs. Nonprescription drugs and drugs used in alternative treatments are not covered by any insurer.

For more information on what insurers do and do not pay for, see chapter 9.

Experimental Drugs and Clinical Trials

Drugs become accepted by physicians and the FDA on the basis of scientific proof of their effectiveness and safety. Scientific proof is obtained through a series of tests called a *clinical trial*. A clinical trial involves the combined efforts of the pharmaceutical company that makes the drug; the independent investigators who test the drug; and the FDA, which licenses the drug. Testing drugs through clinical trials has been standard for over four decades and has provided the foundation for most of the recommended treatments in traditional medicine.

While a drug is being tested in a clinical trial, it is considered experimental. If the drug proves effective and is not too toxic, it is then licensed and made available to the public.

For people with HIV infection, participating in clinical trials has both advantages and disadvantages. Clinical trials are experiments with human lives, and special safeguards are necessary to guard both the people and the scientific procedure. These safeguards, plus the options and aspects of participation in a clinical trial, are spelled out to the participant in painstaking detail. Some trials can be seen as especially risky: they involve taking a drug with unclear benefit in place of a standard drug with established merit. With other trials—for instance, the comparison of two drugs, both of which are known to work, to find out which works better—the risk is lower. The motivation to participate is an individual decision. For further discussion, see below, "Advantages of Participating in a Clinical Trial" and "Disadvantages of Participating in a Clinical Trial."

Anyone worried about the safety of a clinical trial can be reassured that the trials are conducted under the strict supervision of the FDA with substantial safeguards (see below, "Supervision of Clinical Trials"). If the drug being tested proves significantly better or worse than the drugs in standard use, the trial is promptly discontinued. Moreover, a standing rule in all clinical trials is that participants may withdraw from the trial at any time.

The Steps of a Clinical Trial

All drugs used for medical therapy in the United States must first be reviewed and approved by the FDA. The FDA is responsible for assuring that all drugs, before they are sold, are sufficiently safe and effective. Accordingly, the FDA dictates that certain steps be followed from the time a drug is discovered until it is finally licensed. The process of testing drugs has several stages: a drug is tested first in the test tube and in animals, then in a few people for a short time, and then in a larger group of people for a longer time.

Preclinical trials. A new drug is first tested not in people but in test tubes and in animals. These first tests are called preclinical trials because they precede tests with people, which are called clinical trials. Preclinical trials determine the drug's toxicity, its pharmacologic properties, and its effects against certain microbes. Of all the drugs tested in preclinical trials, only about one drug in a thousand is ever tested in people.

If a drug shows promise in the preclinical trials, the FDA grants it the status of an Investigational New Drug (IND). IND status must be granted before the FDA allows the drug to be tested in humans.

Phase one clinical trials. Phase one clinical trials are the first round of tests in humans. Phase one trials are designed to determine the safety and dosage of a new drug. These trials usually involve a relatively small number of people, usually between 20 and 80. The drug is given only for a short time, usually for not more than a few weeks, and sometimes only a single dose is given. Participation in a phase one trial may require staying in a research unit of the hospital, or the participant may visit an outpatient clinic, which carefully monitors the trial. Participants in a phase one trial don't benefit much when the trial is for an infection like HIV because the treatment lasts for such a short time. Therefore, people who participate in phase one trials are often paid for their services, or else they participate for entirely altruistic reasons.

Phase two clinical trials. Phase two clinical trials are the second round of tests in people. Phase two trials usually involve 100 to 300 participants and last for months or years. The purpose of these trials is to determine the schedules for doses, to collect additional information on toxicity, and to test, at least preliminarily, the drug's effectiveness. With HIV infection, the effectiveness of a drug may be determined by the effect on CD4 cell counts, by the numbers of HIV in the blood, by the delay in progression of disease as indicated by medical complications or development of AIDS, and by how the participant feels. People often participate in phase two trials for access to the drug before licensing. Or if the trial is relatively short and benefits to the participant relatively brief, people participate for payment or altruism. With some studies, the distinction between phase one and phase two is blurred, and the resulting classification is phase one/two.

Phase three clinical trials. Phase three clinical trials are the last phase before the FDA reviews a drug for licensing. Phase three trials often include 2,000 to 3,000 or more participants and run for months or years. In this phase, the drug is given to participants in the doses and at the intervals that the FDA is likely to consider acceptable. The purpose of these trials is to get additional information about the safety and effectiveness of the drug. People usually participate in phase three trials for access to the drug before licensing.

NDA review. The next step is to take all the information gathered during the previous steps and submit it in a New Drug Application (NDA) to the FDA. The FDA reviews the NDA and decides whether to license the drug, what the dose should be, how the drug should be administered, which side effects require specific warnings in promotional material, and what conditions the drug is useful for. This and other information is available in the *Physicians' Desk Reference,* or *PDR.* The *PDR* is published each year and is available in most bookstores for $50 to $60. There is also an edition for nonprescription drugs, like ibuprofen, cold remedies, or Dramamine, called *PDR for Nonprescription Drugs.*

It should be noted that the FDA approves drugs for the specific conditions indicated in the package insert and in the *PDR.* Despite this labeling, once a drug is in pharmacies, it may be prescribed for any medical condition. Some physicians are reluctant to prescribe beyond the labeling limits for fear of malpractice suits. The FDA acknowledges the limitations of its labeling, and most physicians believe that "standards of practice" should be the guide. Another potential problem is that some third-party payers limit reimbursement coverage to FDA indications. Such decisions are unusual because most third-party payers do not know a person's medical condition when he or she is an outpatient. When limitations are imposed, it may be possible to appeal the decision. But an appeal requires a fight with bureaucrats who often know little medicine and are paid to keep costs low.

Phase four trials. Phase four trials may be conducted after the drug is licensed in order to determine new dosing schedules, or to collect additional information about effectiveness or toxicity, or to compare the drug to other drugs. People participate in phase four trials of drugs, even though the drugs are already available in the marketplace, in order to have access to the best medical care and (sometimes) in order to receive free care.

Streamlining clinical trials. The process described above has established high standards for determining the safety and effectiveness of new drugs. Unfortunately, the process is also expensive and time-consuming. The average new drug in the United States costs $1 billion to develop and requires an average of twelve years to move from the laboratory to licensing. The FDA has judged HIV/AIDS to be a life-threatening infection for which drugs are necessary. Therefore, the FDA reduces its licensing requirements and uses its fast track to expedite the process: this means that the FDA examines the IND and the NDA more rapidly, the phase three trials require fewer participants (around 300 instead of the usual 2,000 to 3,000), and some drugs are approved at a relatively early stage using criteria that would have been unacceptable in prior years. Drugs also are made available earlier in the testing process through a mechanism called a Treatment IND. Under the Treatment IND classification, the drug can be prescribed by physicians other than the investigators between the time the trial is completed and the time the FDA reviews the complete NDA application.

AZT was the first drug to be evaluated under some of the provisions of this streamlined process. The phase two trial began in February 1986; in September 1986, the first analysis of data showed the drug was clearly beneficial; the drug was then made available to people with AIDS through a Treatment IND, and the drug was licensed in March 1987. The entire process took thirteen months instead of the customary twelve years. The drug was approved based on studies of 282 patients instead of the usual 2,000 to 3,000 patients.

Participating in a Clinical Trial

Most trials are comparisons of one drug versus no drugs, one drug versus another drug, or different doses of one drug. Participants in a clinical trial usually have to meet a specified requirement—they must have a certain CD4 count, for instance, or a certain complication. These requirements are adhered to strictly. Though such strictness is frustrating to both the investigator and the potential participant, it is necessary for the trial to be a valid test of a drug and for the FDA to approve the drug.

Once in the trial, participants are assigned to groups called *treatment arms*. What the treatment arms are depends on what the trial is testing: one treatment arm might be high doses of a drug and another arm low doses; one arm might be one drug and the other arm another drug; one arm might be one drug and another arm no drug at all. In trials involving two or more arms, the participant is assigned to a treatment arm randomly, like flipping a coin. Random assignment is a process over which neither the participant nor the investigator has any control. This is necessary if the trial is to be scientifically credible.

The purpose of a trial is to compare one treatment arm with another. Some trials, called *placebo control trials*, compare a drug with a placebo, a pill that has no effect on the body. Placebo trials are done because people taking any pill, including a placebo, feel better—not necessarily because of the physiological effect of the drug, but because of the psychological effect of taking a drug that might help. For example, 60 percent of the people treated with any drug, placebo or not, for arthritis claim that it improves their symptoms. The necessity for a placebo trial is less when the effects being evaluated are objective: weight, blood counts, tests for the virus, or frequency of medical complications. Some effects, however, are more subjective and cannot easily be measured by scientific yardsticks: the sense of well-being, the level of fatigue, the number of headaches. For these more subjective effects, a placebo control trial is more important. In most trials, the results of a trial are evaluated in terms of both subjective and objective effects.

It should be emphasized that the rule of clinical trials is that, if a drug is known to work, no treatment can be a placebo; in that case, the drug known to work becomes the standard for comparison. Furthermore, once the trial shows a clear benefit, the trial must stop. Thus, in the AZT trials, when the analysis of data in September 1986 showed nineteen deaths in the placebo arm and only one death in the arm receiving AZT, the trial was promptly stopped and everyone was given AZT. Assurance on this point is a matter of medical ethics.

The best way to make the comparison in any trial is to double-blind. Double-blinding means that neither investigator nor participant knows which drug or which dose the participant is receiving. Since both investigator and participant are likely to have biases, double-blinding ensures that results will be evaluated objectively.

Although double-blinding is preferred, in some instances it is simply not realistic. For example, when the trial is to find out which way to administer the drug, by pill or by vein, proper double-blinding would have one treatment arm receive the drug by vein and a placebo by pill, and the other treatment arm receive the drug by pill and placebo by vein. But receiving a drug intravenously is inconvenient and can be risky, and it might be inappropriate for participants to receive placebo by vein simply to maintain the blind.

Not all trials are comparisons: some trials, called *pilot trials* (like pilot TV shows), simply gather enough background information to see if a larger trial would be justified. Other trials compare a new drug with an old drug tested previously—called a historical control. Many times, in an effort to gather additional information, the drug is just given with no second arm for comparison.

Advantages of Participating in a Clinical Trial

The advantages of participating in trials usually include the following:

1. New drugs: Usually, people have access to a new and unlicensed drug only by participating in a clinical trial. For people who have had sequential treatment failures and many resistance mutations, participation in a clinical trial is the only way to have access to drugs likely to be effective.

2. Good medical care: In clinical trials, the participant is monitored extensively in order to evaluate the drug's effectiveness and toxicity. The advantage to the participant is the quality of medical care that accompanies monitoring. Moreover, the research groups that conduct clinical trials are usually composed of health care providers who are devoted to controlling this disease and who are important sources of new information. Participants in clinical trials may find comfort in receiving care from health care providers who have such credentials and clear commitment, and who are working at the cutting edge of the field.

3. Free care: Most participants in clinical trials receive drugs and medical care related to the trial free of charge. The costs are usually covered by the research grant that supports the trial or by the manufacturer, who is interested either in FDA approval or in favorable publicity. However, the participant should not assume that all costs of medical care associated with HIV infection are likely to be included. Most trials provide the drug, the cost of monitoring for safety and effectiveness, and the cost of managing toxicity ascribed to the experimental drug. They do not provide the cost of care for any complications of HIV infection. Some trials are designed to provide the drug and the cost of monitoring only if the participants are not covered by insurance.

4. Altruism: The advantages listed so far provide direct benefits to the person participating. Participating in a clinical trial also serves a greater need. Medical scientists, people with HIV infection, and people at risk for HIV infection all need more information about new drugs for treating HIV infection. Even the participant who does not benefit directly will nevertheless make a contribution to the welfare of others with or without HIV infection.

Disadvantages of Participating in a Clinical Trial

Several factors might dissuade a person from participating. The most frequent concerns are:

1. Inconvenience: Many trials require extensive testing and frequent visits to the clinic. These requirements should be clearly stated in the informed consent papers (see below, "Informed Consent for the Trial"). These tests and visits can be an enormous inconvenience to the participant.

2. Risk: Clinical trials are scientific experiments. They are carried out because medical scientists need information about the effectiveness and safety of a new drug, or about the safety and effectiveness of an old drug used in a new way. Some of these drugs are potentially toxic, and although trials never test drugs on humans that have not been first tested extensively in the laboratory and in animals, unanticipated side effects are always possible. The degree of risk obviously varies with different drugs and different conditions.

3. Assignment to the "wrong group": For all controlled and double-blinded trials, there is always the risk that the participant will receive the placebo, the less effective drug, the more toxic drug, or the less effective dose. Some participants attempt to break the blind and find out what drug or dose they are taking through a variety of mechanisms. The investigators understand participants' reasons for doing this, but breaking the blind destroys the scientific credibility of the trials. If enough people break the blind, the trial might as well not be done.

4. Costs: Usually drugs and costs for monitoring are provided at no expense to the participant. Some drug trials, however, expect reimbursement from the participants for the cost of medical care. You will need to establish what costs, if any, are involved before you agree to participate. In addition, if the drug is toxic, you will need to establish who pays the cost of care for any side effects.

5. Restrictions on other options for treatment: Most trials require that someone who is participating in one trial not participate at the same time in other trials. Some trials exclude people who have received other experimental drugs. Other trials prohibit the participant from using certain drugs or from receiving certain treatments. You should carefully review any such restrictions before agreeing to participate in clinical trials. A reassurance: any participant in a trial can withdraw from participation at any time.

Supervision of Clinical Trials

To be sure that the potential benefits of a trial are larger than its potential risk, the FDA requires that all trials be supervised by an independent review panel. This review panel, called the Institutional Review Board (IRB), must be composed of representatives from both the medical field and the nonmedical public. Most IRBs include representatives from law, nursing, medicine, and the clergy, as well as researchers who are expert in clinical trials. This group has the job of watching out for the participants' interests, seeing that scientific standards are upheld, and protecting medical ethics. At periodic intervals during the course of the trial, the IRB reviews the results. Any serious or unexpected toxicity must be reported immediately to both the IRB and the FDA. If the toxicity is serious and is thought to be related to the drug, all participants in the trial must be notified, and the informed consent form must be revised accordingly.

Many trials, and especially those at multiple medical centers dealing with treatments of serious conditions such as HIV infection, are also supervised by a Data Safety Monitoring Board, which scrutinizes the data from the trials every six to twelve months. The Data Safety Monitoring Board, made up of experts in the field who are not involved in the trial, is also privy to unblinded results. This board is different from the IRB because it has access to data from all centers participating in the trial, not just the local center. The board's purpose is to stop the trial as soon as valid results combined from all centers emerge about the drug's effectiveness or toxicity. Six months into the phase two trials of AZT, the Data Safety Monitoring Board's review of the unblinded data convinced it to stop the trial and give all participants AZT. One year into the second big AZT trial, the data showed that the drug was beneficial when the CD4 count was below 500, and that it was less toxic at low doses; the trial was stopped and all participants with low CD4 counts were given low doses of AZT.

Informed Consent for the Trial

The most important safeguard in protecting the rights of participants in clinical trials is the informed consent process. All participants in clinical trials in the United States (and in most areas of the world) are required to sign an informed consent document. In the event that the participant is not competent to sign, this responsibility is assigned to the spouse, parent, an adult child, or a brother or sister (in that order). The informed consent document must also be signed by a witness and by the investigator.

Information in the consent form usually includes the following:

Purpose of the trial. The informed consent document must include an explanation of the scientific question the trial is to answer. It must also include an explanation of why the participant qualifies for the trial.

Procedures. Informed consent must include an explanation of the trial's design, that is, exactly how the trial will proceed. The explanation will include the nature of the treatment arms; the method by which participants are assigned to a specific arm; the requirements for participation, including the number of clinic visits or the duration of hospitalization; the frequency and types of tests that will be done; the amount of blood that will be required; the duration of the trial; and the end point of the trial.

Risks. Informed consent must include an explanation of the drug's side effects, including their anticipated frequency and severity. It is unrealistic to list every possible side effect, or even all of the side effects that have occurred in previous trials. But certainly the most severe and the most frequent side effects should be noted.

Benefits. Informed consent must include a statement of whether the participant has any realistic likelihood of benefiting from participation. Expenses for the drugs or for monitoring, and any payment to the participant, should also be explained.

Alternatives to participation. Informed consent must include the various options people have if they choose not to participate. This generally includes the statement that a decision not to participate will not affect your care. In other words, no one at the center offering the trial will bear a grudge if you choose not to participate.

Confidentiality of records. People with HIV infection are often concerned about the confidentiality of their trial records. Some trials are done without identifiers, that is without the names, addresses, hospital numbers, or Social Security numbers that would connect the data to a specific person. Trials done without identifiers essentially guarantee anonymity for the participant.

Unfortunately, it is often impractical and undesirable for clinical trials that collect clinically useful data over a prolonged period to be done without identifiers. The next best option to guarantee confidentiality is to keep the records in a locked file with limited access. The FDA and the drug company that sponsors the trial can require access to these locked files, but we are not aware that this access has ever resulted in a participant's name being revealed to inappropriate persons.

In many instances, data obtained in the trial are also recorded in the participant's medical record: such data can be relevant to medical treatment. Occasionally, participants object to what they view as an unnecessary dispersal of sensitive information. The best advice is to read the consent form carefully for an explanation of how data from the trial are handled and who has access to the record. If such an explanation is not included in the consent form, ask for further information.

Further information. No consent form can provide all the information desired by all the participants. And consent forms often include technical information and medical terms that may be difficult to understand. It is expected that most participants will need to discuss any questions not answered or points not clarified with a member of the investigating team. If, either before or after signing the consent form, you have questions about toxicity, alternatives to drugs, possible participation in other studies, or compensation for injury as a result of participation, they should be answered to your satisfaction. You should not sign the consent form until you are satisfied and have no further questions. One option is to take the consent form home and list the questions you have after you have reviewed the form and discussed it with others. In addition, most consent forms include the name and phone number of an appropriate person to contact if the participant has any further questions after participation begins.

Withdrawal of consent. Informed consent continues throughout the course of the trial, but withdrawal of consent at any time is the participant's right. Withdrawal must not have any repercussions for the participant. Withdrawal may not interfere with the availability of care.

Participation. To find the nearest clinical trial, call the hotline of the federally sponsored AIDS Clinical Trial Information Service: 1-800-TRIALS-A. The same information is available on its Web site: www.actis .org.

Chapter 9

Practical Matters: Making Legal, Financial, and Medical Decisions

---

- Legal rights and obligations
- Financing medical care
- Using the social service system
- Putting your affairs in order: advance directives

Many people find dealing with the practical aspects of having HIV infection almost as troublesome as the infection itself. People worry about money; about confidentiality; about dealing with the legal, medical, and social service systems; about writing wills; about removing burdens from those they love; about the possibility of becoming incompetent. Such questions about practical matters are generally best answered by two categories of professionals.

One category is composed of social workers. Social workers are found in most community agencies that deal with HIV infection: mental health centers, state and local social service agencies, AIDS-advocacy organizations, some churches, and virtually all hospitals. Hospital social workers also understand the medical system and can help you navigate it. Their job is usually to help you make plans for the short term, especially plans for leaving the hospital and returning home (see chapter 7).

The other category is composed of lawyers. To find a lawyer, check with people you know who have lawyers they trust, with your state's bar association, or with local AIDS-advocacy agencies. Related professionals (these are often lawyers, too) handle complaints about discrimination. They can be found in your state's human relations or civil rights commission. Check in the telephone book's yellow or blue pages under the name of your state, or under social service organizations. Or get in touch with the American Bar Association's AIDS Coordination Project, which, among other services, publishes a free, downloadable booklet called *The Directory of Legal Resources for People with HIV/AIDS* from its Web site, www.abanet.org/AIDS/home.html. You can also reach the organization at 740 15th Street, N.W., Washington, D.C. 20005-1009; or at 1-202-662-1030 or 1-202-662-1025.

Legal Rights and Obligations

Federal Laws That Apply to HIV Infection

Section 504 of the Rehabilitation Act of 1973 protects all citizens of the United States against discrimination on grounds of disability. *Disability* includes AIDS, and people with AIDS are consequently protected from discrimination. This antidiscrimination law applies to all service providers and organizations—employers, providers of health care, and providers of social services—that receive federal funds either directly or through state and local agencies. The Americans with Disabilities Act of 1990 extends federal protection against discrimination to all people with HIV infection, whether or not they meet the definition of having AIDS. This law applies to all service providers and organizations, regardless of whether they receive federal funds or not.

Your rights to employment under federal law include protection against discrimination in recruitment, hiring, job assignment, sick leave, or other benefits. You also have the right to request that your employer provide you with reasonable accommodations on the job. Reasonable accommodations are aids, services, and job modifications designed to allow you to carry out the essential functions of your job. For a person with HIV infection, reasonable accommodations may include flexible work hours, rest periods on the job to accommodate fatigue, and time off for medical treatments.

Your rights to health care include protection against discrimination in services offered by hospitals, nursing homes, hospices, or other health care providers. Your rights to social services include protection against discrimination in receiving welfare, Medicaid, Medicare, and other social service programs.

Additional information about civil rights under federal law may be obtained by writing or calling the following (if you phone, be prepared to wait on the line a long time):

U.S. Department of Justice
Civil Rights Division
950 Pennsylvania Avenue, N.W.
Disability Rights Section—NYAV
Washington, D.C. 20530
Voice: 1-800-514-0301
TTY/TTD: 1-800-514-0383
www.ada.gov/adahom1.htm

U.S. Equal Employment Opportunity Commission
1801 L Street, N.W.
Washington, D.C. 20507
Voice: 1-800-849-4230
TTY/TTD: 1-202-663-7002

U.S. Department of Health and Human Services
Office for Civil Rights
200 Independence Avenue, S.W.
Washington, D.C. 20201
Voice: 1-800-368-1019
TTY/TTD: 1-800-537-7697
http://hhs.gov/ocr/

People who feel that their rights under the federal antidiscrimination laws have been violated should file a complaint within 180 days with the Office for Civil Rights, U.S. Department of Health and Human Services, 200 Independence Avenue, S.W., Washington, D.C. 20201; this office will then forward your complaint to the civil rights office in your region. You can also file a complaint online at http://hhs.gov/ocr/discrimhowtofile.html, or by e-mail to OCRcomplaint@hhs.gov. Or you can write directly to your regional office; find the address of your regional office by calling 1-800-368-1019 or online at http://hhs.gov/ocr/discrimhowtofile.html. Complaints should include

• Your name, address, and telephone number.

• If you are filing a complaint for someone else, include that person's name, address, and telephone number.

• The name and address of the organization or person you believe discriminated against you.

• How, why, and when you believe you (or the person on whose behalf you are filing the complaint) were discriminated against.

• Any other information that would help OCR understand your complaint.

The representative of the Office for Civil Rights will begin an investigation. If discrimination is found, the Office for Civil Rights will ask the service provider or organization to correct the complaint voluntarily. If this request is unsuccessful, the service provider or organization may have its federal funding terminated, or other legal action will be pursued. If the complaint is not covered by law, the representative of the Office for Civil Rights will attempt to refer the complaint to the appropriate agency.

On December 1, 1991, the federal government passed a law called the Patient Self-Determination Act. This law requires hospitals to educate every patient admitted into the hospital, into home care, or into a long-term care facility about advance directives. Advance directives include living wills and durable powers of attorney. Living wills and durable powers of attorney are documents written by you when you are mentally competent to provide for your medical care should you become incapable of making your own health care decisions. (See "Putting Your Affairs in Order," below.) The exact advance directives that are available to you depend on which state you live in; the federal law requires only that you be informed of those advance directives that your state happens to recognize. Check with your hospital or your lawyer about which advance directives your state has and which are best for you. Also check with your hospital about their policies about advance directives.

State Laws That Apply to HIV Infection

Most states also have laws that protect their citizens against discrimination on grounds of handicap. Whether HIV infection is included in a state's definition of handicap depends on the state: the laws that apply to people with HIV infection, needless to say, vary from state to state. The state laws against discrimination on grounds of handicap are sometimes different from the federal laws. Some people with HIV infection find it useful to pursue claims of discrimination under either federal or state laws, or both.

(Note: Some laws use the word *handicap;* others use the word *disability.* The two words mean the same thing.)

In general, state laws against discrimination govern such issues as your right to public accommodations, your right to housing and employment, your right to confidentiality, and your medical rights.

Your right to public accommodations. Public accommodations are more important than they sound. A public accommodation is any place open to and serving the public. Exactly which places are defined as public accommodations vary from state to state: some states include doctors' offices, for instance, and some do not. Depending on the state, then, public accommodations can include schools, doctors' offices, hospitals, hospices, barber and beauty shops, nursing homes, funeral homes, public transportation, restaurants, and hotels. Any place defined as a public accommodation cannot discriminate according to race, sex, creed, color, or (depending on the state) handicap. In most states, AIDS is defined as a handicap. In some states, having HIV infection but not AIDS may also be defined as a handicap.

Although all laws governing the right to public accommodations are similar, they will differ in detail according to the state. In some states, for instance, beauty shops are not allowed to treat someone with a contagious disease, and since HIV infection is contagious, those states could conceivably bar a person with that virus from a beauty shop. This is, however, an obviously unrealistic use of the word *contagious,* since the type of exposure that occurs in beauty shops carries no risk of transmitting HIV.

To find out the laws in your state, ask a lawyer. Lawyers can also draw up wills and help sort out problems with the Social Security system and with insurance companies.

Another source of information about discrimination is an agency called, in some states, the state human relations commission, and in other states, the state civil rights commission. If you think you have been denied public accommodations because of your HIV status, file a complaint with the state human relations or civil rights commission, and they will investigate. You will not need a lawyer to file a complaint. You will, however, need to be a pest, because agencies move slowly. You also need to remember that filing such a complaint will involve giving up the confidentiality of your HIV status.

Your rights to housing and employment. Your rights to housing and employment are the same as your right to public accommodations. In general, you have a right to whatever housing you can afford and whatever job you can carry out. In most states, refusing someone housing or employment because they have AIDS is illegal. Most states have laws forbidding discrimination on grounds of disability; and, in most states, AIDS is defined as a disability. Whether HIV infection is also defined as a disability depends on the state: ask a lawyer. Therefore you may not be refused housing because of the disabling effects of AIDS. As long as you can carry out your job, you may not be refused employment or fired because of the disabling effects of AIDS.

You also have a right to expect your employer to make reasonable accommodations to your disability. If your job involves heavy lifting, for instance, and you tire easily, you can ask your employer to reassign you to a less strenuous job. The general principle is that you have a right to expect your employer to modify your job in ways that do not compromise your usefulness to the job. Again, as with public accommodations, if you think you have been forced out of a job or housing because of your HIV status, file a complaint with the state human relations or civil rights commission. If the complaint involves employment discrimination, and if you win, you are entitled to back pay, attorney's fees, and damages.

Your right to confidentiality, your right to privacy, and your obligation to disclose. The Health Insurance Portability and Accountability Act, or HIPAA, states that your medical record, including your HIV status, is confidential. Your physician must protect your confidentiality; physicians can disclose information about patients only under certain conditions. In fact, except for physicians, no one with access to your HIV status—laboratory staff, hospital staff, nurses, secretaries—is allowed to reveal your name. Your name can be revealed only if you sign an authorization (unless for some reason your records are subpoenaed). The one exception, as stated below, is that some states require physicians to report all cases of certain diseases, by name, to state health departments. Otherwise, revealing your name without signed authorization is grounds for suit. If your name has been revealed, you can bring a civil lawsuit against the person who revealed it. If the person was a physician, the state board that licenses physicians and the physician's professional society can review the incident.

As with any law, your right to the confidentiality of your medical records has conditions. When you apply for insurance, you usually authorize the company to request release of your medical records. Your HIV status must be included in those records: medical records are, by definition, complete medical records.

If you check into a hospital, you implicitly authorize access to your medical records by all your health care providers at that hospital, including other physicians, nurses, dentists, social workers, and physician's assistants. If your physician refers you to a specialist and you accept the referral, you implicitly grant the specialist access to your medical records.

If you apply for a job, depending on the state, your prospective employer might be able to request your medical records, but your records will be released only if you authorize it in writing. Prospective employers may not require you to authorize release.

Physicians must report every case of AIDS they treat to the state public health department. Some states require physicians to report all blood tests positive for HIV infection. Most states require that this reporting be done either by name or by such other identifiers as Social Security number. The state public health departments are prohibited from revealing your name. In the unlikely event that your name is revealed, most states give you some sort of legal recourse—to a lawsuit, for instance. States are required to report cases of AIDS to the federal government, but to report the cases as statistics, not by name.

HIV infection also confers certain obligations on you. You have a moral and legal obligation to notify anyone you have put at risk for contracting HIV infection. In general, this includes sex partners and people with whom you have shared needles. Health care workers might be obliged to inform the institutions in which they work. If you refuse to notify those you have put at risk, or continue to place others at risk without due warning, they can sue you.

If you refuse to inform anyone you put at risk for infection, your physician may be required to inform him or her. The American Medical Association has advised physicians of that obligation. In many states, the physician's obligation to inform is law; other states may leave it to the discretion of the physician. Thus, whether your physician is required to reveal your name and diagnosis without your authorization depends on the circumstances and varies from state to state.

Once the obligation to inform those placed at risk is discharged, however, you have no further legal or moral obligation to tell anyone else about your HIV status. You have no obligation to tell your employer, your landlord, your psychologist or psychiatrist, your family, your friends, your co-workers, or your neighbors. Lawyers often advise their clients who have HIV infection to tell as few people as possible. Except for those whom you are obliged to tell, tell only the people you love and who will help you and respect your privacy. No one else needs to know.

Your medical rights. One of your principal medical rights is to informed consent. That is, you have a right to an explanation of any treatment or procedure before it is performed on you, an explanation of the risks of that treatment or procedure, and an explanation of the alternatives to that treatment or procedure. "Treatment or procedure" means any drugs, any tests, researches, or surgeries—anything that involves something foreign entering your body. "Risks" means material risks, that is, anything that can reasonably be expected to happen. Your doctor is not necessarily obligated to inform you of an improbable risk, a one-in-a-million chance.

Informed consent also means that you may refuse any treatment or procedure. Anyone who attempts the treatment or procedure without your consent—assuming you are mentally competent to give consent—can be sued on grounds of battery. You have a right to refuse food and water. You also have the right to refuse medication. Your right to refuse treatments, procedures, or medication can be overruled only if you are incompetent. *Incompetent* means that you are unable to comprehend what you have been told and are therefore unable to make decisions. In principle, the courts, guided by the advice of the physician, decide when someone is incompetent. In practice, the court system takes a long time, and competence is decided by two concurring physicians, one of whom is your physician-of-record.

You may request treatments, procedures, or medication, but you may not demand them. You may request transfer to another physician or different medical facility. You have a right to see your medical records. Your medical records are, however, the property of the hospital. As such, the hospital may dictate under what circumstances and in whose presence you may see your medical records. You have a right to a copy of your medical records. You may not remove the original records from the hospital without the hospital's consent. In accordance with the Health Insurance Portability and Accountability Act, or HIPAA, you have the right to make additions or corrections to your medical records.

Hospitals, as public accommodations, may not refuse to treat you on the grounds that you have HIV infection. Some hospitals, however, limit the kinds of treatment they offer and may refuse to treat anyone who requires services they do not offer. Any managed care organization or health maintenance organization (HMO) to which you belong has a legal contract with you that outlines the rights and obligations of both parties.

In a hospital, you may request to be assigned another physician. If other physicians are available, the hospital is obliged to grant your request.

Some states have laws that prohibit a physician from refusing patients on the basis of race, sex, creed, color, or disability. In most states, HIV infection is defined as a disability. However, many physicians do not consider themselves competent to care for people with HIV infection and will refuse care—rightly—on this basis. Others are simply too busy to accept new patients. The first time you see a private physician, he or she may refuse to treat you. If you have previously been accepted as a patient by that physician for other medical conditions and the two of you have an ongoing relationship, she or he may still refuse to treat you, but may not abandon you. Not abandoning you means that your physician must help you find another physician who can provide the care needed.

Similar rules apply to dental care. Many dentists are uncomfortable caring for people with HIV infection. The ethics of dental practice and most state dental practice acts dictate that the dentist is obliged to provide continuing care to established patients, or at least refer them to another dentist who can provide more specialized care.

A Note on Lawsuits

The right to file lawsuits is a right no one can take away from you. But lawsuits often take years to settle. Some people decide not to file a suit because they do not want to take the time. Others decide not to file because their HIV status would then become public record. Many people go ahead and fight and win suits.

Financing Medical Care

People with HIV infection report that among their biggest worries are the problems of financing medical care. Unfortunately, many of their worries are justified. Although the average medical bill for the care of HIV infection is no greater than the average bill for most other serious medical conditions, people with HIV infection should be prepared for expensive medical care.

The average cost of medical care for HIV infection was about $15,000 per year in 1995 and is still about the same in 2006, even when cost is adjusted for inflation. Where those costs are, though, has shifted dramatically. The major cost in 1995 was hospital care; the major cost in 2006, and for the foreseeable future, is at the pharmacy. The average cost of HAART is $10,000 to $15,000 per year.

One factor that greatly affects the cost of HIV care is the stage of the disease. The stage of the disease means the CD4 cell count and its impact on the need for antiretroviral drugs and for hospitalization. The costs of HIV care are modest in the early stages when the CD4 cell count is above 350 and antiretroviral drugs are not necessary: the only costs at this stage are for office visits and laboratory tests. During the second stage, when antiretroviral drugs become necessary but HIV is not causing any of its complications, the costs are primarily for the pharmacy. The most expensive stage of the disease is the late stage, when the CD4 cell count is below 50 or 100 and HIV-related complications require hospitalization. The costs are especially high when the complications cause long-term disability, requiring substantial time in hospitals and chronic care facilities. In addition, many people in the late stages have intolerance or resistance problems with antiretroviral drugs and need increasingly complex drug regimens with many and newer drugs. The newer drugs always cost more, and the combined cost for HIV drugs alone can double. HIV infection, like many other medical conditions, is characteristically imbalanced: 10 percent of the patients account for over 50 percent of the costs.

The second factor that increases the cost of care is the presence of any conditions other than HIV infection. The co-occurring condition that's particularly important is hepatitis C infection, which has its own costs; it also can indicate substance abuse, which carries substantial costs as well.

The mechanisms for financing medical care in the United States are phenomenally complicated and full of jargon. People finance their medical care either by themselves (called self-pay), or through private insurance, or through publicly funded state and federal programs. Private insurance and public programs are together called third-party payers. Most people finance their care through a combination of self-pay and third-party payers.

Private third-party payers include commercial insurance companies, managed care organizations or health maintenance organizations (HMOs), and the nonprofit conglomerate that is Blue Cross/Blue Shield. The main public third-party payers include Medicare, Medicaid, and the Veterans Administration. Medicare accounts for 17 percent of the financing for all health care in the United States; Medicaid for 10 percent; other government agencies for 14 percent; private insurance for 31 percent; self-pay for 25 percent; and private sponsors for 3 percent. An estimated nearly 46 million Americans are uninsured.

Several aspects of financing medical care are unique to HIV infection:

1. Federal spending accounts for most HIV care. This totaled about $5.5 billion in 2000, divided as follows: Medicaid (federal share is about 60 percent of the total), $2.1 billion; Medicare, $1.5 billion; Ryan White Care Act, $1.4 billion; and VA care, $0.4 billion.

2. Medicaid is the third-party payer for 14 percent of Americans and about 53 percent of those with AIDS. The reason is that this disease has, in recent years, moved more and more into disfranchised populations, including drug users, racial minorities, and the impoverished.

3. Medicare accounts for an increasing number of AIDS patients because many more are now surviving the twenty-nine months required to qualify for disability.

4. The Ryan White Care Act has created a safety net for all people with HIV infection who are impoverished and uninsured. The act covers the lion's share of outpatient care and outpatient medications for these people.

5. Most nonfederal third-party payers will not reimburse the full range of services commonly required for people with HIV infection; services that are reimbursed insufficiently or not reimbursed at all include home care, long-term care facilities, hospice care, and prescription drugs.

For more on paying for drugs, see chapter 8.

The following sections go into what may strike you as tiresome detail about financing medical care. But the more you know about what is standard or required or forbidden, the better you will be able to control your options for financing care.

Private, Third-Party Payers for Financing Health Care

All private, third-party payers—managed care organizations or health maintenance organizations (HMOs), Blue Cross/Blue Shield, and commercial insurance companies—offer two kinds of plans for financing medical care: group plans and individual plans. Group plans are offered by the third-party payer to an employer, and then by the employer to the employees. Individual plans are offered by the third party directly to the individual.

Group plans. Blue Cross/Blue Shield, managed care organizations or HMOs, and a large number of commercial insurance companies all sell group plans to employers. Commercial insurance companies are often national businesses that offer similar group plans to all employers throughout the country. Blue Cross/Blue Shield is a group of 77 not-for-profit, regional insurers who offer different group plans in each of their different regions. Managed care organizations or HMOs, whose rules for group plans are different from those of commercial companies and Blue Cross/Blue Shield, are discussed below.

Group plans held by companies with large numbers of employees usually do not require you to have a medical examination or to submit your medical records. Anyone with HIV infection currently working for a large company with a group plan will be covered by that plan. Smaller companies, however, are more likely to have group plans that require the employers to answer health questions about their employees.

If you are hired for a new job in a large company, the group insurance will often have a rule about preexisting conditions. To rule out people who take out insurance only when they become sick (called having a preexisting condition—see below, under "Individual Plans"), insurance companies sometimes enforce a waiting period—usually a matter of months—between the time of application and the time coverage begins. If you are hired for a new job and you have been diagnosed with HIV infection, the insurance company will usually wait for the period set by the preexisting conditions rule before covering you. This rule applies to all preexisting conditions.

Blue Cross/Blue Shield, which has a group plan offered by many employers, does not usually transfer from one employer to another. Each employer negotiates its own individual contract with the local Blue Cross/Blue Shield company. If you transfer from one employer to another, preexisting condition rules will now apply under the second employer's policy.

The insurer (whether a commercial insurance company or Blue Cross/Blue Shield) always sets limits on what the group plan covers. One of the limits is that group plans generally cover only some fraction of your medical expenses. They often cover around 80 percent of hospital expenses and about 60 percent of physicians' expenses. In addition, most of the Blue Cross/Blue Shield group plans also cover home health care, the majority also cover hospice care, and about 30 percent also cover prescription drugs.

That part of the medical bill left over after the insurer has paid its fraction is called your *co-pay.* Co-pay is done two ways, by co-insurance and by deductibles. Co-insurance is usually stated as a percentage of an annual bill; you are usually responsible for 20 percent of eligible medical expenses each year. After that, the company pays all eligible medical expenses. Deductibles are usually stated as an amount of money that you must pay before the insurance company can be billed: you might pay, for instance, the first $25 of any bill.

A second limit on what group plans cover is that they will pay only for what they consider to be the customary charge for a service. For example, an office visit may be billed at $50, the customary charge (based on area charges by physicians for comparable services) may be $40, and the coverage may be 80 percent of the customary charge, or $32; so your co-pay for this bill will be $18. Customary charges can vary from place to place.

A third limit is not so much a limit as an incentive: some plans from Blue Cross/Blue Shield provide you financial incentives to choose specific "participating physicians" or Preferred Provider Organizations (PPOs). In other words, certain physicians or groups of physicians agree to lower their fees, thereby also reducing the cost to you. In general, however, the group plans offered by both commercial insurance companies and Blue Cross/Blue Shield allow you considerable freedom of choice: you can choose your own physician and hospital.

A fourth limit: most group plans limit—or cap—total lifetime payments at $1 million or $2 million.

A fifth limit is on prescription drugs. Most plans require a co-payment. Many have a ceiling on coverage; if the ceiling is $3,000 per year, this will cover about three months' worth of the drugs commonly needed for HAART.

Most insurers periodically renew their policies with employers. Most policies are conditionally renewable, meaning that insurers can refuse an employer's request to renew the policy only if the insurer refuses to renew all similar policies in that state. This means that an employer cannot be refused a renewed policy because some employees have HIV infection. They may, however, increase the rates charged for coverage of the same services.

In spite of the limits, being enrolled in a group plan through your place of employment is obviously desirable. Because group plans spread coverage over many people, many of whom make few insurance claims, insurers can afford to cover you without requiring that you give evidence of insurability (see below, under "Uninsurability").

Managed care organizations or HMOs also offer group plans. These organizations provide comprehensive services for a fixed, prepaid fee. In other words, when you join a group plan offered by the organization, you pay a flat, fixed fee for all your health care bills, regardless of how much health care you actually get. The good news about the organizations is that they finance nearly all medical care. In particular, Kaiser, the largest HMO in the United States, provides a comprehensive program of services for people with HIV infection.

The bad news about the organizations is that, unlike commercial insurance companies and Blue Cross/Blue Shield, these organizations allow little choice in physicians or hospitals. Because competition among the organizations for employer contracts is fierce, costs must be kept low. Consequently, the organization must carefully regulate hospital admissions, expensive drugs, and expensive procedures and must pre-approve any consultation or procedure done outside the resources of the organization. If your physician refers you to a specialist outside your organization, for instance, the organization may rigorously review the referral and often deny payment. As a result, many participants lack confidence in the quality of the health care providers and are disappointed in the range of services the organization provides. Do not be persuaded by organizations' advertisements that emphasize the services offered; in practice, many organizations choose saving money over offering services.

You can find out the details of group plans by reading the policy or by talking to the claims and benefits office of the insurer that offers the policy. For details about group plans offered by managed care organizations or HMOs, often the best source of information is the other people who use the organization, especially those whose health care needs are complicated.

Continuing group plans if you can't work. A person who has been covered previously under a group plan but who can no longer work, may have the option of continuing in the group plan for eighteen months under the Consolidated Omnibus Budget Reconciliation Act of 1985 (COBRA). Under COBRA, the former employee would pay a premium that is 102 percent of the premium previously paid by the employer—the extra 2 percent is for administrative fees. Some states will pay these premiums for you, to delay Medicaid coverage (see below). Requirements for coverage under COBRA are as follows: COBRA applies only to businesses with twenty or more employees; the former employee must pay the premiums; the former employee must be ineligible for Medicare (see below); the employer must continue the group plan for continuing employees; and the former employee cannot join another plan.

People who are eligible for Social Security disability benefits (see below, under "Help with Income and Medical Bills") when employment ends may obtain eleven months of additional coverage (for a total of twenty-nine months) with the same insurer, although the premium may now be 150 percent for the additional eleven months. And some states have programs that extend COBRA for people with HIV infection.

People who are not eligible for COBRA because they worked for a company with fewer than twenty employees may still be protected under the Continuation of Comprehensive Benefits laws in thirty-five states; the duration of coverage of the employer's group policy varies with different states, and ranges from three to eighteen months.

The alternative to COBRA, if COBRA is not available or if it runs out, is a conversion policy: the former employee converts the group policy to a type of individual policy. Conversion policies cover less than group plans and cost more. Thirty-five states require employers to offer conversion policies to former employees when COBRA benefits run out. Premium rates tend to be high, since most people who buy conversion policies are in poor health. Nevertheless, the person with a serious disease might have few other options, and conversion policies are available regardless of health status or preexisting conditions. The remaining option is an individual plan, which costs even more than a conversion policy.

Individual plans. Individual plans are offered by third-party payers directly to individuals. About 15 million Americans have individual plans; approximately 10 million of them have individual plans with commercial companies, 4 million with Blue Cross/Blue Shield, and 1 million with managed care organizations or HMOs.

Individual plans offer four basic kinds of policies: major medical policies, hospital-surgical policies, hospital indemnity policies, and dread disease policies. The best coverage is under major medical policies: they typically pay for hospital care, physicians' fees, laboratory tests, drugs, ambulance services, and skilled nursing facilities. Hospital-surgical policies pay for hospital and surgical services only. Hospital indemnity policies pay a fixed amount only while a person is hospitalized. Since a typical amount paid is $75 a day, and since the average hospital charge per day is ten times higher, hospital indemnity policies are regarded as a rip-off. Dread disease policies will generally not provide coverage for people who already have the dread disease.

Individual plans have different requirements for eligibility, cover different services, and reimburse at different rates than group plans. Generally, an insurer will cover some percentage of your medical costs if you continue to meet certain conditions: if you pay your premiums; if you have not reached some (usually extremely high) upper limit or cap on expenses; if you ask the company to pay for only those items they contracted to pay for; and if you do not seem to pose to them an unacceptably high risk.

For commercial insurance companies and Blue Cross/Blue Shield, risks are classified as standard, for which the insurer will supply standard coverage at the usual rates, or substandard, for which the insurer will supply coverage at increased rates or will exclude coverage for some medical conditions; if the insurer considers the risk excessive, the application will be denied, and the insurer will supply no coverage (see "Uninsurability," below). For managed care organizations or HMOs, risks are either acceptable or unacceptable: that is, the organizations will either accept you at the usual rate or they will deny your application. For insurers, virtually all people with HIV infection, cancer, coronary artery disease, and diabetes pose unacceptably high risks.

To assess the risk you pose, all private, third-party payers (that is, all private insurers) use similar mechanisms. You must fill out an application, which includes a health questionnaire. Nearly all health questionnaires include questions about HIV infection: for example, Have you ever had AIDS or tested positive for HIV infection? Other questions may ask whether you have or ever had symptoms of HIV infection. Still other questions may be about drug abuse, age, and occupation: these questions are triggers for the insurer to scrutinize the application further. Questions about sexual orientation are also triggers, despite the fact that such questions violate the guidelines of the National Association of Insurance Commissioners.

When you apply for an individual plan, the insurer will request your medical records. Everyone applying for individual insurance must authorize the insurer to request medical records. The insurer might also request a statement, called an Attending Physician Statement, from your physician. Your medical records must be complete, including HIV status. Withholding or falsifying any information on a medical record is grounds for the insurer to deny payment and cancel the policy. Most insurers also require the applicant to take a medical examination.

Whether an insurer can require you to take an HIV antibody test is still a matter of legal argument. Some insurers require HIV antibody tests for all applicants for individual plans; most will require the tests if the answers on your health questionnaire merit the test. California and Washington, D.C., have banned HIV antibody testing for insurance purposes but allow insurers to use CD4 counts instead.

What insurers want to rule out with all these questions and tests and checks is what they call a *preexisting condition*. A preexisting condition is defined by the National Association of Insurance Commissioners as "the existence of symptoms which would cause an ordinarily prudent person to seek diagnosis, care, or treatment," or as "a condition for which medical advice or treatment was recommended by a physician or received from a physician within a five-year period preceding the effective date of coverage." In short, a preexisting condition is a medical condition for which you have received advice or treatment (assuming you are an ordinarily prudent person) from a physician within the last five years. Some insurers will accept an applicant with certain preexisting conditions as a substandard risk; others will deny the application for the same condition.

To be certain the applicant does not have a preexisting condition that has escaped everyone's notice, insurers usually enforce a waiting period—usually a matter of months—between the time of application and the time coverage begins. If, during the waiting period, the applicant shows no evidence of a preexisting condition, the company will accept the application and will pay eligible medical benefits. If you develop AIDS well after you enrolled in an individual plan with the insurer, that company is ethically obligated not to drop you. The company could, however, legally contest that obligation.

The bottom line: An asymptomatic person with a positive HIV blood test does not fit the definition of having a preexisting condition. Insurers nevertheless will often deny the applications for individual plans from people with HIV infection. Some of these denials have been contested in court.

Note that the preexisting condition rule affects people who apply for individual plans with a new insurer. For this reason, people with HIV infection who have a long-time plan with an insurer are often advised to stay with that insurer.

You can find out the details of individual plans by reading your policy or by talking to your insurance agent.

Uninsurability. About 8 percent of the applicants for individual plans are denied. Those whose applications are denied include virtually all people with HIV infection, cancer, coronary artery disease, and diabetes. This and other health-related information obtained by insurers is recorded in the Medical Information Bureau in Boston, an insurance industry clearinghouse. Most people with preexisting conditions will find their access to individual insurance coverage limited unless that coverage comes through what is called an exclusion rider or unless they pay extremely high premiums.

People unable to purchase insurance because of preexisting conditions may have access to high-risk pool insurance at inflated prices. Pool policies are provided in twenty-three states. Requirements for eligibility include residency in the state for at least six months and a notice from an insurance company of rejection, of a high-risk rate, or of an exclusion rider. Problems with the pool policies are that only twenty-three states carry them, that waiting lists are long, and that premiums are high. Information about pool policies can be obtained from state insurance departments.

Another option is the open enrollment policies periodically available in some Blue Cross/Blue Shield plans in thirteen states. Open enrollment means that any applicant, including anyone with HIV infection, is granted insurance regardless of health status. Not surprisingly, the premiums are higher, the waiting period for preexisting conditions is longer, and some preexisting conditions have limits on their coverage.

Public Programs for Financing Health Care

Help with financing health care is offered by both state and federal governments. One kind of help, called Medicaid, is available to those who are indigent; that is, people who are unable to support themselves. The other kind of help with finances is called Medicare. Medicare is an add-on to Social Security benefits. Therefore, if you are over 65 years old, or are disabled by Social Security standards, and if you are eligible for Social Security benefits, you should qualify for Medicare.

Medicaid. Medicaid is a combination of state and federal programs for medical care of those who are indigent. Both state and federal governments therefore dictate the requirements for eligibility and for benefits. Medicaid is the major third-party payer for people with HIV infection. Whether you qualify as indigent, what services are available, and what services will be reimbursed, all vary from state to state. Most state Medicaid programs are moving toward requiring that all members belong to a managed care organization or HMO. The purpose of the requirement is to control costs of publicly funded health care. The benefits covered are variable, especially the benefits for mental health care, dental care, long term care, hospice care, substance abuse treatment.

The definition of indigence is, in general, stringent. It ranges from an income that is 23 percent of the poverty level in South Dakota to one that is 97 percent of the poverty level in California; in thirty-four states, the definition is 50 percent of the poverty level. In other words, if the poverty level is around $7,000 per year for one person, then most states will find you eligible for Medicaid if your income is $3,500 per year or less. Some states have a definition of indigence with a higher income level for people with AIDS; that is, people with AIDS can qualify for financial help from public funds and still be relatively able to support themselves. Some states also have definitions of indigence that are substantially higher for women who are pregnant and for children.

In defining indigence, Medicaid also considers resources you have other than income. To be considered indigent, you may have liquid assets (for instance, a savings account), a car, a house, or other property only if their values are below a certain level. What that level is differs in different states.

Medicaid pays for most medical necessities but pays relatively little for each one, especially for physicians' fees. Depending on the state, it may pay for inpatient services, outpatient services, and time-limited skilled nursing home services. In some states, Medicaid also pays for home health care, private nursing, and drugs. Some states pay for as few as fourteen days of hospital care; some states have no limit. Some have special programs for people with HIV infection. Professional fees such as physicians' bills are usually reimbursed at only a small fraction of the physicians' customary charges. As a result, unfortunately, many physicians do not accept patients who are on Medicaid. Home care, hospital care, and chronic care are also reimbursed at low rates, and some facilities will reject Medicaid patients on similar grounds.

Medicaid restricts payment to drugs that the FDA has approved and sometimes pays only for conditions the drug is specifically approved for. In the case of protease inhibitors, many state Medicaid programs cover all protease inhibitors that are FDA approved. Some state Medicaid programs will cover only some of these drugs. This means that if a clinical trial shows a drug is useful, Medicaid will not pay for the drug until the

FDA has approved it. If the FDA has approved the drug but has not approved it specifically for a certain condition, Medicaid may deny payment until the drug is approved for this condition.

Requiring that recipients join managed care organizations will have a profound impact on HIV care: 53 percent of people with AIDS receive Medicaid, and the reimbursement rate will be a small fraction of the health care costs. The reason for the low reimbursement is the lack of any adjustment of rates for people with AIDS—obviously a high-cost population. This means that most AIDS care units in the United States will have substantial financial losses if they care for people who receive Medicaid.

Medicare. Medicare, unlike Medicaid, is funded entirely by the federal government. The various eligibility requirements and services do not vary from state to state but are uniform over the whole country.

Medicare is primarily for the aged, but it is also for the disabled and those with severe kidney disease. To receive Medicare, you must have contributed to Social Security, but you need not be indigent. Most of the people with HIV infection who are eligible for Medicare are over 65 years old or are disabled. You receive Medicare after applying for Social Security Disability Income (see below, "Help with Income and Medical Bills"). After you apply, Medicare enforces a waiting period of a total of twenty-nine months. During these twenty-nine months, you may also qualify for Medicaid, depending on your income and illness; if so, you will usually but not always lose Medicaid when Medicare finally kicks in.

Medicare pays for hospitalization and physicians at rates that compare with the rates of private third-party payers; it asks you to co-pay for these services. It pays little for long-term care: it will pay for 100 days a year in a skilled nursing facility (see chapter 7). After the 100 days, you must self-pay or spend down until you are eligible for Medicaid.

As of January 2006, Medicare cooperates with pharmacies and insurance companies to pay for drugs. A prescription drug plan is available to anyone with Medicare. Different plans with different pharmacies cover different drugs, offer different discounts, and require different monthly premiums. You sign up for the plan that best meets your needs. More information is online at www.cms.hhs.gov/partnerships/.

Veterans Administration (VA). About 30 million Americans are veterans and are potentially eligible for care through the Veterans Administration, or VA. The VA hospital system is the largest health care system in the United States: it has 171 acute care hospitals, 133 of which are affiliated with medical schools.

Eligibility for the services of a VA hospital includes having spent time in the armed services, plus having a disability connected with that service or an income below the poverty level—for the VA, poverty level is around $18,000 for a couple. Eligibility for HIV services includes only having spent time in the armed services and having an honorable discharge. HIV infection does *not* have to be service-connected.

The VA provides a comprehensive program of services, including hospital care, outpatient care, and medications. The VA does not require any co-pay.

The budget for the VA has not kept pace with the rising costs of medical care, so the VA has made a rigorous effort to reduce costs. The result is a corresponding reduction in services. The best quality of care is provided in the VA hospitals affiliated with medical schools, though most of this care is supervised by medical residents.

Some VA hospitals have comprehensive programs for people with HIV infection. Like most health care, the availability of resources and expertise varies in different locations.

Using the Social Service System

If you have been denied insurance, or if you have exceeded the limits of your insurance policy, you can turn to the social service system. The social service system gives financial help to the elderly, to children, to the poor, and to the disabled. You are disabled if you have a diagnosis of AIDS *and* if you are also unable to work. Social service money is a benefit, paid by federal and state governments, to which you are entitled as a citizen.

A problem is that many people with HIV infection are severely disabled but do not have AIDS. Therefore, they are not eligible for many benefits that are based almost exclusively on this diagnosis.

To get into the social service system, begin by calling your city or county or state social service agencies. These agencies are listed under *social services* in the telephone book's yellow or blue pages. Or start with a social worker at your hospital, clinic, church, or AIDS-advocacy agency.

Help with Income and Medical Bills

The social service system offers several kinds of help with income. What kind of help you can get, and how much, depends on several factors. If you have worked in the past but are disabled and cannot work now, and you need financial help, you qualify for disability income. Some people get disability income as part of their job benefits. If not, the same Social

Security that insures your retirement also gives you disability income, called Social Security Disability Income, or SSDI. Whether you are qualified for SSDI depends on whether you have paid into Social Security for a minimum number of annual quarters. How much you can collect depends on how long you have worked and what your salary has been. Whether you are qualified for SSDI also depends on whether the Social Security Administration thinks you are disabled. The criterion for disability is that the person is unable to do any work because of medical conditions that can be demonstrated by medical documentation. For more information or for a booklet on SSDI and HIV infection, call 1-800-772-1213; expect to wait on the line.

If you are disabled, cannot work, and need financial help, you may also get Supplemental Security Income, called SSI. Whether you are qualified for SSI depends on your means, that is, on your income plus all your assets, everything you own. How much you can collect from SSI also depends on your means. In other words, the government says you are entitled to a certain minimum income. SSI will add up whatever you get on your own, whatever your family can give you, and whatever you get from SSDI; then they will pay you the difference between that sum and the minimum income. If you have no income and no outside means of support, SSI will pay you the entire amount of the minimum income.

If you need financial help, you may qualify for general public assistance, called welfare or GPA. GPA, which is offered through the states, will differ from state to state. Some states do not offer GPA at all. Other states offer it if you need financial help and if you are disabled and cannot work. Some states also offer GPA if you need financial help and are disabled only temporarily; in this case, a person with early symptomatic HIV infection who is unable to work might be able to get financial help, though only for a limited time. And some states are replacing GPA with programs that offer loans. In any case, the amount of money you can collect from GPA is small and depends on your means.

If you have children and need financial help to care for them, you may qualify for Temporary Assistance to Needy Families, or TANF. Money from TANF can be used only for caring for your children. Notice that to qualify for TANF, you need not be disabled. The amount of money you can collect from TANF will be related to the size of your family and your income. You can receive income from both SSI and SSDI at the same time. You can also receive income from both GPA and TANF at the same time. But you cannot receive income from both GPA and SSI at the same time.

If you qualify for SSI or GPA, you automatically qualify for help with medical bills. For details, see above, "Public Programs for Financing Health Care."

Some states have pharmaceuticals assistance programs for people who have low incomes and need help paying for drugs, but who do not qualify for Medicaid.

Navigating the Social Service System

Often people with HIV infection are unfamiliar with the large, bureaucratic social service system. They say that getting through the system is a dehumanizing and irritating experience, that the system seems to be geared more toward frustrating than toward helping people. People occasionally become annoyed enough with the system that they give up and forgo their benefits.

Getting through the system requires preparation. In a single, separate file, keep documentation of the following: proof of identity, address, and date of birth (driver's license, passport, birth certificate); Social Security card; records of income, assets, medical expenses, living expenses, and dependents, anyone living with and sharing expenses with you, and a record of who is responsible for you. Take this file with you when going to social services.

Keep another file of every person you talked to at social services, what date and time you talked to them, what you talked about, and what you understood the outcome of the talk to be. Find out the names of the supervisors. If someone sends you away to get more information, ask them to write down what information they want; then, when you bring the information, also bring along what they wrote. Do not try to keep your diagnosis a secret: some branches of social services will speed up the system if you have HIV infection. Some benefits apply only to those with HIV infection.

Take a friend with you, especially if you're tired or ill. Some AIDS-advocacy agencies offer social workers, lawyers, counselors, or buddies who will go with you.

When to Stop Working

Often your qualification for income from social services comes down to a question of legal disability, which involves making a decision about when to stop working. Most people quit when the stress of getting to work, working, and getting home again becomes overwhelming. Some people quit work after their employers have pressed them to quit. Some people quit after they have had a specific mishap, like an assignment done badly or an accident with a machine or while driving. People usually work as long as they can.

Some people quit gradually. They work half-days for a long time, or they arrange for a leave of absence.

The importance of the decision to quit work should not be underestimated. It is one of the most difficult decisions people with HIV infection have to make. Our image of ourselves as competent and useful members of society depends to some extent on our jobs. When no one pays us to do a job, we worry that we are no longer worth anything at all. Caregivers often forget the extent to which people identify themselves with their jobs. Caregivers worry about the people they're caring for and want to protect them against stress and fatigue and accidents. Because of their worries, they sometimes urge the person with HIV infection to quit working before he or she is ready.

Some people welcome the chance to assess whether they really want to work. Some people decide to quit work and manage the transition well. These people see the decision not as whether to quit but as how to change. They believe that life is the process of developing one new identity after another. They want to try a new identity—to be a writer or traveler or teacher or artist or builder or musician or inventor. Many do volunteer work. Many others become AIDS activists (see chapter 11).

Putting Your Affairs in Order: Advance Directives

An advance directive is a statement in which you describe how you want to be cared for should you become incapable of making your own decisions. Specific examples of advance directives are durable powers of attorney, DNR orders, and living wills.

Assigning Durable Power of Attorney/Choosing a Health Care Agent

Many people want to provide for the possibility that they might become unconscious or mentally incapacitated. They worry about their ability to hire help, give medical consent, sign their checks, pay their bills. Such an eventuality can be provided for by naming someone as your agent, giving him or her the power to make decisions for you. This power is called the *durable power of attorney.*

These powers differ according to the state; some states do not accept durable powers of attorney. Usually, however, you can give these powers to anyone you trust who is over 18 years old; that person can be a friend and need not be a spouse or relative. In general, a durable power of attorney gives that person the legal authority to sign on your behalf if you are unable to do so. That authority can cover a broad range of functions, including most financial and medical matters. You may want to assign a durable power of attorney if you have a long-term partner whom you wish to have make decisions; when not otherwise designated, most states recognize family members, rather than friends, as decision makers.

The durable power of attorney begins either when you decide it will—even before you become incompetent—or when you become incompetent. *Incompetence* is defined as it was with the right to informed consent: it is the inability to make informed decisions based on the information available to you. Two physicians decide the point of incompetence. To assign a durable power of attorney, however, you must be in capacity; that is, you must be able to make informed decisions. The durable power of attorney lasts until you die or until you revoke it. Assigning durable power of attorney can be free and the necessary forms can be downloaded from your state government's Web site or obtained from a local hospital. AIDS-advocacy organizations can often help you find free legal help. You can also fill out forms available from the state or your hospital.

There are two kinds of durable power of attorney: durable power of attorney for health care and durable power of attorney for financial matters. The two are not the same. A person to whom you give durable power of attorney for your finances cannot give medical consent. Because you specify what jobs you want the person with durable power of attorney to have, you can give medical and financial powers to the same person or to different people.

Durable power of attorney for health care/health care agent. The person to whom you give a durable power of attorney for health care must be at least 18 years old and willing to serve as your agent. It is recommended that you choose someone who knows you and knows your wishes. Health care professionals—physicians and nurses who are involved in your care—are not considered appropriate.

The document assigning a durable power of attorney for health care generally contains the following: a statement that you are creating a durable power of attorney for your health care; the name of the person and any alternate person to whom you are giving durable power of attorney for health care; the conditions under which this document becomes effective; a statement of what authority you are granting this person; and a list of specific wishes. The durable power of attorney generally takes effect when two physicians, including the physician-of-record, certify that you are not capable of understanding or communicating decisions about your own health; it will apply as long as this condition continues.

This document can give the person with durable power of attorney the authority to withhold or withdraw any treatments or procedures—including mechanical ventilation (respirators or breathing machines), dialysis (artificial kidneys), antibiotics, operations—that sustain life. This document can also include the statement that you in fact do want specific treatments and procedures, such as those mentioned. You should also include a statement about whether your agent has the right to admit you to a psychiatric unit and to consent to psychiatric medication and treatments. The person to whom you give durable power of attorney may have access to your medical records and may place you in a nursing home. The document assigning durable power of attorney can also include a section for any specific instructions you might have. For example, you could write, "In the event that I am in a coma, and have an incurable physical condition or lose my mental capacity, and have little hope of recovery, I do not want treatment that will merely prolong my life." (Also see "Living Wills," below.)

The document assigning durable power of attorney for health care must be dated and signed by you, and by two witnesses who are not interested parties. It is wise to have the document notarized by a notary public; some states may require this.

The original of the document assigning a durable power of attorney for health care should be kept by you or by your lawyer or by someone you trust. Copies of the document should be given to the person to whom you assign durable power of attorney, to any alternate person, to your physician, and to members of your family. You may wish to consult your physician when drawing up the document. Laws on durable power of attorney for health care change often, so it is wise to review the document annually.

Lawyers, hospital legal offices, and the state can provide examples of such documents that meet state laws.

Durable financial power of attorney. Much of what applies to the durable power of attorney for health care also applies to a durable financial power of attorney. One difference between the two is in the responsibilities held by the person with the durable power of attorney.

The person with durable financial power of attorney for you can pursue anything to do with business or banking, including signing checks, opening bank accounts, signing promissory notes, selling property, transferring property, signing proxies, or pursuing lawsuits. The durable financial power of attorney can be limited to any one of these jobs or can include all of them.

As with the durable power of attorney for health care, the durable financial power of attorney is in effect when you decide it should be, or if two physicians declare you incapable of understanding and communicating. It continues in effect only so long as you remain incompetent.

You may revoke either of the above documents at any time by tearing up the document.

DNR Order

A DNR (do not resuscitate) order is an order your physician writes, directing that if you are near death, you are not to be revived. Your physician should discuss this order with you or with your surrogate. People with advanced HIV infection may reach a stage in the disease when either they or their physicians question whether to continue medical treatment. Medical treatment has a great deal to offer people with HIV infection, including those in advanced stages of the disease, but we would deceive you if we implied that people do not sometimes reach a point where the quality of life becomes questionable. For some people, that point might be dementia; for others, it is emaciation, or repeated or incapacitating complications of HIV infection; and for some, it is simply the inability to do the things that make life meaningful.

These are the points at which people consider DNR orders. The word *resuscitate* in DNR specifically means cardiopulmonary resuscitation, or CPR. Cardio (heart) pulmonary (lungs) resuscitation (revival) means reviving a person whose heart stops beating (cardiac arrest) or whose lungs stop breathing (pulmonary arrest). All hospitals and most medical facilities have the equipment—including machines for chest compression and heart shock (defibrillation), drugs, and respirators—to respond instantly to cardiac or pulmonary arrest. The DNR order means, then, that if you have reached the point where you question the quality of life and if you suffer cardiac or pulmonary arrest, you order that you not be revived. A DNR order applies only to CPR; it does not mean that other treatment is not offered or given.

The decision to carry out DNR orders is based on your medical condition and on the quality of your life. Your medical condition is evaluated by your physician and the evaluation is based on the disease, the stage of disease, prior treatment, and the response to that treatment. Your quality of life can be evaluated only by you, based on your own unique values.

The decision about DNR orders should depend on several factors. One is how demanding the medical treatment to be withheld would be. For example, while intravenous fluids and commonly used antibiotics place few demands on either the hospital or the patient, dialysis, respirators, total intravenous nutrition, and major operations are considerably more demanding. Other factors affecting the decision include the likelihood of response, alternate treatment options, and the potential for relieving symptoms like pain. For example, questions that you might raise in the event of lung failure are, What is the likelihood of survival without the respirator? What is the likelihood of being able to get off the respirator once being put on it? What kind of treatments can be offered if you get over this hurdle? Will there be pain either with the respirator or without it? Is it likely that the condition causing lung failure is temporary and can be cured?

If you are medically competent (see above) and are 18 years of age or older, you might consider making a decision about DNR orders. It is probably best to deal with this issue at a time when you and your physician can discuss the whole issue to your satisfaction and when you don't need to make fast decisions in compromised circumstances. Physicians are encouraged to discuss DNR orders with anyone who has a serious medical condition, but many are understandably reluctant to do this. If your physician does not discuss DNR orders with you, you might wish to bring up the subject.

If you are not conscious or have been declared medically incompetent by two physicians, then your representative can discuss DNR orders with your physician. Who your representative is varies from state to state. Typically, your representative will be, in rank order, your durable power of attorney/health care agent, your guardian, your spouse, your children aged 18 or older, your parent, or your brother or sister. Your representative should make decisions about DNR orders based on your anticipated desires, not on his or her own desires.

Most people have strong opinions about such decisions, and they worry that they will not be able to make rational choices at the time the choices need to be made. Two ways of dealing with such decisions in advance are to assign a durable power of attorney for health care (see above) and to make health care instructions (see below).

Living Wills and Other Health Care Instructions

A living will is a legal document outlining your decisions about treatment to sustain your life should you be unconscious or incompetent. Laws about living wills vary from state to state. The living will is somewhat different from the durable power of attorney for health care: the person with your durable power of attorney for health care, when faced with the decision of whether to prolong your life, will usually decide to prolong life. The living will or health care instruction provides that person with your specific instructions for making this decision. The person with your durable power of attorney for health care can also make decisions that may not have been foreseen in your living will.

Living wills, unlike regular wills, apply only to medical treatments. The actual form and scope of a living will is established by state laws. In general, living wills specify which types of treatment you wish to have or wish not to have. Living wills also specify the physical and mental states in which you do or do not want these treatments. These treatments include transfusions, support on a respirator, operations, and resuscitation. Some states have no provision for living wills. Other states that do provide for living wills do not allow any restrictions on food and water.

In most cases, a living will applies only after the person becomes incompetent and has a terminal condition. In some states, a living will applies to both terminal conditions and a kind of permanent coma called a vegetative state; in other states, a living will applies only to terminal conditions.

A living will might be written as follows:

> In the event that I have an incurable disease and I am certified to be in a terminal condition by two physicians who have personally examined me—including one who shall be my attending physician—and these physicians have determined that my death is imminent and will occur whether or not life-sustaining procedures are used; and where application of such procedures would serve only to artificially prolong the dying process, I direct that these procedures be withheld or withdrawn, and that I be permitted to die naturally with only the administration of medication, food, and water, and any additional procedure necessary to give comfort and alleviate pain. In the absence of my ability to give directions regarding the use of such life-sustaining procedures, it is my intention that this declaration shall be honored by my family and physicians as the final expression of my right to control my medical care and treatment.

To make a living will, obtain a sample document from your lawyer, from your state attorney general's office, from a hospital legal office, or from a social worker. The content of the living will may be discussed with your physician to assure the use of proper terms and to include likely decisions. The living will must be dated and signed by you and by two witnesses. You must be at least 18 years old and competent. The witnesses must be at least 18 years old, must not be related to you, must not be financially responsible for your care, and may not be your health care provider; witnesses may, however, be connected with the facility providing your care. You or your representative should give your physician a copy of the living will. You should also forward a copy to the medical records department at the hospital where you receive care, so that the copy can be included in your permanent record. You may revoke the will at any time, preferably by a written statement, but also by destroying the living will and notifying any persons—including the physician—who retain copies.

Stipulating What Happens to Your Property

Most people stipulate what happens to their property by making a will. No one requires that you do so. If you die without a will (called dying *intestate*) your property goes automatically first to your spouse and then to your nearest living relatives. Your property will not go to friends or to unmarried partners. To assign property to friends or unmarried partners, you must make a will.

Wills apply mostly to property—money, house, car, furniture, clothes. Wills do not necessarily legislate any of your other wishes. Life insurance benefits will go to the beneficiary, even if the will states otherwise. In principle, a will may specify what your funeral arrangements are and whether you'd like to be buried or cremated, but in practice, wills are often not read until after the funeral.

Over a certain value, property left in a will is taxable. You can minimize taxes your beneficiaries will pay by setting up trusts or by giving to them a certain amount of money per year while you are still alive. Neither trusts nor gifts under a certain dollar amount are taxable.

Trusts and annual gifts also ensure that you will have property to leave. Some people, rather than use their property to finance their own medical care, decide to put it into trusts or give it to the people they love. Once they are impoverished, their medical bills will be paid by public assistance programs. Leaving your property in trust or as a gift must be done years before you need extensive medical care: Medicaid/Medicare will check to see if money or property has been given away in recent years. To find out how and when to leave your property, see a lawyer or a financial planner. A will can also be used to specify who has control over your body when you die. This may be important to you if you want a friend or companion, rather than your family, to bury you.

A lawyer is the best source of information regarding what happens to your property. Lawyers also often draw up wills. State laws set the forms for wills, however, and if you know the form, you can draw up your own will.

Providing for Hospice Care

Some people want to decide where they will die. Some choose to die at home; some would rather leave their homes as a place for the living, so choose to die elsewhere. In either case, they may choose hospice care.

A hospice can be either a place or a concept, that is, either a building or a program dedicated to care of the dying. Hospice programs can be run through hospitals, nursing homes, or private organizations. Nursing agencies, like the Visiting Nurse Association, often also provide hospice care.

Both private insurance policies and medical assistance provide some level of reimbursement for hospice care, providing the requirements of the hospice are met. To find a hospice or hospice program, ask your doctor or nursing agency or hospital social worker. Your doctor can advise you on when to consider hospice services.

Chapter 10

On Dying: Preparing for and Accepting Death

- Emotional responses to death
- Making decisions about the rest of life
- Other people's reactions to death
- The dying person and the caregiver
- Balancing living and dying
- Death

Helen Parks: I've lost too many friends in too short a time. It gets stronger with each one, closer to home. I haven't been sleeping too well. I get out of bed and look at the moon. I just stand there. I don't know why I do that. I go back to bed but can't sleep. I thought I'd have a longer time. Now I think the time is shorter.

Death is hard to think about, harder to face. The thought of death is slippery, difficult to focus on, surrounded by a cloud of pain and fear. At the same time, the thought is irrepressible; it is impossible to truly ignore. No one with HIV infection ignores the thought of death altogether. "No matter how positive I am, there's a lingering dark cloud," said Alan Madison. "It's tick, tick—your time is running out. It's not like one day it's on your mind, the next day it's not. You think a lot about how it might end."

Emotional Responses to Death

Elisabeth Kübler-Ross is a psychiatrist who wrote the standard book on how all people, regardless of the causes of their deaths, respond emotionally to the fact that they are dying. After interviewing people who were dying, she found they have several responses in common.

One is disbelief and denial that death could happen to them: as Dean Lombard said, "You feel it's not going to happen, though you know it is. You feel emotionless because it can't be real." Another is anger at having been singled out. Another is an impulse to bargain, to push back the inevitable and gain a little time: "I don't think we ever feel as though it's all complete," Steven said, "as though the world owes us nothing else." The next is depression: the loss, pain, and sorrow that come from recognition that death is inescapable. The last is acceptance, coming to terms with death: "The meaning of the diagnosis finally hit me," said Dean. "I might not be here forever. I should make my preparations for death."

Kübler-Ross said the responses to death occurred in stages: first denial, then anger, bargaining, depression, and finally, acceptance. Later, she and subsequent researchers amended the idea, saying that perhaps the word *stages* is misleading. Not everyone has all these responses, or has them in this order. Some have several at once. For others, the responses alternate: anger, then depression, then anger again. And not only the people who are facing death, but also their caregivers, have these responses. Caregivers share the same feelings of denial, anger, depression, bargaining, and acceptance, both on behalf of the people they are taking care of and for themselves.

To anyone who has learned to live with a diagnosis of HIV infection, these responses come as no surprise. They are nearly the same emotions people experience when they learn of their diagnosis of HIV infection. These emotions are also the same as the normal responses to living with HIV infection. Perhaps this means that people with HIV infection have been facing death since the moment of their diagnosis; perhaps it means only that these are the responses people have when faced with any catastrophe.

In any case, the responses to the diagnosis serve as a rehearsal for the thought of death. People who have had these responses before are a little used to them, and know a little about how to handle them. The same strategies—strategies for refusing to fret about what will not change, for finding harmless or even helpful ways of discharging anger, for turning despair into some sort of hope for something or someone, for facing down fears, for distracting yourself with pleasure, for accepting yourself with fondness and your condition without self-hatred, guilt, or blame still work, even against death.

People have other natural responses to the thought of death. One is fear. People are afraid of dying in pain. They fear the moment when life stops. The truth is that dying—the process that leads to the moment of death—sometimes does hurt, but doctors have medications to block the pain.

Death itself seems not to hurt. The body, either quietly or quickly, stops working. No one knows much about the moment of death, but it does seem that a built-in mechanism protects people from physical and psychological pain. As a rule, death comes peacefully.

Most of our fears about death are actually about what will happen before death. This fear is universal; the sixteenth-century French philosopher Michel de Montaigne wrote about it in his *Essays:* "It is not against death that we prepare ourselves. . . . To tell the truth, we prepare ourselves against the preparations for death. . . . It is certain that to most people preparation for death has given more torment than the dying." Montaigne goes on to offer a sort of rough comfort: "If you don't know how to die, don't worry; Nature will tell you what to do on the spot, fully and adequately. She will do this job perfectly for you; don't bother your head about it."

Specifically, people are afraid that while they are dying they will be abandoned. They are afraid of being alone at such a difficult time. They fear they will lose control. They worry that they have been bad and deserve death. They fear physical pain and disfigurement. They worry about the people they will leave, about the relationships left unresolved and business left unfinished.

Another natural reaction to death is confusion. The thought of life ending is new territory, and people are unsure how to think about it or what to do about it. What does it mean to be dying, but alive at the same time? "I don't know how to just let life go on until death comes," Helen Parks said. "I'm between this pole and that pole."

Still another natural reaction is a sense of loss. Through sickness, people lose the bodies they were accustomed to. They lose their abilities to do what they were good at, their competencies. They lose the healthy, active lives they shared with their friends, and to that extent, they lose a commonality with their friends. And because they are aware of dying, they lose their sense of a future, the feeling that limitless time is available to them. Accepting these losses brings anguish.

Some of the anguish in accepting losses comes from knowing that smaller losses are tokens of greater ones, of the loss of life and the entire world. Some is because losing the future also means losing the idealistic, hopeful part of you, your potential, the person you might have become. And some of the anguish is because people want so much to live. "The will to live is so great, you can't even think about it," said Dean. "You feel as though you could beat anything just by wanting to live." The anguish people feel over losing life is in proportion to the intensity with which they want to live. "The inevitability of death has the effect of making you appreciate life more," said Edward Carroll. "The irony is, appreciate it or not, someday it will be taken away from you.

There is a lot of sadness with this. Sadness at leaving people. Sadness at not being able to see the rest of the world."

People facing death also want to settle existential questions about life: What is being human all about? Do I believe in God? What will happen to the world after I die? What will happen to me after I die? They turn to religion or spirituality or philosophy, and they think about the same questions people have been asking for centuries. Lisa's husband was not unusual in becoming religious before he died, reading the Bible and writing his thoughts in a journal. Edward had similar impulses: "If there's a God and if there's a Judgment Day, as I believe there might be," he said, "you want to face that knowing that your life hasn't been wasted. I do think we're put on this earth to work and be productive. One of the reasons I've worked so hard over the last eight or ten years is so I could look back and say I'd got something done. I'd like to think that what I've done has been useful to other people, that maybe if I haven't accomplished what I set out to, that at least I got well on the way."

For all the feelings and worries that dying people have in common, their progress through these feelings and worries is individual. People experience these emotions in fits and starts and at their own paces. Sometimes they want to face death, sometimes they do not. Sometimes they want to make plans and see people, sometimes they do not. Sometimes they want to take control and make decisions, sometimes they do not. Sometimes they want to talk about their feelings, sometimes they do not: Lisa's husband said, "I don't always want to talk about dying. Sometimes I want to have days when I'm just living."

Emotional Responses to Death from HIV Infection

Most of the responses to death described above are shared by all people who have time to contemplate dying, regardless of the cause of death. What makes HIV infection different is death at an early age in the midst of the deaths of many friends. Most people who die of HIV infection are in their thirties. Someone who has HIV infection probably knows many others with the disease.

Because they are young, they have worries about dying that older people do not. Young people have less time to get used to death gradually. They are not yet tired of living. They have not slowly come to see themselves as dispensable and mortal. They do not understand what to do about mortality, how to sum up and conclude their lives. "I have to face my own mortality," said Dean, "which I didn't expect to face until I was 80." They look at their relatively short lives and ask questions they are not used to asking. "Usually people ask in their sixties, 'What have

I accomplished?'" Alan said. "Maybe I'm going to have to ask that earlier." They often feel resentful that they must ask these questions so early, and they feel unready to supply the answers.

They also worry about dying before their parents. They want to be able to help their parents out as their parents age. "Now I'm looking at dying before my parents," said Dean. "That changes the natural process. It hurts."

Because people with HIV infection often know others who are dying of the disease, they have concrete images of what will happen to them. They visit their friends in the hospital and think, "Is this what will happen to me? Is this what I will look like? Is this what I will feel?" "I know what the last few months are," said Alan, "and I wish I hadn't seen the suffering. Knowing what it looks like is difficult." Dean lost twenty friends in two years. "It gets stronger with each one," he said. "Closer to home." People with HIV infection say too much death surrounds them. "I have so many friends who are disappearing," Steven said. "In one year, I went to twenty-six funerals. I sit at the funerals and think how wonderful the person was, and how they looked before the end, and how long will it be before I'm there." For that reason, some, like Steven, no longer go to funerals. Alan said, "I've been to forty-seven funerals. That's my limit."

Making Decisions about the Rest of Life

People who are facing death begin gradually to make decisions about the rest of their lives. They look inside themselves for reference points, for what is important to them: Which people mean the most to me? What kinds of things should I be involved in? Where should I live? They also find outside references: people, poetry, spirituality, support groups, music, books. They often talk with counselors who can help them make decisions and handle their overwhelming emotions. What they finally do is decide whom to spend their time with, and how to spend it.

Some people begin by summing up their lives. Part of what Dean called his preparation for death was to look at what he had accomplished and decide what his legacy would be. Dean runs a small newspaper, and he is arranging for the smooth transfer of the business to his partners. He also thinks of the paper as his legacy: "I have to have something that says, 'Dean was here.' I'd like people to read today's newspaper in fifty years and say, 'Oh that's what it was like then.' My paper is going to go on, and people after me are going to benefit from it." Lisa's husband began talking more about an earlier marriage that had ended in divorce, how sad he was that the family hadn't been able to stay together, and for the first time in twenty years, he invited all his children to come home at the same time.

Some people decide to do the things they have always wanted to do. Dean had always wanted a personal computer with which to keep track of household expenses and could never justify the cost; finally he bought one. A friend of Dean's decided he wanted to travel because he never had. He arranged his trip, arranged his sources of medical care and medicine, sold his house, and took off.

People often want to resolve relationships. They work hard to get on more comfortable terms with their parents, children, brothers and sisters, spouses, friends. Lisa's husband and his family had for a long time been unhappy with each other. When the family understood Lisa's husband was dying, Lisa said, "Everyone realized all the things they had gotten wired up about were garbage. All he had ever wanted was to be accepted for the person he was, and that's what they fought about. Finally either he let it rest, or they did, and they all seemed to accept each other. The acceptance showed as much in what they didn't talk about as what they did."

Often the person with HIV infection makes the first step toward resolution. Some people who are approached for this purpose do not react positively. Resolving a relationship with a dying person means admitting death's inevitability, and some people are intimidated by the thought of death. Sometimes they only want time to get used to the idea, and they react more positively when they are approached again a little later. In general, people with HIV infection and the people they talk to both want the same things. They want to reminisce and think about what good times they had. They both want to know they're loved; they want to be accepted for who they are. They want to feel comfort and warmth in each other's company. People who are dying also want reassurance that the people they love will be watched over and cared for.

Some people decide what should happen to their property. Helen said, "Finally I sat down and decided who was getting what, and wrote it down. I considered giving stuff to the people that most hated it. Then I decided not to do that." Some people decide they are uninterested in having a say about the disposal of their property, so they don't bother with it.

Some people consider suicide. Thoughts of suicide most commonly occur early in the course of the disease. People often devise concrete plans: at what point they will decide to end their lives, what method they will use, how they will keep the burden of guilt off their survivors. Mental health professionals recommend that people talk to a professional about their decision, then give it a while before doing anything.

Some people who are dying and their caregivers want to know what to anticipate clinically. They find that knowing what their bodies might do and what the treatment will be takes the mystery out of the process. They say that the more they know, the less they invent to worry about. For these people, a book called *How We Die,* by Sherwin Nuland, might be helpful. Other people do not want to know, and would like to distance themselves a little from the physical aspects of being sick and dying. Still others want to know a little at a time. Learn the facts only if you want, and only when you want to.

Often people decide under what conditions they would like to be allowed to die. Some refuse medication or procedures they think would prolong a life that has become distressing. A friend of Dean's who had become blind, deaf, and incontinent refused transfusions and drugs with painful side effects that might prolong his life, and accepted only pain-relieving medication. Dean's friend saw this not as giving up but as making his last days comfortable. Others refuse life support systems. Lisa spent nights at the hospital with her husband toward the end of his life. He refused the respirator, so Lisa brought him home. He lived ten days, then died as he had wished, at home. Like Lisa's husband, many people would like to die where they feel a sense of control and privacy, in their own beds. Many others feel their homes should remain a place of life and would rather die in a hospital or hospice. And some people do not want to choose beforehand but simply wait and see how they feel at the end.

Some people who are dying make funeral arrangements with the help of their caregivers. Some want to make sure their caregivers find a funeral home that won't refuse to offer services because of AIDS. Others want to give their caregivers some moral support. "I asked my partner his opinion on a cemetery plot," said Dean. "The reason is, once when I had to go away for six months, he was very upset. I helped him through that by doing everything—my planning and packing—with him. That's what I'm doing now, helping him by doing everything with him."

Other People's Reactions to Death

We are raised to think of death not as a necessity but as an enemy. When people who are still healthy are confronted with someone who is dying, they are intensely uncomfortable. They are frightened of losing the dying person, of their own deaths, and of death's finality. "Death isn't like breaking up with someone and time heals it," said Helen. "Death is death, period, and no one wants to deal."

Sometimes their discomfort, their not wanting to "deal," makes people appear insensitive. Helen was in a mall, shopping, and someone she knew came up and asked, "Why have you got all those shopping bags? Aren't you dying soon?" Helen snapped back, "How soon are *you* dying?" but she was surprised and confused and hurt by her friend's question. Dean had a friend who habitually made a joke of looking around at Dean's furnishings and saying, "Oh, that's new. Leave it to me in your will." Dean finally replied, "Okay, that's fine. Do you want the kitchen chairs too?" After that, the friend dropped the joke. Such remarks sound insensitive, as though the person is taunting you with life and health. But they are not; no one is this callous. Insensitivity is the method some people use to deal with their own pain and fear. The method is certainly inappropriate. Both Helen and Dean let their friends understand how inappropriate their remarks were and that they should be more careful in the future.

Sometimes people's discomfort with the reality of death isolates those who are dying. People facing death often find that other people are friendly and sympathetic but want to talk only about easy, comfortable subjects. When the subject of death comes up, they talk instead about what they've done recently, or about the future: "I can't wait until we get you to a ballgame." They also sugarcoat the subject: "Remember how sick you thought you were before, and a month later you were off on a trip." This is hard on people facing death. They may be happy enough to talk about the weather, the news, or sports, or to gossip about mutual friends. But being prohibited from talking about the things that are of most concern makes them feel isolated and sad.

But everyone facing death also knows some people who will "deal." Perhaps it is someone who also faces death or someone who has lost a person they loved, or a professional who has had training in helping people handle the emotions and problems of dying. Often it is someone who loves the dying person and is less afraid than other people of the reality of death. These people tell the person who is dying that they will not leave, they will stay as long as they can. With Helen's young nephew, that message is reversed. Helen's nephew worries about Helen's death, and Helen tries to help by telling him he won't be abandoned: "My nephew cries when he thinks about it," Helen said. "I tell him, 'I'm not going to give up easily and I'm going to try to be there for your graduation. Don't be disappointed if I can't, but I'll try.'"

The Dying Person and the Caregiver

People who are dying and the people caring for them ask difficult questions of each other, and say things they always meant to say to each other, and cry together. They find these things comforting—people feel better knowing someone else is concerned or is having the same feelings. Both the people who are dying and their caregivers find it a relief when someone sincerely asks them, "How are you?" Dying people and their caregivers want attention and companionship. They want to be taken seriously. They want to know that they need not be alone. People facing death together often grow closer.

This is not to say that their interests always converge. They have to solve some real problems. One is that they may be experiencing different "Kübler-Ross" responses at the same time. When, for instance, one person is accepting death and the other is denying it, they will probably feel alienated from each other and find communication difficult. They may solve this by accepting that the other person's feelings are as compelling as their own. They try to treat the other person's feelings as facts, at least temporary ones, that require respect. In extreme circumstances like these, people have only the feelings they can afford to have, and they feel things only when they are ready. Sometimes they have had enough of HIV infection and death, and they need to take a break for a while. Sometimes they are ready to think and feel and talk about what is happening to them.

Another problem for the caregiver is knowing when the dying person wants to talk about what is happening and when he or she needs to ignore it. The best the caregiver can do is listen for cues. Cues are when the person begins talking about his troubles or what he has read about dying or how tired she is or that she is frightened or how to deal with the business of leaving the world. Then the caregiver can say, "How can I help? What would you like to do?"

A third problem is that the normal balance of the relationship begins to change. Dean is not yet close to death, though he and his partner are aware that he could die and they discuss it. "My partner is going through a hard time right now," said Dean. "Not only is he concerned about me, but he also just had to put his mother in a nursing home, and he doesn't get along with his father and sister. So now he's telling me, 'I need you. Don't go anywhere for a while.'"

When Lisa was in distress because her husband was dying, she found herself asking him for comfort. From the outside, this seems odd: surely the caregiver should not ask for help from the dying. But in fact, it is an entirely natural extension of the relationship between people who care for each other. People in a relationship normally take turns. Sometimes one is the comforter, the helper, the listener, sometimes the other is. The problem is that for the person close to death, this sort of give-and-take becomes too heavy a burden. When death is imminent, the balance of responsibility begins to shift to the caregiver.

Caregivers need to begin to forgo the luxury of asking for help with their own fears and worries. They need to gradually stop coming to the dying person with both minor irritations and profound troubles. They listen. They ask questions: "Are you comfortable enough? Are you upset? What do you fear?" They let the dying person cry, and are silent or cry with him. They let the dying person express her fears and fantasies, and help test fears against reality. They say, "I will try to do what you like. How can I help?" They hold and touch the dying person whenever they can and as often as the person wants.

A common ground rule is that the dying person calls the shots: when to stop working, when to get another X-ray, whether to answer the phone, which friends to see and when, whether to make decisions, when and where to talk about their feelings about what is happening to them. The caregiver can argue, but the decision rests with the person who is dying.

Balancing Living and Dying

In general, people facing death continue the process they began in response to depression and fatigue. They concentrate their energies on what is possible. They let go of some things they had wanted, mostly long-term career goals. They take control of their own attitudes: they decide how to live with their limits in life and still feel satisfied. In short, they balance living and dying.

In a way, they seem both to live and to die at once. Not only did Helen plan her trip to the beach the following summer and buy beach clothes, she also celebrated Mother's Day in December—"In case I wasn't here," she said. Alan says his life is "back to normal," and he doesn't "sit around waiting to get sick," but he doesn't "order things that will take a year to get," either. Dean says, "I'm keeping myself healthy and trying to keep the disease from getting worse"; he also says, "I won't enroll in night school, I'm afraid I couldn't finish."

These people are not contradicting themselves. They are dealing with two facts; one is that they are dying, and the other is that they are still alive. They have to live recognizing both death and life. "I might need some help dying," said Edward. "But I also need help with living until I die, graciously and with dignity."

In fact, people have always had to learn to do this. Everyone has to figure out how to stay alive and still be ready for death, how to approach dying and still live the rest of their lives.

Eventually people say that they have always known how. At some time in their lives, they have had to accept the inevitable with courage and grace. "If we have not known how to live," wrote Montaigne, "it is wrong to teach us how to die, and make the end inconsistent with the whole. If we have known how to live steadfastly and tranquilly, we shall know how to die in the same way." Lisa's husband said the same thing, that he would die as he lived, by paraphrasing the Bible: "I know I came into this world naked and I will go out naked." The person who has lived is the same as the person who will die. If you know yourself at all, you know how you will die.

Death

Because we have to, we accept the conditions of mortality: having means losing, being here means leaving. Seneca, a Roman philosopher, wrote to his old friend Lucilius, in *Moral Letters to Lucilius:* "You will die, not because you are ill, but because you are alive." The idea, though people have known it forever, always comes as a surprise. We want life never to end; we want those we love never to die.

But we have never been able to have everything we want. The fact that we want what we cannot have is only a fact, not a surprise, not cause for despair. Sooner or later, we find ways to accept it. Edward's way is to think about his friends' future: "Each person who has fought this disease does it with his own weapons. When the people die, they leave their weapons behind. When I die, my friends are going to pick up my weapons." Like Edward, people who are dying are often calm and talk quietly about death and their lives.

For the caregiver, this hurts badly. Caregivers want to resist the pain by trying to keep the dying person alive as long as possible. Lisa said, "I was fighting to keep my husband alive. I just didn't want to give up. He said to me, 'Don't you know, Lisa, it's just one sickness after another.' I said, 'Never mind. Just keep fighting.'" After a time, caregivers become a little better used to the death, and know they must let go. Lisa said, "I stopped fighting about two weeks before he died. I finally let him go, said to myself if he had to die, that would be okay. I didn't want him to die. But I would not cling to him."

At the end, people who are dying should be able to have with them the people they love. People who love someone who is dying should be able to be with that person. Lisa sat with her husband while he was dying: "I held his hands and talked to him. I think he could hear, even though he seemed unconscious. I told him who I was and that I wouldn't leave. I just kept talking, I said, 'I love you. I don't want you to suffer any more. I'll take care of the kids. It'll be fine. Let go if you want.' I did all I could. I think I helped him die."

People tell those who are dying, "I won't leave you. If I go away, I'll come back soon." They say prayers. They read aloud, often their Bibles. Some sing: a woman Dean knew sang gospel songs to her son while he died. Some, like Lisa, just talk, lovingly and reassuringly. When they find nothing to say, they sit quietly. Most importantly, they hold, touch, caress, hold hands. For both the dying and those left behind, the physical presence of another person eases loss and loneliness. One hospital clergyman said that at death, the physical presence of another person amounts to a sacrament.

Maybe death is not so bad. We know so little about it. Why should it be worse than sleep? Socrates, a Greek philosopher who lived in the fifth century, was ordered by the leaders of his state to kill himself for insubordination. Socrates acquiesced, and he died after drinking poison. Before he died, he talked about death: "Perhaps death is something indifferent, perhaps desirable. It is likely, however, that if it is a transmigration from one place to another, it is an improvement to go and live with so many great persons who have passed on and to be exempt from having any more to do with unjust and corrupt judges."

"If it is an annihilation of our being," Socrates continued, "it is still an improvement to enter upon a long and peaceful night. We feel nothing sweeter in life than a deep and tranquil rest and sleep, without dreams."

Chapter 11

On Living:
Tactics for Preserving
Mental Health

- Sources of support
- Taking control

This chapter is about how to live with this disease and stay in one piece. It is about how to face uncertainty and still preserve emotional health. Preserving emotional health in the face of HIV infection is heroic, and people do it all the time, using all sorts of tricks. The tricks allow people to function in their daily lives, to endure uncertainty, to choose how to live, and to find real satisfaction and pleasure in the process.

A great variety of such tricks are successful. People use different tricks at different times, depending on their needs. Many of the tricks even seem to contradict one another: sometimes people need to confront what the disease might bring; other times they need to take a break from that. Some tricks might work for you; some you might need to modify. You will almost certainly make up new ones for yourself.

Some tricks come from mental health professionals, though these professionals have no firm rules for maintaining emotional wholeness. Most tricks come from the rich imaginations and enormous inner resources of the people affected by HIV infection.

These people are proud of their toughness and resourcefulness, and so they should be. Steven Charles said, "I have to deal with this whether I want to or not. Six or seven years have gone by since I was diagnosed with the virus. How have I come through it? I think I've come through it admirably." Neither Steven nor anyone else feels they have been admirable every minute: "It's hard to do seven days a week," he says. But on the whole, everyone who uses these tricks says that life is better.

The tricks seem to fall into two broad categories. The first is: use your sources of support. The second is: as far as you are able, take control of your life.

Sources of Support

Over and over, people affected by HIV infection say they could not manage to preserve their emotional health without a sister or a certain friend or support group or aunt or doctor or counselor. In fact, they go further and say that without these people, they would no longer know how to live.

This is not an absolute. Some people are more private than others, or would rather rely on their own resources. All people have times when they would rather be alone. Nor are other people always a treat; they can be boring or irritating or demanding or cause outright pain. Even the best of friends can get tiresome. But in general, the people who do best with this or any other disease are those who have the support of their family and friends.

The principal sources of support for people with HIV infection are their partners, parents, husbands and wives, brothers and sisters, aunts and uncles, cousins, grandparents, friends, neighbors. Other sources of support are other relatives, volunteer buddies from advocacy agencies, co-workers, church members, and members of any other groups to which they belong. Still other sources are the professionals who tend the mental health of those affected by HIV infection: psychiatrists, psychologists, social workers, counselors, religious leaders—therapists of all kinds.

Helen says of a team at her clinic who treat her like family: "The strong-willed person they thought I was, I wasn't. I wanted to die. They just don't know how important their friendship is. They kept me alive."

In general, supporters find ways to get people out of themselves. Supporters touch them and let them know they're valued. Supporters talk about themselves and by doing that, give tacit permission to the person affected by HIV infection to talk as well. Supporters listen—without criticism, without advice, without too many suggestions for improvement, and with kindness.

What follows are examples of the ways family, friends, religious leaders, AIDS-advocacy organizations, and mental health professionals have provided support. The examples can give caregivers some ideas of what support to offer and how vital that support is. The examples can also give people with the virus some notions of what support might be possible and where to get it, and perhaps a recognition of the support they already have. This is not a representative sample of all the kinds of support. People are endlessly inventive, and the ways to provide support must be nearly infinite.

Family

Families can provide a unique kind of support and some of the closest relationships people ever have. For some people, this closeness seems to make them feel as though they and their families are arms and legs of the same body. The exact kind of support families provide is not always concrete, and sometimes it is a little mysterious. Steven's face shines when he talks about his family: "Sometimes when I feel pretty much alone and discouraged, my family overpowers me. They just overpower me." And Rebecca says, "I feel all the more 'me' around my family."

One of the most important things that members of the family do is bring with them a sense of a shared past. Families reminisce, talk about good times, retell old stories. Steven's family remind him of the time he fell out of the tree onto the picnic table and got his mother's potato salad all over him. With such stories about the past comes a sense of being part of both the past and the future, a sense of who you are and what your roots are, a sense of continuity. Feeling a part of something larger is a deep comfort to people affected by HIV infection. Perhaps that is what Steven means when he says his family just "overpowers" him.

Families also make people feel cared about. "My husband has been really, really great," said Rebecca Wolfe. "My whole family has all been great. This disease can become so overwhelming—you feel like you'll never be like anyone else. But my parents are very proud of me, of how hard I'm trying. How awful it must be for people who don't have the support."

People affected by HIV infection seem to feel most free with their brothers and sisters. They often find it easier to tell their brothers and sisters about the diagnosis in the first place. They feel their brothers and sisters understand them and accept them as they are. "I've been able to talk and let loose my feelings with my sister," Dean said. Helen's stepmother did the same thing: "My stepmother brought her little kids to visit me when I was in the hospital. I told her not to, there are germs here. But she just said, 'You're sick. We're coming.'"

Not everyone whom people consider family is a blood relative. People who are distant from their families make substitute families out of their friends. They celebrate holidays and birthdays together, give each other presents, stay in touch, travel together, help each other out. Steven has an old teacher who took him into her family, introduced him to her friends, and takes him on trips and out to dinner: "She's extended family to me," he said. A friend of Alan's has a mother who, Alan said, "is like another mother to me." Family also needn't be exclusively human; many people find comfort in their pets. "My cat meets me at the door every night," said Alan. "One night, he didn't, and I missed him. I realized how much I appreciated that he usually did."

In some families, the same closeness makes them expect more of each other than they would of other people: they feel that members of their family should not be gay or use drugs, should not be depressed or even sick. Such expectations are difficult and often impossible to meet, and both sides feel disappointed and frustrated. For some people, then, the family is unable to provide much help. "My husband's family couldn't deal with his being sick," Lisa said. "For a long time, they wouldn't call, wouldn't come to visit. When they finally did come, they talked only about routine things." Notice, however, that Lisa's in-laws did come to visit, and did provide what small comfort they could by talking about routine things. Though Lisa wished they could have done more, both for her and for her husband, she recognized they had been a help. "All the same," she said, "it helped him just to hear from them."

Probably, even if your family cannot provide as much support and comfort as you would like, they nevertheless wish they could. They probably feel they should be able to make all your problems go away, and they feel guilty and helpless when they cannot. Perhaps the best thing to do is what Lisa finally did: accept what they are able to offer, and find the comfort in it.

Families are also prime sources of well-meant and unasked-for advice. Such advice can be hard to listen to, especially because the adviser rarely has experience with the kinds of problems HIV infection presents. As a result, the advice can sound annoying or distrustful or condescending or just wrong. The same principle that applies to disappointed expectations also applies to unwanted advice: ignore it, or explain that you'll have to agree to disagree, and find comfort in the adviser's good intentions and concern. Dean said his rule with his family is, "No criticisms, no advice."

Friends

Another vital source of support is friends—anyone from a partner, lover, or confidant to a person to have fun with, a neighbor, a co-worker, another person affected by HIV infection, or anyone who shares interests. Sometimes, because some of these people feel less intimately connected to you than family, they actually find it easier to be good companions and sources of support.

Sometimes friends are also less intimidating to talk to than family. You choose your friends in the first place for what you have in common, and because they will not judge what you say. People commonly say of a friend, "I can say anything to her." Alan is quiet and not especially talkative, but he gets together with other people who have HIV infection and listens to them talk. "It helps to hear other people talk," Alan said. "They say your feelings for you. You relate to people who think the way you do."

Even co-workers can be a support: some people feel the people they work with are a kind of family. When Edward was hospitalized, a co-worker called his hospital social worker and asked what she and other colleagues could do. The social worker's answer was a good one to give anyone who asks such a question: "Don't leave him alone. Give him openings to talk but don't push. And stick around and don't head for the hills."

Religion

People's religions offer them two sources of support, one human, one spiritual. Priests, rabbis, ministers, nuns, pastors of all religions give the same sort of help as social workers and psychologists, but they talk particularly to people who want to talk about God. They offer advice, company, and comfort. A hospital chaplain who deals largely with people with HIV infection says, "I start by asking, 'What do you want me to pray for?' They tell me, and we talk about that. I think my presence as a representative of the church brings a sense of hope and warmth and comfort."

A pastor in a large city church, when she celebrates the Eucharist at church, consecrates extra wafers and takes them along for celebration of the Eucharist at the hospital. "That's become important," she said. "The people in the hospital are getting the wafers that were consecrated when everybody has gathered together to celebrate the Eucharist. That connection becomes very important to sick people."

The spiritual comfort of religion can be separate from the human comfort. Dean's faith brings him strength: "My greatest source of support is my church," said Dean. "It's spiritual support, having God who is greater and could intervene. I don't believe God creates these things; I don't believe any of that stuff about plagues. I do a lot of communicating with God. I say, 'Okay, I'll work it out with you.' It has a healing effect. God gives us the strength to meet each day and live it to the fullest."

Helen's faith brings her reassurance: "God loves me so much. Even when I fail in my own eyes, I don't fail in God's. God is a good parent. If someone is hungry, God sees to it that they're fed."

AIDS-Advocacy Organizations

What this book calls AIDS-advocacy organizations are organizations in the community, sometimes only local, sometimes affiliated with a national organization, that offer a huge variety of services to people with HIV infection and to their caregivers. The services these organizations offer include buddies, counselors, information on treatments, education about HIV infection, help with financial problems, home health care, help with housing problems, help with legal problems, legal services, reports on the latest medical research, support groups, political action, and transportation—to name a few.

Many of these organizations also run hotlines, which are toll-free phone numbers to call for information on HIV infection and for referrals to the organizations and services available in your local community.

To find out what's available in your community, check the phone book's yellow pages under AIDS or HIV, or the phone book's government blue pages under Health or AIDS or HIV. Or call the hotlines of national AIDS-advocacy organizations. Your physician or hospital social worker is also a good source for the resources in your own community.

For more information, and for addresses and phone numbers of national organizations and hotlines, see Appendix A, "Resources."

Support and Therapy Groups

Some of the best support for people affected by HIV infection comes through organized support and therapy groups. People often resist joining such groups because, they say, their families and friends and religion are sufficient, or they are embarrassed to turn to strangers, or they just don't like joining groups. Once they join a group, however, they find that talking to people who share the same experiences allows them to open up and say things they could not otherwise say. For people whose family and friends are unable to be much help, support and therapy groups are lifesavers.

Talking to people who share your situation can reduce your sense of isolation and give you a feeling of community. Listening to them talk can also give you a different perspective on your own problems. Seeing what works for other people, and what does not, helps you decide what might work for you. Hearing your problems described by someone else as their problems is somehow reassuring, calming—you don't feel alone with your problems; you're in good company. People say that groups give them a sense of relief from their own problems, and a sense of hope. People like the thought that they might be helping others in their group.

Support and therapy groups are found everywhere (see Appendix A, "Resources"): hospitals, clinics, churches, AIDS-advocacy organizations, to name a few. Groups are composed of people with common situations. Some groups are for people who have the virus but no symptoms; some are for people with HIV infection, some for people with AIDS; some are for caregivers; some are for the people with HIV infection or AIDS and their caregivers; some are for women with HIV infection; some are for black men with HIV infection; some are for gay men; some are for injection drug users.

Though the difference between support and therapy groups is not always clear-cut, support groups tend to be for company and comfort, therapy groups for solving specific problems. The goals of support groups often include learning to reduce isolation, to share experiences, to see what works for others, to express things you might not express elsewhere, to feel accepted. Those who choose a support group are principally looking for a safe place in which to be themselves and to be less isolated. The goals of therapy groups are the same, but also include learning to confront patterns in people's lives with which they are unhappy: they feel they are always lonely, for instance, or that they pick the wrong sorts of partners. These are not necessarily problems specific to HIV infection, though everyone else in the group should also be dealing with HIV infection. Both types of groups should be small, usually from five to eight people. Both groups are usually led, more or less loosely, by a qualified, experienced mental health professional.

Alan began going to a support group when his counselor recommended it: "The group has had a big effect on me. One of the worst things about the virus is not talking about it. When I talk to the group, my feeling of isolation is gone. The group also helps me release stress and anger. Plus you get a perspective on HIV, that it's no big thing, though I'm logical enough to know it is a big thing. But the perspective helps me not paralyze myself and not get into self-fulfilling prophecies. The group has been such a support."

Steven found that his group helped him feel hope and courage: "It's uplifting at the meetings. You get encouraged to keep trying to find help, to pursue all avenues. You learn that someone is out there no matter how bad it is. You learn you're entitled to help."

Support groups help people understand themselves better and find connections with other people. "Sometimes, when you finally verbalize the things that are pretty far down," Alan said, "they become a permanent part of you. I have always felt pretty isolated, and I was able to say that. One time the group leader said that we will realize the people we love, love us. I found some people who love me that I hadn't even realized did love me. That opens me up to a nonsexual loving relationship."

Mental Health Professionals

Some mental health professionals—psychiatrists, psychologists, social workers, psychiatric nurses, counselors—deal primarily with people affected by HIV infection. Psychiatrists are physicians who have specialized in psychiatry—that is, in disorders of mood and thinking; psychiatrists can prescribe medication. Psychologists have doctoral degrees, either a Ph.D. or an Ed.D., in psychology; psychologists can test and diagnose. Social workers have master's degrees plus supervised training. Psychiatric nurses have master's degrees plus supervised training. And counselors can be pastors or others who counsel people. All these professionals should be certified by the certifying boards of their respective professions. The certifying boards for counselors are variable, some good, some not so good, and as a result, counselors are not as tightly monitored as the other mental health professionals.

To overgeneralize, these professionals offer two kinds of therapy— talk therapy and medical therapy. All of them offer talk therapy. They can help you express and understand and resolve painful feelings, analyze and solve problems with other people, gain a sense of who you are as a whole person. They will work with problems that range from the specific and practical to the fundamental and philosophical. You can say anything to them. Psychiatrists alone can also offer medical therapy, drugs that restore sleep, appetite, and mood. Probably the best advice is to begin with talk therapy, but you will want to ask the professional to refer you for medical therapy if necessary. The professional who is unwilling to do this is best avoided.

If you do not know who the mental health professionals are, begin by asking medical professionals—doctors, nurses, physician's assistants—whom you do know. If they cannot help, they will surely refer you to someone who can. Local AIDS-advocacy groups, the gay community, local mental health associations, and state mental health agencies all have lists of qualified, experienced mental health professionals.

Taking Control

At some level, everyone knows that, as Robert Burton wrote in *The Anatomy of Melancholy,* "[In this life, we are] subject to infirmities, miseries, interrupt, tossed & tumbled up and down, carried about with every small blast, often molested & disquieted upon each slender occasion, uncertain, brittle, & so is all that we trust unto."

One of the conditions of life is that we are susceptible and vulnerable, and so is everyone else we depend on. People affected by HIV infection know that their emotions—depression, anger, uncertainty, fear, guilt, dependency—though painful to feel and difficult to admit, are also realistic and perhaps inevitable. They know that despite the comfort of their friends and relatives, they must resolve these painful emotions alone. Their resolutions, though varied, are at bottom the same: somehow or other, they learn to deal with the conditions of life. The twentieth-century poet Randall Jarrell wrote: "'If you are afraid of wolves, do not go into the forest,' the Russian proverb says. We all live in the forest, and there is nothing to do but get used to the wolves."

Getting used to the wolves, for people affected by HIV infection, means that in spite of an inescapable infection and the inevitable accompanying emotions, they're in charge. They make their own decisions and determine their own outlooks. "I'm made of good stuff," Dean said, "and the stuff I'm made of doesn't change because my situation changes." "Facing what I'm up against gives me a new frame of mind," said Alan. "I expected a lot of life that I might not get. But I will do the best for myself and be an inspiration to others. I think we have more control over our lives than even we think we do."

When Alan said adjusting to HIV infection gave him a new frame of mind, he had been living with the infection for six years. Since then, however, he has begun taking new drugs and his world has changed again, giving him an even newer frame of mind. "My CD4 cells were down to 24. Without knowing it, I'd resigned myself to being less of a person, being less responsible, to not working. That meant I wasn't going to live that long. Now my CD4 cells are up to 280, and I'm going back to coping with reality. I started back to work, came home, and cried. This surviving business is nearly as tough as losing everything. In so many ways, I'm the new kid on the block."

Dean's world changed in much the same way: "I got pneumonia. I lost 30 pounds. I had 12 CD4 cells and a half-million viral load. I was on the road to dying and accepting it. I looked God in the face and said, 'Take me, I'm yours.' He didn't. He shoved me right back here on earth. I got all the drugs in the world. That was five months ago. I'm alive now and feeling ok, but I can't stay out and party."

Living with HIV infection is not easy. But easy or not, people do get used to the wolves, do gain a sense of control, do find a new frame of mind. Here are some nice rules that in spite of their simple-mindedness, work.

Consider Changing Your Usual Tactics

Most of the tactics people use to get through their lives are appropriate to normal circumstances. HIV infection, however, is certainly not one of life's normal circumstances. So people occasionally have to consider switching their normal tactics, their usual style of living, the way they normally go about things. Alan has been a successful professional whose success was partly the result of concentrating hard, working persistently, passing tests, and solving problems until he got what he wanted. But HIV infection and his new medication present him with different kinds of problems: his job is now too demanding, and he needs more emotional support. For these problems, Alan's usual tactics—concentration, hard work, and persistence—no longer work. So he's gradually changing his tactics. "I was more aggressive in the workplace than I am now," he said. "For the past ten years, I was a real high producer. Now I won't push myself. It's a tough adjustment going from star to drone. But what options do you have?" Alan asked to be assigned a less demanding job and taught himself not to bring work home. He spends more time with his friends now.

Divide and Conquer

Cut overwhelming and insoluble problems into manageable, solvable ones. People have various ways of doing this.

Divide problems into those that have solutions and those that do not, and focus on the problems that have solutions. Focus on short-term problems. What this tactic comes down to is this: avoid looking at the whole picture and trying to solve everything at once. Steven says he lives from one day to the next, and does only what is necessary to get through each day. He says he solves only small problems, one at a time, and trusts they will add up. Edward Carroll said almost identically, "It really is the old adage of taking each day as it comes—I don't think a whole lot about next week or next year."

Dean says he has learned to stop worrying about overwhelming problems. He tries to change only what he can: "I always tried so hard to change things I couldn't. Realistically I can't change my problems—the only way not to have problems is to be dead. And I can realistically change myself. I forgot I could make myself happy. I am as happy or unhappy as I decide to be. I'm surprised at how happy I am, and it's not in spite of the problems. There are happy people with problems." In short, take it a little at a time.

Expect of yourself only what is reasonable. Try not to borrow trouble or worry about what might happen or cross bridges before you come to them. Be easy on yourself.

Take a Break

"With this disease," says Steven, "you need an escape hatch. Sometimes I zombie out in front of the TV." Lisa goes for long walks, reads what she describes as "trashy love stories," and drives out into the country. People go away for a weekend, plan an evening away at a play, an opera, a concert, a sports event, a movie. For a while, they let themselves drop their worries, they say, and think of nothing except the pleasure of the moment. Some, like Helen, take advantage of the mind's ability to distract itself with pleasant thoughts. She has learned to recognize these moments of pleasure as they occur and to say to herself, "At this minute I happen to be happy, so I'll enjoy this minute."

A lot of people do relaxation exercises; they say relaxation gives them the necessary distance from their problems. Relaxation exercises are part of performing artists' training, some psychotherapies, meditation routines, and yoga practices. All exercises are pretty much the same. Go into a room, maybe your bedroom, and close the door. Ask anyone else in the house to make sure that you are not interrupted. Lie down and get comfortable. Beginning with your feet and working up to your face and scalp, muscle by muscle, first tense the muscle, then relax it. Repeat the tension and relaxation with each muscle several times before going on to the next muscle. Eventually you will notice that you breathe more slowly and regularly, that your body relaxes, and, finally, that your mind relaxes. In this state of relaxation, imagine yourself in a place you know about that is comforting to you, a place you've always wanted to be, a place where you have been free and have felt happy, where you feel safe and calm. Stop the exercise when you feel like it. You can either do this relaxation on your own or buy recorded tapes that direct you through the relaxation or join a group that does the exercises together. In any case, mental health professionals often know where you can get help learning the exercises.

When Edward wants a break, he listens to music: "Music is a great salve for me," he said. "I listen to music that's evocative to me of places and events that I want to remember fondly. I can conjure up places, I can close my eyes and feel things. Those memories are really the sum of my life. The places where I found real joy in life I can revisit. There's a piece by Keith Jarrett called "Köln Concert" that to me is the place I grew up. When I want to go home, I put that on and there I go."

Give Your Feelings Their Due

When you feel bad, go ahead and feel that way. Tell yourself, as Dean does, "I'm just tired of this. I don't see how I can do it any more." Cry, stare into space, refuse to talk, stay in bed, write your terrible feelings in a private journal—go off by yourself and do whatever expresses the bad feelings. "I don't believe in this crap of, 'You've got to be happy all the time,'" says Steven. "I'm not taped together as well as I thought I was, or more likely, the tape was old. Anyway, sometimes I fall apart and just feel awful."

In short, give your feelings their due. This is not giving in. It is acknowledging the reality and size of the problems you face. "This is not the best thing that ever happened to me," said Rebecca. "My life was much better. I feel like I'm being negative, but I'm not necessarily being filled with light." Somehow, such acknowledgment is easier than trying to control how you feel, or going from crisis to crisis and never feeling anything. These feelings, once acknowledged, don't last as long as you might think. They seem to wear themselves out and disappear. "After I've been feeling hopeless for a while," says Dean, "the feeling lightens up, and I feel that I've really got a good road ahead of me. I feel like I'd just like to keep going."

The bad feelings will certainly come back again—Steven says he now knows when he is likely to feel bad and sets aside time for the feelings: "I plan for falling apart," he says. But when the feelings do come back, you will have them in better perspective. That is, you will know that the feelings are both real and temporary. You will know that the situation hasn't changed, only your view of it has. For good reasons, you feel bad; and after a while, for reasons just as good, you will feel better.

Learn to Deal with the Medical System

A crucial part of living well is taking control. A crucial part of taking control, for some people, is learning to deal with the medical system. The medical system is complicated (chapter 7 outlines the system and explains who does what). The best advice we can give the person with HIV infection is to find a doctor who treats HIV infection for a living (see chapter 7). "I was growing concerned with my local doctor, who wasn't keeping up," said Rebecca. "I would read about research in the *Wall Street Journal* and ask him and he wouldn't have heard of it. The writing was on the wall, I'd outgrown my doctor and needed to find an expert." Bluntly put, people with experienced doctors live longer.

The next best advice is to ask questions. One reason that people don't ask questions is because they feel intimidated. Medical people often don't understand that they are intimidating. If you don't ask them questions, they assume you already know the answers, not that you're afraid to ask. Another reason people don't ask questions is because they worry about offending their physicians. Any good physician will not be offended by a question. Neither of these is a good reason not to find out what you want to know.

Ask how to get medical care at night and on weekends. Get pushy if you are in pain; pain is usually unnecessary. Ask what's happening with new treatments. Ask what tests you are being given, what those tests detect, what the alternatives to the tests are. Ask for a second opinion on a diagnosis or an interpretation of a test. People worry especially about asking for second opinions; but this is a reasonable and prudent request, and physicians are not offended by it.

In general, you have a right to know about treatments, medications, and procedures. Patients in hospitals have a whole set of rights; chapter 7 outlines them.

It is a good idea to write questions down before visiting the doctor: most people forget some or most of what they want to ask. Questions about medical care are best addressed to your doctors. Questions about the medical system and resources for medical care in general are best addressed to a social worker.

Edward Carroll, a long-time activist who writes columns on AIDS research, has had to teach himself the relevant medicine. "You have to understand enough of what the doctor is telling you," he says, "so you can make a rational decision about your care. I think good patients with good doctors survive longer and live better than bad patients with good doctors."

Relabel the Negative; Focus on the Positive

Relabeling means redefining a troubling situation so that it seems more benign (see chapter 5). Relabeling is related to thinking positively: any situation, no matter how bad, also contains the possibility for something good. The idea is to focus on the possibilities for good and define the situation in those terms. "If I approach it with the right attitude," says Steven, "I can see the blessings."

Call something a challenge rather than a struggle, a preference rather than a need, an opportunity rather than a problem. Alan says even though life "is tough or difficult, if I look at it from a different angle it's just grace. I have a good life and it's by my design." And some people manage the near-miracle of relabeling HIV infection itself. "This infection gave my life purpose," said Edward. "I never aspired to much of anything, I just sort of poked along at life. I always worked hard, but never with any goal in mind. And this infection gave me the opportunity to do good and useful work. In very many ways, it's the best thing that ever happened to me. I've done my best work. I've met the best people I've ever known. Who can complain about that?"

Shakespeare's Hamlet says, "For there is nothing either good or bad, but thinking makes it so." With relabeling, people come to feel they're in control, they're calling the shots, they're in charge of how they're affected and what their reactions are. By relabeling they shape the character and quality of their own lives.

Eat Well

In general, people with HIV infection should be careful about their nutrition; a balanced diet including all the food groups is important. For specific advice, ask a registered dietitian. (A registered dietitian is usually trained and licensed in nutrition and problems of nutrition; nutritionists need not be either trained or licensed.) Registered dietitians can be found at hospitals, clinics, and county health departments, and in private practice.

Dietitians often advise people with HIV infection on issues related to lipodystrophy. The main benefit to dietary advice is when blood lipids—cholesterol and triglycerides—are too high. Dietitians can't usually give useful advice about fat redistribution. Sometimes, dietitians' advice also helps people avoid infection by microbes like *Salmonella* that live in perishable food. Such infections occur only rarely in people with HIV infection. If you want to be extra cautious, however, the microbes' growth can be inhibited by very hot and very cold temperatures, and by cleanliness. Keep hot food hot: cook at 165 degrees F to 212 degrees F, keep warm at 140 degrees F to 165 degrees F. Keep cold foods cold: refrigerate at 40 degrees F, freeze at 0 degrees F. Keep everything clean: wash fresh fruit and vegetables. Do not eat moldy food. Do not eat rare meat, raw fish, or raw meat, and do not drink unpasteurized milk. Thaw meat in the refrigerator, not at room temperature. Do not eat raw eggs; cook eggs thoroughly.

Encourage Yourself

Protect your physical health. Eat well, sleep enough, cut alcohol and smoking down or out. Exercise reasonably and regularly; just going for a walk is great exercise. Relax when you can: read, watch a movie, do relaxation exercises. Take good care of your body; give your body a chance to fight the infection.

Be kind to yourself emotionally. Steven gives himself pep talks: "When I feel good," he says, "I let myself know that. I tell myself, 'Steve, you feel great today.'" Dean says that every day he rates how he feels on a scale of one to ten: "It's mostly nines and tens," he says.

Helen says that her best support is herself. "Basically, it comes down to me," she says. "I have to support myself, and when I do something well, I pat myself on the back." You can pat yourself on the back for the littlest things: "You certainly did a good job of polishing your shoes," you can say, or "My, but those fingernails are clean." The reason for the pat is less important than the pat itself. The pep talks Rebecca gives herself are more like inspirational lectures: "Every moment of my day is to lift myself up," she said. "Throughout the day I say, 'Jesus is healing me.' I tell myself I am healed, I am healed. I don't accept this illness at all. I talk to this virus and tell it to get out of my body. I'm going to beat this."

If an emotional problem seems too severe or does not go away, or if you are seriously considering suicide, or if you simply want someone to whom you can express all your feelings, see a mental health professional.

Confront the Possibilities a Little at a Time

Once, when Dean was in the hospital, he roomed for a while with a man who was in the advanced stages of AIDS. "I was glad to get out of that room," Dean said. "As long as I was there, I needed to confront the possibility that what happened to him would happen to me. But confronting that possibility seemed necessary, to deal with this disease as positively as I am."

Confronting the possibilities means, for Dean and others like him, understanding and admitting that the fact of HIV infection cannot be annulled. Steven said, "I have to deal with this whether I want to or not." It is now a part of life. So are the possibilities of clinical appointments, physical discomfort, and complicated and unforgiving drug regimens. And so are the emotional reactions to all this. "HIV makes me face things I didn't think I'd have to face," Helen said.

Confronting everything all at once, however, is overwhelming and unnecessary. Face what you are ready to face, and only when you are ready. When you are tired of thinking or feeling, stop and rest. Do not push yourself because you or someone else thinks you ought to be facing things. Face a little at a time.

Positive Denial

Denial has a negative sound, as though you weren't facing facts. But whether denial is positive or negative depends on what you are denying. Denial is negative only if people deny the facts of their infection and live inappropriately: drink too much, ignore their drug regimen, practice unsafe sex, or avoid seeing a doctor.

Denial that admits both the realities of today and the unpredictability of tomorrow is positive. No one knows what new treatments will come along. No one knows how any one person's body will handle HIV infection.

Positive denial is nearly essential in dealing with this disease. "Friends ask me how I deal with the diagnosis," said Rebecca. "I tell them I don't deal with it. I'm not denying the illness, I'm denying it access to take over my life."

Your life has many aspects, many parts to it, many things you are interested in, many things and people you love; and HIV, though important, is only one aspect of your life. "I'm not denying I'm sick," Dean said. "But I've made up my mind not to act sick, not to just sit around being a sick person."

Positive denial also helps people feel feisty about the disease. They feel like they are not just victims of some virus; they are people who have some say in how their lives are run. "Steven Charles is much bigger than this infection," said Steven. "I'm not letting the illness be that big a deal. I'll be changed—it will always be a big part of who I am. But I haven't lost control. It makes me feel good every day, the things I do to heal myself. I think, this is going to pay off, this is going to pay off."

Find Comforts and Interests in Things Outside Yourself

"Don't lock yourself in," says Steven, "get yourself out." The world is full of pleasures, beauty, people to get to know, wrongs that need to be righted, jobs that need to be done, places to visit, adventures to be had. People find, in things outside themselves, anything from a trivial and momentary distraction to a profound interest in living. The possibilities are limitless.

Some people make their surroundings beautiful and comforting. Helen says she tries to make the place where she spends her time a space she enjoys: "I like brass and glass. I like plants—they're another life. I like a little elegance. Things should be as fine as they can be." Rebecca repainted her house: "I've made it warm, restful, and interesting with colors. These colors reflect a color of light that looks good on people. People look wonderful in my house. And my own house is a comfort to me."

Some people find things they like to do, or things they have always wanted to do but have never done. Helen gardens: "I crave being out there. I put all these bulbs in, and now I have next year to look forward to. Plus I also have a room I want to redecorate." Dean plays music and reads: "Thinking about HIV is stressful and if I can drive it out of my mind, that's relief. I play music, the guitar. I'm in a band and we perform once or twice a month. It's a great distraction, very fulfilling. Mostly I read. Dickens is the best. If you've got HIV, just go out and get the Dickens library."

Some people teach themselves new things because learning, they say, takes them out of themselves. Steven became interested in archaeology and astronomy: "Maybe, in the light of ancient history and the immense universe," he says, "my disability insurance isn't all that important. Now I wonder why people worry about things that don't matter all that much." Alan had decided to make a career in banking, but his training was in music. As he's relaxed his focus on his career, he has turned back to his music. "My viral load is undetectable," he said. "I'm going to buy a new instrument—which is like buying a car. I could make a living in a professional orchestra. Maybe now I can do what I need to do, what my heart tells me to do. It's here, the fire is still burning, I'll do what it takes. I deserve to make a good penny making music."

Some people spend more time with people they love and enjoy. Some people become activists. Lisa was going to run for city council, but decided instead that she could do more putting out a newsletter, so she raised money and started one: "I think you should speak up, be visible, be yourself." Steven began doing public speaking and recommends it to others: "Get interested in legislation," he said, "in outreach; contact speakers' bureaus, call people up. I've gone from being a passive type to being a real civil disobedient type." Edward is doing all this and more: he taught himself immunology, helps run a money-raising organization for which he single-handedly puts out a newsletter on AIDS research, and is editor of a local newspaper for which he writes a regular column on AIDS. Dean is writing a book about his experiences with AIDS, and says the book gives him a positive attitude: "It's leaving my mark. It's doing what will help other people."

Some people help others in different ways. Many become buddies through AIDS-advocacy programs. Dean volunteered in a hospital on a floor for children with cancer. "It was hard on me to see those kids so sick," he said, "but it put things in perspective for me. I thought, 'Who am I to complain? They're so good and so happy.'" Helen is less ambitious but no less helpful: "I visit the woman who used to be my roommate in the hospital. She won't eat anything. I make her get out of bed, sit in a chair, go for a walk, and then I give her jellybeans."

Maintain Equilibrium

Living with HIV infection requires balancing hope and uncertainty, confidence and worry, courage and despair. The balance is tricky, and many people with HIV infection, whether or not their health has improved, manage it by consciously lowering the amount of stress in their lives.

"I take my time, nap, read, I try not to get upset any more," said Dean. "Also I get a massage twice a week. I don't drink or smoke. I get eight to nine hours of sleep a day. I eat three good meals a day. I work out, though I don't exhaust myself. I live more cautiously, take a sweater when I go out, things I wouldn't have done before. People in my life I had problems with before, I started contacting them—they were very open, very friendly. I just try to be nicer to people than I was before. It makes you just feel good."

Rebecca has to contend not only with the same balance but with side effects of the drugs. "I look normal but I get tired. And I can throw up very easily. A good day is when everything is in symphony, when I keep everything down, don't feel tired. One bad day—even just emotionally bad—and I can't rebound. I walk a fine line every day. If I have my routine and don't push myself, then I can allow this illness. I can deal with it. I tell myself, 'Don't rush, don't rush.' I've had to stop being so achievement oriented. I've always had a goal, but stress sets me up for being sick. I stay at my house and do things my way. I want so much to have a normal day every day. Maintaining equilibrium requires a lot of work."

By not pushing themselves, Rebecca and Dean maintain an equilibrium, which allows them to not be overwhelmed by their problems and to enjoy life. Rebecca's days are balanced: "I walk my dog, clean the house, exercise. I go for a power walk. I watch re-runs of Andy Griffith's show; I love that Barney. They all care about each other. Sometimes I'll buy a soft t-shirt. I walk through this development and look at the grass, the flowers. There's so much beauty around us. I feel so much better— I see God, see goodness. This is something I never would have done before."

A Positive Attitude

People affected by HIV infection agree on this, that the single most important thing they can do is to keep a positive attitude.

"I've become more conscious of the quality of life," Dean says. "Now I'm concerned with living before I die, and living *every* minute. Sometimes it's like a violent smack: wake up and enjoy life."

Steven has feelings that are almost identical: "I don't know where my ability to enjoy life comes from. I love life so much, I want every minute. I keep myself occupied and my mind working. I compare myself to other people—I still have advantages others don't. I've been fortunate."

Keeping a positive attitude can change the way people think of themselves. They think of themselves less as people with a disease and more as people who are alive. They say they know how to be alive and will live their lives the way they know how. They come to trust their own resources, to trust themselves. Sometimes they even become different people: "I've never liked telling anyone what's going on with me," said Alan, "but dealing with this disease has made me more open than any time in my life. I'm voicing my opinion more, am more self-confident."

Keeping a positive attitude can also change the way people see other people. Helen said HIV infection had changed her, too, then added: "I really want to do something to help people, not just people with HIV and AIDS. Maybe through my trials and while I'm still here, I can just be an example. We're all connected and if you do good for others, you do good for yourself."

And finally, keeping a positive attitude can also change the way people feel about the future. "I'm not going anywhere any time soon," Alan said. "I'm thinking about the future and I'm not talking 5 or 10 years, I'm talking old age." Dean's partner said the same: "Sometimes I see us being old together." "I'm alive and I'm well, so I'm brave enough to look down the road to the future," said Rebecca. "Who knows, maybe my husband and I can have kids. I'd really like that." And Helen, whose viral load is still detectable, says she doesn't know what the future holds but she won't give up: "I've worked too hard, I'm a good person, and I have a will power that won't quit. I want to make something positive out of something negative."

Dean has a motto he uses to keep himself active and interested in life: "A body at rest stays at rest," he says, "and a body in motion stays in motion." He borrowed the idea from his high-school physics class and, he says, "I say it over and over. I use it to think myself well."

People come to believe that life need not be perfect or infinite or certain to be good and that hope can come in little packets and delight can come from little things. "I've been able to cope and feel happy and delighted about living," said Steven. "A lot has to do with your attitude toward life. You like it or you don't."

Chapter 12

What's Ahead

The history of HIV is brief but dense. It is filled with aggressive debates, politics, human tragedy, a rich vein of research in medical science, and a dramatic change in drugs and tests in 1996 that translated immediately into better health and longer life.

AIDS was first described in 1981. The first report, of a small number of gay men with pneumocystis pneumonia, was relegated to the second page of the Centers for Disease Control's weekly bulletin. The virus that causes AIDS was identified two years later, in 1983; by then, epidemiologic studies had already identified virtually all mechanisms of transmission. Once the virus was found, the next conquest was a diagnostic test, which by 1985 had become a part of medical care. During the next ten years, researchers traced the infection's path through the body and worked hard to defeat the virus. By now, HIV infection has emerged as arguably the most important epidemic of the twentieth century. And at the beginning of the twenty-first century, it is the world's most common cause of death from a microbe.

AIDS is following the same history as the other newly detected microbes of the past twenty-five years—Legionnaires' disease, toxic shock syndrome, *Helicobacter pylori*, and Lyme disease. In each case, the disease was described, the responsible microbe identified, the diagnostic test created, preventive strategies developed, and treatment, usually with an antibiotic, found. With the same approach and with the help of public health, many older infectious diseases have lost their menace. These diseases have been some of the great epidemics in the history of medicine: diphtheria, measles, mumps, whooping cough, polio, tetanus, rheumatic fever, tuberculosis, nephritis, cholera, and typhoid fever. Twenty years ago, smallpox was eradicated throughout the world. This incredible success story, however, may have established an unrealistic expectation that faced with a new microbe, modern medicine wins easily. Still, the precedent is established, and if the plague is bad enough, the combined efforts of public health, medical research, and medical care will succeed.

HIV has turned out to be a formidable enemy. To begin with, many features of HIV infection are unique. One unique feature is its persistence. Once HIV is incorporated into the body's genes, it stays there for the rest of life. Other viral infections—the herpes viruses, for instance—are also persistent, but unlike HIV, they are usually dormant. HIV is usually in a state of constant growth.

Another unique feature is that HIV infection is primarily transmitted by sexual intercourse and injection drug use at a time when injection drug use is an epidemic and attitudes about sexual experiences are liberal. Asking people to modify their sexual behavior is a form of disease control that has never been successful. Asking people to stop their drug abuse is another sad tale.

Still another unique feature is that HIV attacks the very system designed to protect the body against attack. As a result, people with HIV infection are not usually sick because of the virus, but because of other infections that seize the opportunity presented by weakened immune defenses. In addition to these unique features, HIV is also formidable because it has an extraordinary rate of mutation. By midstage in the infection, the average person has a million different forms of the virus; by late stage, over 100 billion different forms. Any virus with this property changes its appearance so fast that no single vaccine or drug is likely to target all variants; influenza virus has the same property and therefore requires a new vaccine each year. The highly-publicized problem with antibiotic resistance happens with HIV just as it does with common bacteria. Thus, some of those mutant strains of the virus will be resistant to a drug designed to kill them and will flourish in its presence. The result is that many or most drugs directed against HIV are likely to be effective only temporarily. The same problem of resistance applies to potential vaccines.

In fact, most of medicine's success in controlling infections with drugs has been with bacterial infections rather than viral infections. Literally thousands of viruses infect people, but the only viral infections that can be treated successfully with drugs are influenza, herpes, shingles, cytomegalovirus, and some forms of hepatitis. For some reason, bacteria appear to be much easier targets.

Despite these difficulties, however, progress in the war on AIDS has been substantial. The first drug, AZT, was found effective in 1986 and approved shortly thereafter, in 1987. In the next few years, a series of related drugs followed: ddI, ddC, d4T, and 3TC. All these drugs worked, but only temporarily: clinical trials between 1986 and 1994 showed that these drugs extended life by six to twelve months at best. Further trials between 1993 and 1995 showed that two of these drugs taken together worked better than one. But progress was clearly slow, the available drugs flawed, and the challenge high. Professional meetings on HIV infection were filled with smug satisfaction about progress in preventing complications and with boring and somewhat unconvincing presentations about drugs named with letters and numbers.

So in 1996, with the stunning changes in managing HIV infection, the optimism was unprecedented. Three interrelated developments came in rapid sequence. First was the demonstration that in the average person, HIV produced 10 billion new viruses every day. This demonstration not only clarified the central role of the virus in causing AIDS and its complications, but it also implied that the virus had to be the target of any therapeutic attack. The second development was viral load testing, a new method of determining prognosis and response to treatment. The viral load test meant that physicians no longer had to wait until their patients got drastic decreases in CD4 counts or pneumocystis pneumonia or wasting or even died to find out if the treatment was not working. With viral load testing, the physician could tell within two to four weeks whether the drug was knocking back the virus. The third development was new drugs that, though requiring a complex regimen, were far more potent than their predecessors. At the end of 1996, AIDS researcher David Ho, of the Aaron Diamond AIDS Research Center, was *Time* magazine's Man of the Year and protease inhibitors were *Science* magazine's Breakthrough of the Year.

By 1997, the real progress of 1996 was obvious, and in cases of HIV infection followed to 2000, this progress continued. For the first time in the history of the disease, death rates from AIDS in the United States were down by 60 to 70 percent. Rates of hospitalization and rates of progression to AIDS were down by 60 to 80 percent. Rates of transmission of HIV from mother to baby were way down. AIDS wards throughout the country were running at 30 to 50 percent occupancy. And one life insurance company was bold enough to offer life insurance to people with HIV infection.

To a physician working in an HIV clinic, the shift of events was dramatic. The typical office visit of 1995 was occupied largely by warnings: about complications, about the importance of preventing complications, about using CD4 counts to track the rate of decline. In 1996, the typical office visit was an explanation of progress in the field, a description of treatment options, a discussion about when to start therapy, a review of drug toxicities, and viral load testing. For many of us, the new treatment was as close to a miracle as medicine ever gets. One patient had a CD4 count of 9, a late-stage complication with MAC bacteremia, and a life prognosis of six months; he now has a CD4 count of over 500 and has returned to work. Another patient who had wasting and had lost 50 pounds is now a weight-lifter. A young woman with PCP and a CD4 count of 4 in 1995 decided, despite her odds, to go on a respirator; she now has a CD4 count of 500, has had no detectable virus for eight years, and lives a healthy life.

These are not isolated exceptions. A statistical analysis in 2006 of a large population of people with HIV infection shows that on average, HAART lengthens life by 179 months, or about fifteen years. On average, coronary by-pass surgery adds 20 months to a person's life; cancer chemotherapy, 10 months. It's fair to say that treatment of HIV infection has made more progress in the past twenty years than treatment for any other widespread serious disease.

What will come next is hard to predict for any human endeavor, but especially for the field of HIV infection. When the virus was first discovered in 1983, the idea that a virus could become an integral part of a human gene seemed highly unlikely. Even though we now know that's true, still we're able to control the virus. But we face big challenges.

- We have no cure. No one with HIV has ever eradicated the virus, either spontaneously or with antiviral drugs.

- The drugs are potent, but their regimens all require three or four drugs and a level of adherence not required in any other field of medicine.

- The drugs have side effects—fat redistribution, blood lipid problems, diabetes—that can be long-term and that were a complete surprise and are still not understood.

- Resistance to drugs limits the treatment of every other infectious disease—pneumonia, sinusitis, tuberculosis, malaria, influenza, as well as HIV infection. By 2005 about 10 to 25 percent of new HIV infections were with strains of HIV that had at least one major resistance mutation.

- Everyone agrees that prevention is a high priority. We also have good evidence that so far, prevention efforts have failed. Although progress in treatment has been extraordinarily successful, progress in prevention has not. In the United States, the estimated number of new infections in 1990 was 40,000; in 2005 it was also 40,000. The rest of the world is no better: the global burden of HIV disease is now double what the World Health Organization thought in 1990 that it would be by now. About one-third of people with HIV infection in the United States don't know they have it and therefore continue risking transmission of the infection. Preventing transmission by tracing the sexual contacts of people with the infection is standard practice for nearly all sexually transmitted diseases except this one. Preventing transmission by drug abusers (who make up 25 percent of people with HIV infection) by needle exchange programs is known to work, but is mired in politics. Prevention efforts currently target the middle period of HIV infection, which accounts for only 30 percent of the transmission; the other 70 percent of transmissions take place during the first and last weeks of infection when the viral load is very high. This mismatch needs to be addressed with a more serious and focused public health effort.

Even though the future remains unpredictable, some high-priority developments are in process and are likely to change the field.

- Treatment simplification: Therapy will get easier. The first-line treatment will likely be reduced to one or two pills per day, and each pill will contain two or three drugs.

- Testing: Testing will get easier. The blood test to detect HIV, the CD4 cell counts, and the viral load tests are about as accurate as they can get, but they should become cheaper and faster. The resistance test still needs work: interpreting it requires special expertise, and even then, the experts disagree. The current tests for "minority species"—that is, viruses that are hidden in the body that can cause trouble in the presence of the right drug—find only the dominant 80 percent and are being refined so they will find the other 20 percent.

- Drug side effects: We are likely to find the cause of the "metabolic syndrome"—the fat redistribution, the lipid problems, and diabetes—and will find drugs without those side effects. We'll also develop effective methods for predicting who gets those side effects.

- Genetics: With the identification of the human genome, the field of genetics has exploded. So far, the explosion has not translated into the windfall of diagnostic tests and therapeutic drugs that geneticists promised, but fulfilling the promise is just a matter of time. For the field of HIV infection, genetics should eventually be able to explain why some people never get HIV despite hundreds or thousands of exposures; why some people who go untreated progress through the infection rapidly and others remain apparently well for twenty years; why some people have the metabolic syndrome side effect with certain protease inhibitors and others don't; why 5 percent of people with HIV infection have unusual reactions to the drugs, like the abacavir hypersensitivity reaction, or the serious liver disease that can accompany nevirapine. Genetics determines the extent to which the immune system and drugs control HIV. So understanding genetics should dramatically improve the prospects for both a therapeutic vaccine and antiretroviral therapy.

• Therapeutic vaccine: Since HIV infection first surfaced, efforts to develop a vaccine to prevent it have been extensive and well-funded. The effort has attracted the best immunologic scientists in the world and has resulted in amazing discoveries in immunology and vaccine strategies. But apparently the prospects for a preventive vaccine are little better now than they were in 1985. Hopes for a therapeutic vaccine—a vaccine not to prevent HIV infection but to control it—are much higher. A therapeutic vaccine would control HIV much the way the immune system does, once it recognizes the virus. A good therapeutic vaccine would augment the immune response, and though it would not cure HIV infection, it would reduce or even eliminate the need for pills and the accompanying nuisances of remembering them and suffering the side effects.

• New antiviral drugs: HIV therapy began in 1987 with one drug, AZT, and now has over twenty; and the pipeline is rich with new drugs. Particularly important are the new classes of drugs, drugs that the virus has never seen and for which it has no resistance. The classes attracting the most attention are integrase inhibitors and attachment inhibitors.

Appendix A

Resources: Where to Go for Help

- Types of services
- Selected national resources
- Finding local services

Many organizations offer help of different types to people affected by HIV. The list of these resources, however, is a moving target. Any such list—and there are many—gets outdated fast. New organizations spring up, and old organizations change the services they offer, change their addresses and phone numbers, expand, merge, or go out of business. Most lists of resources are updated every few months.

Given that, the best thing this book can do is list the types of services that can be available to people affected by HIV, list a few national resources that offer these services, and offer advice on how to find resources that are local.

Types of Services

The types of services an organization offers will depend on, among other things, the purpose of the organization and its geographical location. The range of services is immense, from problems specific to some people (e.g., Spanish-speaking educational counselors) to problems shared by everyone with HIV infection (education on preventing transmission). If the organizations do not offer the services themselves, they will recommend other organizations that do offer the services.

The following is a list of the services organizations may offer. If you need any of these services, call a national organization (see below) to find who in your local area offers the services. Or find a local resource (see below) that offers them.

Alcoholism: the national organization Alcoholics Anonymous (AA) has information on which of its local branches offer groups specific to people with HIV infection who also have problems with alcohol.

Buddy systems: buddies are volunteers, sometimes trained, who provide services that range from filling prescriptions and driving you to the grocery store to cleaning the refrigerator and holding hands.

Children with HIV infection

Counseling: can be individual or group counseling (see below, "Support groups")

Drug use and HIV infection

Financial problems

Government reports

HIV testing

Home health care

Hospice care

Hotlines: toll-free phone numbers, either community, state, or national. Ask any questions about HIV infection and about services available to people with HIV infection.

Housing problems

Insurance problems

Legal services

Minorities and HIV infection, including organizations with Spanish-speaking counselors

Nursing homes

Physician referral

Political action, speakers' bureaus

Preventing transmission of HIV

Religious counseling

Safer sex

Scientific research reports

Sexually transmitted disease testing and treatment

Social workers help with plans for recuperating at home, with plans for finances and insurance, with recommendations to different organizations. They are hired by mental health centers, churches, social service agencies, and virtually all hospitals.

Support groups: groups can be specifically for women, gays, drug users, couples, caregivers, spouses, the worried well, and people who are HIV-positive, or who have AIDS.

Transportation

Visiting nurse programs

Women and HIV infection

Selected National Resources

The following is a list of national resources, selected because they are good sources of information, whether in print, by phone, or online. These organizations sometimes change their telephone numbers. If you call and get a message that the number is not in service, try directory assistance. For 800 numbers, the directory assistance number is 1-800-555-1212. These organizations also change their Web sites. If you get an error message, try an Internet search with, say, Google, on the organization's name. The Web sites can be difficult to navigate. Try clicking on About Us, or Contact Us, or Site Map.

AIDS Clinical Trials Groups (ACTGs). These are the medical centers (discussed in chapter 8) that are part of a national program of the National Institute of Allergy and Infectious Diseases (NIAID) to test new treatments for HIV infection and all its complications. ACTGs need people to participate in these clinical trials. ACTGs are also superb sources of information about treatment. They also have information specific to HIV-infected women and children. The list of ACTGs changes with time, so the best way to find the ACTG nearest you is online at www.aactg.org/, though this Web site makes information difficult to find. A better site is http://aidsinfo.nih.gov/clinical_trials/. Or call 1-800-448-0440, TTY 1-888-480-3739, Monday to Friday, 12 noon to 5 P.M., Eastern Standard Time. Or e-mail ContactUs@aidsinfo.nih.gov. Or write to AIDSinfo, P.O. Box 6303, Rockville, Md. 20849-6303. For real-time, online help Monday to Friday, 12 noon to 4 P.M. Eastern Standard Time, go to http://aidsinfo.nih.gov/live_help/. All information, whether online or by phone, is available in Spanish as well as English.

AIDS Treatment News, 1233 Locust Street, 5th floor, Philadelphia, Pa. 19107, 1-800-873-2812. This is a free online newsletter on the latest HIV infection treatments, traditional and alternative, plus related legal and policy news. The newsletter is also available in print form, but for a negotiable subscription price. Web site: www.aids news.org/.

American Foundation for AIDS Research (amfAR), 120 Wall Street, 13th Floor, New York, N.Y. 10005. Phone: 1-212-806-1600 or 1-800-39AMFAR. Fax: 1-212-806-1601. AmfAR funds basic biomedical and clinical research, efforts in prevention and education, and the development of AIDS-related public policy. In addition, it publishes print news about treatments, prevention, and policies. To subscribe, write to Public Information at amfAR's address or e-mail publications@amfar.org. Web site: www.amfar.org.

CDC National Prevention Information Network, 1-800-458-5231 (Monday–Friday, 9 A.M. to 6 P.M., Eastern Standard Time), or www .cdcnpin.org. This is a resource for both print and electronic materials, run by the Centers for Disease Control and Prevention, offering information on HIV infection, prevention, treatment, medical care, and local organizations. All information is also available in Spanish. To find current information about organizations, or to talk to a Health Information Specialist, call 1-800-458-5231, TTY 1-800-243-7012, Monday through Friday, 9 A.M. to 6 P.M., Eastern Standard Time. Or e-mail info@cdcnpin.org. Or write CDC NPIN, P.O. Box 6003, Rockville, Md. 20849-6003. Or talk online with an NPIN Information Specialist, www.cdcnpin.org, Monday through Friday, 2 P.M. to 4 P.M., Eastern Standard Time.

Gay Men's Health Crisis (GMHC), 119 W. 24th Street, New York, N.Y. 10011, 1-212-367-1000. GMHC publishes *Treatment Issues,* a monthly newsletter on HIV therapies; also available free online. GMHC also publishes a number of booklets on specific safer sex practices. GMHC has a hotline for AIDS information and for peer counseling: 1-212-807-6655 or 1-800-AIDS-NYC. The Web site, also available in Spanish, is www.gmhc.org.

National Association of People with AIDS (NAPWA), 8401 Colesville Road, Suite 750, Silver Spring, Md. 20910, 1-240-247-0880, info@napwa.org. A national AIDS-advocacy organization, with advice on education in treatment and prevention, on organizing community-based support services, and on policy issues. Publishes guides to dealing with managed care, Medicare/Medicaid, and health insurance, and offers an online newsletter. Web site: www .napwa.org.

National Institute of Allergy and Infectious Diseases (NIAID), a branch of the National Institutes of Health in the U.S. government's Department of Health and Human Services. NIAID is the source of the latest federally approved information about HIV/AIDS. It has an excellent Web site on HIV/AIDS that provides information on drugs, guidelines for treatment, preventive and therapeutic vaccines, clinical trials, and general information at http://aidsinfo.nih.gov/. It also offers real-time online help, Monday to Friday, 12 noon to 4 P.M., Eastern Standard Time, at http://aidsinfo.nih.gov/live_help/. Or call 1-800-448-0440, TTY 1-888-480-3739, Monday to Friday, 12 noon to 5 P.M., Eastern Standard Time. Or e-mail ContactUs @aidsinfo.nih.gov. Or write to AIDSinfo, P.O. Box 6303, Rockville, Md. 20849-6303. All information, whether online or by phone, is available in both Spanish and English.

The National Institute on Drug Abuse is another branch of the government's National Institutes of Health. Its Web site has information on preventing and treating drug or alcohol abuse in people with HIV infection: http://hiv.drugabuse.gov/. For your local resources on general HIV/AIDS information or on HIV testing, call the National AIDS Hotline at 1-800-342-2437; or in Spanish, 1-800-344-7432; or TTY 1-800-243-7889. Or call the National Prevention Information Network at 1-800-458-5231. Or write P.O. Box 6003, Rockville, Md. 20849-6003.

National STD and AIDS Hotline, 1-800-342-AIDS (1-800-342-2437). This is a 24-hour-a-day, 7-day-a-week hotline, contracted through the Centers for Disease Control and Prevention. Ask them questions about types of services, about general information, and about what services are available in your local area. For Spanish-speaking callers, the number is 1-800-344-SIDA (1-800-344-7432). The TTY number is 1-800-243-7889.

Pharmaceutical Research and Manufacturers of America (PhRMA), Communications Division, Suite 900, 1100 15th Street, N.W., Washington, D.C. 20005, 1-202-835-3400. It publishes *New Medicines in Development for AIDS*, a chart of drugs, diagnostic tests, and vaccines available online at www.phrma.org/newmedicines/aids/.

Project Inform: National hotline with information about treatment for HIV and AIDS. Its Web site provides information about AIDS policy and advocacy. Call 1-800-822-7422 (treatment hotline) Monday–Friday, 9 A.M. to 4 P.M., and on Tuesdays until 7 P.M., Pacific Standard Time. Web site: www.projectinform.org.

San Francisco AIDS Foundation, P.O. Box 426182, San Francisco, Calif. 94142-6182, or One Sixth Street, San Francisco, Calif. 94103; main number: 1-415-487-3000. It publishes *BETA, Bulletin of Experimental Treatments for AIDS,* a newsletter about experimental treatments of HIV infection, updated quarterly; no subscription price, but a donation is requested. The Foundation's AIDS information hotline is 1-415-863-AIDS. The Web site has some issues of *BETA* online at http://sfaf.org/beta/, and good links to other sites: www.sfaf.org.

Other Resources on the Internet

The Internet is a highly varied junk shop. The best sites are extraordinarily helpful, offer up-to-date and accurate information from respected sources, and are linked to a variety of other, sometimes more specific, sites. The worst sites offer speculation as though it were fact. No one assures the quality of any site on the Internet, so, as always, let the buyer beware.

Besides the sites listed in the section above, the following are sites of general interest that we know to be good. Other sites that we don't yet know about might be just as good. See also the Web sites of the other resources cited here.

AIDS.org: The Web site of the publishers of *Treatment News,* it provides extensive information, including basic information, frequently asked questions, treatment recommendations, public policy issues, relevant news items, community issues, and summaries of medical conferences. www.aids.org.

The Body: Aimed at people affected by HIV infection. A searchable site, covering treatments, HIV/AIDS news, prevention, lists of local resources, quality-of-life issues, policy issues, professional meetings, lists of hotlines, many links to other sites. Information is in the form of articles, mostly taken from the newsletters of community-based organizations. www.thebody.com.

HIVInSite, University of California, San Francisco, Center for AIDS Prevention Studies: Aimed at caregivers but readable by anyone. A searchable site, covering treatment, prevention, research, statistics, trials, drugs, professional meetings, policy, and legislation. http://hivinsite.ucsf.edu.

Johns Hopkins AIDS Service: Aimed at caregivers but readable by anyone. A searchable site covering medical management, treatment guide, research, epidemiology, trials, and case conferences with freely downloadable publications, a question-and-answer section that allows you to ask questions, and archives of previous answers. www .hopkins-aids.edu.

National Center for HIV, STD, and TB Prevention; CDC Division of HIV/AIDS Prevention: An official government Web site with extensive data on HIV/AIDS statistics, guidelines for management, federal funding, frequently asked questions, prevention, HIV testing, publications, and fact sheets for consumers. www.cdc.gov/hiv/.

National Library of Medicine, another branch of the National Institutes of Health: The world's largest medical library, containing research articles, encyclopedias, dictionaries, drug information, and directories. The Web site includes PubMed, public access to biomedical research, at www.ncbi.nlm.nih.gov/ and click on "PubMed Central." The Web site also includes Medline Plus, an all-purpose site on HIV/AIDS news and information that can also be reached separately at http://medlineplus.gov or www.nlm.nih.gov/medline plus/aids.html.

Finding Local Services

These organizations sometimes change their telephone numbers. If you call and get a message that the number is not in service, try directory assistance. For 800 numbers, the directory assistance number is 1-800-555-1212.

To find the services nearest to you, call or write:

Your state, county, or city health department. Find their phone numbers in the blue government pages of the phone book under Health. Departments of health offer varying services but usually know what's available locally, including local and state hotline numbers; all state health departments have AIDS education departments.

National STD and AIDS Hotline, 1-800-342-AIDS. This is a 24-hour-a-day, 7-day-a-week hotline, contracted through the Centers for Disease Control and Prevention. For Spanish-speaking callers, the number is 1-800-344-SIDA. The TTY number is 1-800-243-7889. Even though it is a national hotline, they have information on the services available in your local area, including local and state hotline numbers.

Local and state hotlines. They know local resources; to find hotline numbers, call the National AIDS Hotline or look up AIDS in the index to your phone book's yellow pages, or look up Health in the blue government pages of the phone book.

Your physician should also know about local resources; so should a social worker.

Appendix B

Understanding Tests for HIV

- The tests
- Who should get tested
- Confidentiality of medical records
- What the test results mean

In 1983, the virus that came to be called the human immunodeficiency virus (HIV) was discovered in human blood samples. Two years later, researchers developed a test to detect HIV in the blood. At that time, the best use of the test was to screen people who wanted to donate blood so that blood transfusions and the blood supply would be free of HIV.

Medical researchers were reluctant to use the screening test to identify people with HIV infection. First, although the test was one of the most accurate tests of its kind, occasional errors in its results created a lot of anxiety. Someone whose test result was positive might not have HIV, while someone whose test result was negative couldn't be certain that HIV was not present. Second, at that time, the public was not ready to accept people with HIV infection, and the newspapers were full of stories of discrimination against these people. This public response was partly due to fear and partly to our uncertainty about how the virus was transmitted. The third reason, and the most important, was that physicians had little to offer anyone who tested positive. As a result, recommendations from the medical profession and from others concerned with the epidemic about whether to get tested for HIV were ambiguous. That is, no one knew whether testing for HIV made sense or not.

Since these early times, the accuracy of the test has improved substantially, public understanding has progressed somewhat, and medical research has made a gigantic leap forward in the treatment of HIV infection. Recommendations have changed accordingly. The purpose of this appendix is to discuss the screening tests themselves and their accuracy, make recommendations about who should be tested, discuss the confidentiality of the tests, and help interpret the results.

The Tests

There are two general tests that detect HIV infection. Both tests are done with blood, although tests using saliva and urine are also available. One blood test detects the antibody to the virus; the other detects evidence of the virus itself.

Tests for Antibodies to HIV

The standard test to detect HIV actually detects the antibody to HIV. Antibodies are proteins the body makes to kill any microbe that invades human tissues. If antibodies are present, the microbe also is, or has been, present. Testing has been done to identify antibodies to many microbes for several decades; it is a common method for finding the microbes that cause a multitude of infectious diseases.

Virtually everyone with HIV has a positive test. The only exception is that the time between infection with the virus and formation of the antibodies can be 3 to 6 weeks, or even (rarely) up to 24 weeks. The result is that some people with recent infection will not show antibodies to HIV, and will not have positive results, despite having HIV. When we suspect this might be the case, we usually repeat the test in 2 to 3 months; or if it's important to know the results immediately, we test for the virus itself.

People with a positive antibody test nearly always have HIV infection. The usual exception is human error—such as a mix-up in the report of the results or in the tubes of blood. If someone tests positive and the positive results don't make sense, we repeat the antibody test.

Some test methods offer special advantages (see table 10); some avoid a needlestick by using not blood but urine or saliva; rapid tests give results not in one to two weeks but in less than an hour; and self-tests allow complete anonymity. These tests are all approved by the FDA, but they vary somewhat in accuracy. They all use standard scientific methods to detect antibodies to HIV—just as the standard blood test used since 1985 does.

Tests for HIV

Tests that measure "quantitative HIV" or "viral load" detect not antibodies to the virus, but the virus itself and its concentration in the blood.

Table 10. Tests for HIV Antibody

Test	Cost	Comment
Home kits		
Home Access Express (1-800-HIV-TEST)	$35–$50 or, by Federal Express, $50– $55	A tiny incision is made on the finger with a small, sharp lancet, and a drop of blood is absorbed on a filter. The filter is put into a protective envelope, along with an anonymous code, and then mailed. Results take about 3 days. Accuracy compared to standard test is nearly 100%. Results are anonymous.
Rapid tests	$9	Advantage is that test results are available in 20 to 40 minutes. You take a drop of blood, which is then tested for HIV antibodies. The test can be done with no special equipment and the results are usually clearly positive or negative. The test is easily done in a clinic or almost any place with someone qualified to read the results. If the test is negative, the result is as reliable as that of any antibody test we have, and you are told the result. If the test is positive, it needs to be confirmed with a standard test. This test has revolutionized our ability to detect HIV rapidly.
Saliva test		
OraSure (1-800-ORA-SURE) (1-800-672-7873) www.orasure.com	$33	This is a device for collecting saliva by placing a specially treated pad between the gum and the lower cheek for 2 to 5 minutes. The pad is put in a vial and sent by mail to a laboratory, where it is tested using

(*continued*)

Table 10. (*Continued*)

Test	Cost	Comment
		the standard HIV antibody tests. The kits are available in some health departments or AIDS service organizations, or can be obtained by calling the company. Results are available by phone or fax within 3 days and are anonymous.
Urine test Calypte HIV-1 Urine EIA (1-800-428-4007) www.calypte.com	$4	Available to physicians. Uses the same technology as the standard blood test, so results are comparable in validity. Advantage is that blood is not required. Disadvantages are that it is available only through physicians and that positive tests require confirmation with a standard test.

Although the test is done on blood, most of the HIV is in other places in the body, mostly in the lymph nodes. Nevertheless, the test on blood does accurately represent the amount of HIV in the body.

The viral load tests commonly used give results in "copies per milliliter of blood," or "copies/ml." One "copy" is one virus. The test will measure between about 500 copies/ml and 750,000 copies/ml. So-called ultra-sensitive tests will detect as few as 50 copies/ml. People with untreated HIV infection have a wide range of viral loads, but the average is about 30,000 copies/ml.

The highest viral loads occur in the first three to four weeks of infection, before the person's antibodies have had time to kick in. After that, the viral load drops to a "set point" where, if the person doesn't get treatment, it stays for years. If the set point is high, the infection progresses rapidly—that is, the CD4 count declines quickly and the time before HIV complications set in is short. People in this situation are called "rapid progressors." If the set point is low, the infection progresses slowly; these people are called "chronic non-progressors."

The difference between rapid progressors and chronic non-progressors may lie either in the virulence of the virus or in the quality of the person's immune system—the latter probably being more important. Don't confuse the quality of the immune system's response to HIV with its response to other infections. The immune system's ability to control HIV has nothing to do with its ability to control other infections. A person who seems to catch every circulating flu bug is as likely to be a chronic non-progressor as someone who never seems to get sick.

The goal of HAART is to kill the virus, that is, to get the viral load as low as possible for as long as possible. Our target is usually a viral load of less than 50 copies/ml, or "undetectable," within six months of starting the therapy. This target is virtually always possible, but it has three caveats. (1) The virus must be susceptible to three drugs in the HAART regimen. (2) The person taking the drugs must stick closely to the regimen. (3) The HAART drug must have no side effects or interactions with other drugs that keep them from getting to where the virus is.

A medical rule is, the viral load dictates the probability of transmission. In other words, the more virus, the more likely the transmission to others. This is true of all infections, not just HIV: the larger the number of microbes, the more likely the infection is to be transmitted. The implication is that reducing the viral load with HIV treatment may reduce the probability of transmission. A further implication is that the amount of the reduction in transmission may depend directly on the amount of reduction in viral load. The bottom line is, "no detectable virus" is good and markedly reduces the probability of transmission but never completely eliminates it.

Who Should Get Tested

All pregnant women.

People at increased risk for HIV infection. Factors associated with increased risk are:

- age between 15 and 54 years

- homosexual or bisexual sex

- injection drug use

- commercial sex work (prostitution)

- multiple sex partners

- sexually transmitted diseases like gonorrhea, chlamydia, or syphilis

- sex with people who have any of the above factors, or who are known to have HIV infection

People with medical conditions commonly associated with HIV:

- thrush

- any AIDS-defining condition

- active tuberculosis, that is, not just a positive skin test, but active disease with a cough, fever, and weight loss

People who have been exposed to the blood or bloody body fluids of someone known to have HIV infection or suspected of having tuberculosis. The exposure should be to blood on mucous membranes in the mouth or eyes, on skin with cuts or acne or any other openings, or from injections with a needle.

Confidentiality of Medical Records

Once a person consults a physician about a positive HIV blood test, the results of that test become part of the person's medical record. Simply excluding the result of HIV blood tests from a medical record is not possible: the results are too important a part of the medical record. But these results, if made public, may conceivably affect a person's job, housing, insurance status, personal relationships, and social standing. The obvious questions are, Who has access to this information? And how is it guarded? The answers to these questions differ for different institutions, different states, and sometimes even for different physicians.

In general, medical records can be reviewed by certain medical personnel. Various authorities also have the legal right to review medical records: third-party payers (such as insurance companies), professional review groups, and the like. Although this sounds alarming to someone worried about breach of confidentiality, the actual number of cases in which confidentiality has been breached is nil. The reason is that the people who have access to medical records are well aware that they have ethical as well as legal responsibilities to prevent unnecessary or unwarranted disclosure.

Similar rules apply to health departments that maintain such information. All people with AIDS are reported to health authorities by law. Some states require reporting everyone with a positive blood test. To our knowledge, reporting to state or federal health authorities has never once been the source of inappropriate disclosure of the information (see also chapter 9).

In New York State, anyone with a positive test is asked to identify people whom they have placed at risk by sex or shared injection drug use. The health department then contacts the people identified and advises them to obtain testing but does not reveal the source of information about their exposure. The exception in this policy is a situation in which such disclosure may lead to domestic violence. People with positive tests obviously control this situation by giving only the names they select. But the goal here is simply good public health. The policy is designed to counsel those who are infected to stop further transmission and to get people into care at a time when care is highly effective.

What the Test Results Mean

To repeat, the HIV test is designed to determine the presence of HIV infection—that is, it is designed to detect antibodies to the virus. Antibodies to the virus are present in virtually all people who are infected and absent in people who are not infected. Test results are usually either positive, meaning the antibodies are present, or negative, meaning they are absent. Occasionally test results are indeterminate, meaning that the results were neither clearly positive nor clearly negative. In this case, the test should be retaken.

Inaccurate or false test results are extremely rare. Nevertheless, as discussed above, the test is not always positive in people who are infected and not always negative in those who are not infected.

Negative Test Results

A negative result of the test generally means the virus is not present. In rare cases, as noted above, the negative result can be false. This can happen if the test is taken during the three-to-four-week period (or occasionally longer) between the time of infection and the time when antibodies develop. For the person who is concerned about false negative results, the usual recommendation is to repeat the blood test after two to three months.

Indeterminate Test Results

The virus is either present or not present—there is no middle ground. But like all tests in medicine, the test for antibodies to HIV does not always give decisive positive or negative results. Indeterminate test results are a gray zone, and they are an obvious source of anguish for the person tested. They could mean that the person is early in the course of infection and in the process of manufacturing antibodies to the virus. Or they could mean that the body has produced some miscellaneous protein that is unrelated to HIV. Or indeterminate results could mean that the body has produced antibodies to a virus related to HIV but still somewhat different. Certain rare strains of HIV in Africa are occasionally seen in the United States. These rare strains, known as HIV-2 or type M, don't give clear-cut results on the standard HIV test. Most rare strains turn out to be HIV-2, for which we now have tests.

People with indeterminate results are usually told to be tested again in two to three months. If the person with an indeterminate result has been exposed to the virus recently, the results of the second test may be positive. If the person has not recently acquired HIV infection, the results of the second test are usually indeterminate again. The reason for this is unknown. Almost invariably, however, these people do not have HIV infection. The indeterminate results are never explained and have no consequences.

As noted above, alternative tests may be used to detect the virus instead of antibodies to the virus. These tests, however, are not as well standardized as the antibody tests.

The usual recommendation is to repeat the test for antibodies in three months. While all this gets sorted out, the person being tested is advised to take precautions to prevent transmission, just as if the test were positive.

Positive Test Results

A positive test means that antibodies to HIV are present. If the antibodies are present, the virus is also present. The person with positive results can transmit the virus to others and needs regular medical attention and access to therapy.

Over 99 percent of the people with positive tests know how they became infected; for a small portion of people, the source of the infection is unknown or claimed to be unknown. Because false-positive tests occur occasionally (rarely), the person with a positive test who has no reason for it may request that the test be repeated. People with a positive test will understandably be upset, will need psychological counseling, will need medical care, will need to know how to prevent transmission, may need ongoing psychological support, and will certainly need the support and friendship of the people they love. All this, of course, is what this book is about.

Glossary

Abacavir (Ziagen, ABC): A nucleoside like AZT, and the most potent drug in its class. The main side effect is a serious allergic reaction with high fever, gastrointestinal upset, and a rash, usually during the first 30 days of treatment. If these symptoms occur, the drug should be stopped and should not be taken again. If you think you're having these reactions, always check with your doctor.

ACTU: ACTU stands for AIDS clinical trial unit. ACTUs are a consortium of medical centers throughout the United States that conduct clinical trials of drugs for treating people with HIV infection. Specifically, the drugs are for treating HIV itself, for treating complications (opportunistic infections or tumors), and for stimulating the immune system. The entire consortium of ACTUs is called ACTG; the G stands for *group*. The ACTG is funded federally, at about $60 million yearly, through the National Institutes of Health. The ACTG has two components: AACTG (adult ACTG) and PACTG (pediatric ACTG). The ACTG is the largest clinical trials group for HIV infection in the world: it has the largest budget, the largest number of investigators, and the largest number of participants.

Acute HIV infection, or *acute retroviral syndrome:* Acute HIV infection refers to the first illness that occurs after infection with HIV. Symptoms show up about one to three weeks after infection. Typical symptoms are sore throat, fatigue, headache, fever, and a rash. The illness precedes seroconversion, when the standard blood test for antibodies to HIV first turns positive. The illness lasts about one to two weeks. During this period, the risk of transmission is great. Avoid sex and get medical attention.

Acyclovir (Zovirax): A drug used for infections caused by herpes simplex (genital herpes or "fever blisters" or "cold sores") or herpes zoster (shingles). Acyclovir is available as a cream, a pill, or for intravenous administration. It has been used in millions of patients since 1982 and has nearly no side effects. Acyclovir not only treats herpes outbreaks, but when taken daily, it also prevents them from recurring.

ADAP, or AIDS Drug Assistance Program: A provision in the Ryan White Care Act that makes HIV drugs available to people who can't afford them with their own income plus assets or with their health care plans.

Adenopathy: Enlargement of lymph nodes, which can be felt in the neck, armpit, or groin; or seen on a CT scan of the chest or abdomen. Enlarged lymph nodes usually mean infection of some sort or, less commonly, a tumor like lymphoma. See *Lymphadenopathy.*

Adherence: The ability to adhere to or comply with something. In the context of HIV infection, adherence means the ability to stay on the regimen of antiretroviral drugs. Good adherence means taking 70 to 95 percent of HIV drugs at the right time.

Adverse event: Medical term for a complication of a drug—allergic reactions, side effects, toxicities.

AIDS: AIDS stands for acquired immune deficiency syndrome. AIDS is the late stage of an infection caused by the human immunodeficiency virus, or HIV. The virus infects the CD4 cell (also called a T4 cell, a T4 lymphocyte, and a T-helper cell), which is critical to immune defenses. As the numbers of these cells decrease, the immune system weakens until it becomes susceptible to what are called *opportunistic infections* and *opportunistic tumors.* These infections and tumors are called opportunistic because the microbes that cause them are opportunists, taking advantage of a weakened immune system. A person with HIV infection has AIDS if he or she has a CD4 cell count below 200 or one or more of certain specific opportunistic infections or tumors, called *AIDS-defining diagnoses,* that go along with a severely weakened immune system. The list of AIDS-defining diagnoses was drawn up by the Centers for Disease Control and Prevention (CDC) in 1986 and has been modified twice, once in 1987 and again in 1993. The CDC's latest definition of AIDS includes all the old criteria and adds a CD4 count of less than 200.

AIDS-advocacy organizations: See *Community-based organizations.*

AIDS-defining diagnosis: A person with an AIDS-defining diagnosis has HIV infection plus any one of a number of common infections that result from a specific defect caused by HIV. According to the Centers for Disease Control and Prevention, the complications included as AIDS-defining diagnoses are, in order of frequency, pneumocystis pneumonia, wasting, candidal esophagitis, tuberculosis, CMV infection, Kaposi's sarcoma, *Mycobacterium avium* complex infection, chronic herpes simplex, HIV dementia, toxoplasmosis, and cryptococcal meningitis. These are not the only AIDS-defining diagnoses, but they are the most common. The CD4 count is usually, but not necessarily, below 200. In fact, the average CD4 count for most people with AIDS-defining diagnoses is 50 or less.

AIDS dementia complex: See *HIV-associated dementia.*

AIDS-related complex: See *ARC.*

Alprazolam (Xanax): See *Benzodiazepines.*

Alternative medicine: The alternatives to traditional medicine. Alternative medicine can include use of herbs, acupuncture, Chinese medicine, meditation, and a variety of other approaches to medical care. *Complementary medicine* is another name for alternative medicine. Alternative medicine generally does not have scientific verification of its effectiveness; if it did, it would be traditional medicine. Most physicians don't object to their patients using alternative medicine, as long as the alternative medicine is not being used in place of drugs known to work, or causing interactions with those drugs, or causing harm.

Amitriptyline: Amitriptyline hydrochloride (or, e.g., Elavil) is one of a group of drugs called *tricyclic antidepressants* that are grouped together because of their chemical similarities. Other tricyclic antidepressants include amoxapine (or Asendin), desipramine hydrochloride (or Pertofrane or Norpramin), doxepin hydrochloride (or Adapin or Sinequan), imipramine hydrochloride (or Tofranil), and nortriptyline hydrochloride (or Aventyl Hydrochloride or Pamelor). Tricyclic antidepressants are used to treat depression and the peripheral neuropathy that causes painful feet. In many cases, the dose is arbitrary: many people start on a low dose and have the dose increased as necessary. Side effects are common, but usually not severe enough to stop treatment. The main side effects are drowsiness, weakness, and fatigue; dry mouth; constipation; and low blood pressure and dizziness. Some people gain weight or have decreased libido. All of these side effects are dose-related, meaning the higher the dose, the more common and severe the side effect. Because the drugs cause drowsiness, they are often given before bedtime.

Amphotericin B: The antibiotic amphotericin B is the standard treatment for many infections caused by fungi, including most of the fungi that affect people with HIV infection: *Candida, Cryptococcus, Histoplasma, Coccidioides,* and *Aspergillus.* Amphotericin B, which is usually given by vein, is highly effective. Unfortunately, it is also one of the most toxic antibiotics known. The most important side effects include kidney damage, *anemia* (see below), disturbances in the balance of electrolytes, nausea and vomiting, fever and chills, and phlebitis or inflammation of the vein into which the drug is injected. Many of these side effects can be lessened or eliminated by stopping the drug, or by concurrently taking medicines to combat the side effects, or by taking new preparations of amphotericin that are much more expensive but much easier to take. Because of amphotericin B's toxicity, other drugs, like ketoconazole, itraconazole, voriconazole, and fluconazole, are given when they are considered to be as effective or sometimes even more effective. Another option to beat the side effects of amphotericin is to use a special formulation called AmBisome, which does everything amphotericin does (in most cases) with a fraction of the side effects. The problem with AmBisome is that it costs $1,500 per day, compared to amphotericin's cost of $16 per day.

Anemia: Anemia means that the number of red cells in the blood is reduced. Red blood cells are responsible for delivering oxygen to all parts of the body. When the reduction is severe, the result is fatigue. Anemia can be caused by HIV infection itself, by a complication, or by several of the drugs commonly taken by people with AIDS. Drugs often responsible include trimethoprim-sulfamethoxazole, other sulfa drugs, pentamidine, amphotericin B, and AZT. When the anemia is severe, it can be corrected with transfusions or a drug called erythropoietin (EPO). When drugs are responsible, the drugs can be reduced in dose or discontinued.

Antibiotics: Antibiotics are drugs made from natural substances (as opposed to drugs made artificially) that inhibit the growth of certain microbes. Antibiotics may be effective against any of the classes of microbes—including bacteria, fungi, parasites, and viruses—that cause infections.

Antibody: Antibodies are proteins and are the part of the complex immune system that attacks any substance—protein or microbe—that is foreign to the body. Certain cells called *B lymphocytes* recognize these substances as foreign and manufacture antibodies that inactivate or eliminate the foreign substance. The foreign substance that the antibodies attack is called an *antigen* (see below). For most antigens, the B lymphocytes take one or two weeks to produce antibodies; for HIV, however, the time required may be months. Antibodies are the means by which vaccines work.

Antigen: Antigens are foreign material, including microbes or vaccines, that the immune system responds to by manufacturing antibodies.

Antiretroviral: HIV is a retrovirus, and drugs that inhibit it are antiretroviral drugs. These drugs come in four classes: two reverse transcriptase inhibitors (nucleosides and nonnucleosides), protease inhibitors, and entry inhibitors. Examples of nucleoside reverse transcriptase inhibitors are AZT, ddI, ddC, d4T, 3TC, TDF, FTC, and ABC. Examples of nonnucleoside reverse transcriptase inhibitors are efavirenz and nevirapine. Examples of protease inhibitors are saquinavir, ritonavir, nelfinavir, indinavir, fosamprenavir, lopinavir, atazanavir, and tipranavir. The entry inhibitors include enfuvirtide and several others still in development. See table 4 in chapter 3.

Aphthous ulcer: Aphthous ulcers are ulcers or sores in the mouth and occasionally in the esophagus. They are often extremely painful, they have no clear cause, and they are often cleared up by *corticosteroids* (see below) or other medications.

ARC: ARC stands for AIDS-related complex. ARC is a collection of conditions associated with HIV infection that do not meet the diagnostic definition of AIDS. There is no official definition of ARC, and most people in the field no longer use the term.

Aspergillus: A fungus found in nature that occasionally causes a chronic infection of the lungs in late symptomatic HIV infection. Treatment is amphotericin B or itraconazole.

Asymptomatic: Asymptomatic means the absence of symptoms. The asymptomatic person feels healthy.

Atazanavir (ATV, Reyataz): A protease inhibitor, or PI, that may or may not be taken with ritonavir to boost its levels in the body. Atazanavir is highly active against HIV but, like all HIV drugs, needs to be combined with at least two other drugs. One of its special advantages is that, unlike other PIs, it doesn't increase levels of blood lipids like cholesterol. Another of its advantages is that it can be taken once daily. Its disadvantages are that it needs to be taken with food and that it needs stomach acid. So always take it with a meal and never take it with drugs—like prilosec, omeprazole, Maalox, Pepto-Bismol—that neutralize stomach acid.

Atovaquone (Mepron): A drug to prevent or treat pneumocystis pneumonia. The drug is a liquid with a bad taste. It is taken twice daily and must be taken with food.

B lymphocytes: B lymphocytes are the white blood cells—called lymphocytes—responsible for producing antibodies. B lymphocytes are distinct from T lymphocytes (including CD4 cells, also called T4 cells), which are also part of the immune system, but which work against a different group of microbes using different mechanisms.

Baclofen: Baclofen is a drug used to control muscle spasms. The most common side effect is drowsiness and, in large doses, severe sedation, lack of coordination, and lowered functioning of the heart and lungs.

Bactrim: See *Trimethoprim-sulfamethoxazole.*

Barbiturates: Barbiturates are drugs commonly used to treat insomnia, anxiety, and seizures. Examples of barbiturates are amobarbital (or Amytal), pentobarbital (or Nembutal), phenobarbital, and secobarbital. All barbiturates affect the central nervous system: low doses cause mild sedation, and high doses can lead to deep coma. When barbiturates are used for sedation, they remain effective for only about two weeks. As a result, alternative drugs are generally preferred to treat insomnia. Barbiturates' most important role may be for controlling anxiety.

The major side effects are symptoms of central nervous system depression, including drowsiness, depression, lethargy, and hangovers. People who take barbiturates should be aware that the drug may impair their ability to perform hazardous activities. Prolonged use of high doses of the drug can cause physical dependence, psychological dependence, and tolerance (that is, higher doses of the drug are required to produce a similar effect). Discontinuing barbiturates can cause withdrawal symptoms that are similar to the withdrawal symptoms an alcoholic has when abruptly discontinuing alcohol. Other side effects include stomach pain, allergic reactions, and fever.

Benzodiazepines: Benzodiazepines are a class of drugs commonly used to treat anxiety, insomnia, seizures, and painful muscles. Examples of benzodiazepines include alprazolam (or Xanax), diazepam, flurazepam hydrochloride (or Dalmane), lorazepam (or Ativan), midazolam maleate, oxazepam (or Serax), prazepam (or Centrax), temazepam (or Restoril), and triazolam (or Halcion). In general, all benzodiazepines act in similar ways and seem to be equally effective.

Most physicians prefer benzodiazepines for treating anxiety and tension. Compared to barbiturates and meprobamate, and when given at the doses that relieve anxiety, they are less addictive and produce less sedation. The major side effects are drowsiness, loss of coordination, confusion, dizziness, hangover, and fainting. People taking benzodiazepines should be aware that the drug may impair their ability to perform activities that require mental alertness and physical coordination. Using alcohol and other mind-altering drugs will make these symptoms worse. Benzodiazepines can also cause physical dependence and symptoms of severe withdrawal if the drug is stopped suddenly after being used regularly for a long time. If taken in high doses for long periods, it should be withdrawn slowly under a physician's guidance.

Biopsy: Biopsy is a procedure for obtaining a piece of tissue for examination under the microscope. The microscopic changes in tissue often provide a diagnosis, and stains and cultures for microbes will often reveal the infecting organism. The biopsy may be obtained using lidocaine to deaden the skin to avoid pain. The biopsy may be performed on an outpatient basis when the area to be biopsied is near the surface or when it is in the lungs or gastrointestinal tract and can be reached through an endoscope, an instrument passed through the mouth or anus. Alternatively, the biopsy of organs deep within the body may require an operating room procedure.

Bleach: Chlorine bleach is highly effective in killing HIV within minutes. It is available at most grocery stores and is commonly recommended for killing any virus or other microbe that may be in such body fluids as blood or saliva, or in stool. Bleach is usually diluted 1:10, or one part of bleach in ten parts of water. This dilution can be applied to surfaces or in the washing machine for clothes.

Blood count: Blood is composed of red blood cells (erythrocytes), which carry oxygen to all parts of the body; white blood cells (leukocytes), which help make up the immune system; and platelets (or thrombocytes), which are required for blood clotting. All three kinds of cells can be counted under a microscope. A low red blood cell count is called *anemia* (see above), a low white blood cell count is called *leukopenia* (see below), and a low platelet count is called *thrombocytopenia* (see below). People with HIV infection commonly have low red counts, low white counts, and low platelet counts. A blood count is a routine procedure for clinical laboratories; it is a relatively simple, inexpensive, and standard test to evaluate people with HIV infection.

Bone marrow: Bone marrow is the tissue in the central portion of many bones where blood is manufactured. Bone marrow can be withdrawn (by placing a needle in the hip bone) and analyzed to detect abnormalities in the production of red blood cells, white blood cells, or platelets. Either HIV infection or drugs can suppress the bone marrow, causing anemia, neutropenia (low white blood cell count), or thrombocytopenia (low platelet count).

Branched chain DNA (bDNA): See *Quantitative virology.*

Bronchoscopy: A procedure done by a lung specialist to look at and collect specimens from the lung. The procedure is done with a long tube that is passed through the nose or mouth and down the bronchus (the breathing tube), using an anesthetic on the surfaces. This is the best method for diagnosing *Pneumocystis jiroveci* pneumonia and other lung conditions.

Buffalo hump: The common term for a collection of fat at the base of the neck or on the upper back. The fat is part of the lipodystrophy syndrome and may be difficult to reverse. Occasionally it occurs with pain. Sometimes it is removed with surgery.

Candida: See *Candidiasis.*

Candidiasis: Candidiasis is an infection caused by the fungus *Candida albicans.* People with HIV infection commonly have candidiasis in the mouth (thrush), in the esophagus (candidal esophagitis), or in the vagina (vaginal candidiasis). Thrush occurs in about 80 percent of the people with CD4 counts less than 200. Candidal esophagitis is the most common cause of difficulty swallowing in the late stages of HIV infection. Vaginal candidiasis, or "yeast infection," is common in women with or without HIV infection. Treatment is with topical drugs (drugs placed in contact with the infection, such as nystatin or clotrimazole) or pills such as ketoconazole, fluconazole, or itraconazole.

CD4 cells: The blood contains several kinds of white cells, each of which plays a specific role in the immune system. CD4 cells (other names are T4 cells and T-helper cells) are the cells that HIV selectively infects. The number of CD4 cells frequently indicates the stage of HIV infection. Healthy people without HIV infection usually have around 1,000 CD4 cells in every milliliter of blood; counts of 200 to 500 are considered abnormally low, but not alarming. People with AIDS usually have counts of less than 200, and this is now considered the threshold for the definition of AIDS. Most people with CD4 counts of 50 to 200 feel well, and many have no complications. Nevertheless, counts of less than 200 suggest severe weakening of the immune system.

In any one person the count varies considerably: the same laboratory performing the test on the same specimen can show counts that vary by as much as 20 percent. This means that if the true count is 500, the lab may report any value between 400 and 600. The CD4 count is also influenced by the time of day it is measured and by other medical conditions independent of HIV infection. As a result, although the CD4 count is frequently used to assess progressive disease, changes in the count are sometimes difficult to interpret, and it is advisable not to attach too much credibility to a single test. The test should be repeated if there are big changes that are not readily explained.

The CD4 count is a relatively expensive test (usually $50 to $100), but it is an important way of monitoring the state of the immune system. Most medical authorities base their recommendations of HIV treatment primarily on the CD4 cell count, and monitor the response to that treatment with the viral load and CD4 cell count together. An average person with HIV infection who is not taking treatments has a decrease in CD4 cell counts of about 50 per year. The same person with a robust response to HAART has an increase in CD4 cell count of 50 to 100 per year.

Centers for Disease Control and Prevention (CDC): The Centers for Disease Control and Prevention is a federally funded institution located in Atlanta, Georgia. It has three responsibilities: to serve as an epidemiologic and public health resource for state and local health departments; to investigate epidemics; and to keep track of contagious diseases and other diseases important to public health. The CDC has about 4,000 employees, including 800 physicians and Ph.D.'s. In the past, the CDC has been responsible for much of what we know about Lyme disease, tuberculosis, Legionnaires' disease, Ebola, and toxic shock syndrome. More to the point, the CDC provided much of the early epidemiologic data that identified the symptoms of HIV infection, the kinds of behavior that risked infection, and how HIV was transmitted—in fact, the CDC was responsible for the name *AIDS*. At present, the CDC is the storehouse for all reported cases of AIDS in the United States. It provides guidelines for disease prevention and gives advice on safety for health care providers. It is responsible for funding state and local agencies that test for HIV, counsel, and collect data.

Chloral hydrate: Chloral hydrate is a sedative used to treat insomnia. It is usually taken fifteen to thirty minutes before bedtime. Using chloral hydrate regularly for more than two weeks often reduces its effectiveness. Major side effects include stomach irritation, residual sedation, or a hangover. Chloral hydrate should be used with great caution in people who are depressed, who may commit suicide, or who have a history of drug abuse.

Chlorhexidine: A mouthwash available without prescription for treating gingivitis, an inflammation of the gums.

Cholesterol: A steroid found in the blood along with its carrier protein, called a lipoprotein. The low-density lipoproteins (LDLs) carry cholesterol from the liver to body tissue. The high-density lipoproteins (HDLs) carry cholesterol to be eliminated. Heart disease is associated with high levels of LDL ("bad cholesterol") and low levels of HDL ("good cholesterol").

Ciprofloxacin (Cipro): An antibiotic with a broad spectrum of uses. It can be taken by mouth or intravenously.

Clarithromycin (Biaxin): An antibiotic used to treat sinusitis, *Mycobacterium avium* complex (MAC) infection, and other infections. It is the best drug for MAC, but must be used with other antibiotics because MAC can become resistant when treated with only one antibiotic. The major side effect is nausea and vomiting.

Clostridium difficile: People who take antibiotics often develop diarrhea as a side effect. A relatively common and sometimes severe cause of this diarrhea is a microbe called *Clostridium difficile.* Almost any antibiotic can cause this complication, but the most frequent causes are ampicillin, amoxicillin, clindamycin; a group of drugs called cephalosporins that includes cefixime (or Suprex), cefotaxime, ceftriaxone, cefuroxime, cephalexin (or Keflex), and cefaclor (or Ceclor); and fluoroquinolones such as ciprofloxacin (Cipro), levofloxacin (Levoquin), moxifloxacin (Avelox), and gatifloxicin (Tequin). People who have diarrhea while taking these or any other antibiotics should stop taking the antibiotics and call their physicians. A test of stool will determine if *Clostridium difficile* is the cause. If it is, it can be treated with metronidazole or vancomycin. Vancomycin is preferred for serious cases of diarrhea, but it costs about $50 to $100. Metronidazole is less expensive—$10 to $20—and equally effective. The authors are fond of *Clostridium difficile* and its connection to antibiotic-associated diarrhea because one of us (J.B.) discovered that connection.

CMV: CMV, which is short for cytomegalovirus, is a virus commonly found in people without HIV infection. Usually the immune system holds CMV in check, and it remains dormant in the body without causing any serious disease. With a severely weakened immune system, however, CMV may cause serious infection. The site of the infection can be in the eye, lung, liver, gastrointestinal tract, bone marrow, brain, or widespread in many of these areas. The virus can be detected by examining tissue and culturing the virus. CMV retinitis, a vision-threatening infection of the eye, was initially a common HIV-associated complication but has now become relatively rare in this era of HAART. Treatment of CMV retinitis and other forms of CMV infection is with valganciclovir, ganciclovir, foscarnet, or cidofovir. The most important treatment, however, is HAART: the immune system, if it is reconstituted, will control CMV itself.

Colon: The gastrointestinal tract—which starts at the mouth and ends at the rectum—includes the esophagus, stomach, small intestine, colon, and rectum. The colon and the small intestine are commonly the sites of infections that cause diarrhea. To diagnose problems in the colon, common procedures are colonoscopy and sigmoidoscopy. These procedures permit visualization and biopsy of the colon by passing a tube through the rectum. Colonoscopy is expensive ($1,200 to $1,800) and is usually done by a specialist called a gastroenterologist.

Combination treatment: Combination treatment means taking two or more drugs against HIV. The goals of combination treatment are to "gang up" on HIV with a double whammy attack; and to prevent resistance, since a microbe can develop resistance most easily to one drug at a time. The downside to combination treatment is that it may be more toxic, and microbes may develop resistance to both drugs and leave fewer options for treatment. All HIV treatment is now combination treatment, usually using three or four different drugs.

Combivir (AZT + 3TC): One of the combinations of *nucleoside analogs* (see below) that are taken as one pill twice daily. The advantage is the reduction in "pill burden," which makes adhering to the drug regimen easier.

Community-based organizations (CBOs): Community-based organizations are also called AIDS-advocacy organizations and AIDS service organizations (ASOs). They are organizations and agencies that provide services to people with HIV infection, as well as education and prevention programs for the whole community. The leaders of community-based organizations are lay people, ordinary people who do not come from the government or from organized medicine—although many community-based organizations have physicians as advisers, and most receive public funds.

Examples of community-based organizations dealing with other diseases are the American Lung Association, the American Heart Association, and the American Cancer Society. There is no similar nationwide organization for people with HIV infection or AIDS. Nevertheless, most cities have one or sometimes several such organizations: examples include Shanti in San Francisco, the Gay Men's Health Clinic in New York City, and HERO in Baltimore. The types of services offered vary but may include counseling, crisis support, financial assistance, case management, a buddy system, transportation, meals, housing, support groups, legal aid, social services, education, psychological support, hotlines, buyers' clubs, and medical services (see Appendix A, "Resources"). Most of these organizations have a paid professional staff but rely heavily on volunteers. Funding usually comes from state governments, corporations, foundations, and local fund-raising events.

Complete blood count (CBC): An inexpensive blood test to measure the numbers of white blood cells, red blood cells, and platelets.

Computerized tomography scan (CT scan): CT scans are a particular kind of X-ray that provide a three-dimensional view of the body. Conventional X-ray tests provide a two-dimensional view of the body; CT scans use computers to stack a series of two-dimensional X-rays together to form a three-dimensional image of the body. CT scans can be done of the entire body or of parts of it. The person receiving a CT scan often receives an injection of what is called contrast material—material that shows up under X-rays. Some people have allergic reactions to contrast materials and should not receive them again. The person receiving the CT scan is next put into a chamber with a scanner that circulates around the body, producing three-dimensional images in parallel sections of about an inch or less. CT scans, first developed in the 1970s, are an excellent method for detecting tumors, infections, or other changes in the anatomy of the brain, chest, abdomen, or other parts of the body. They are also expensive, usually costing around $300 to $800.

Constitutional symptoms: Symptoms caused by the impact of an illness on the entire body or constitution are frequently referred to as constitutional symptoms. Included are fatigue, achiness, weight loss, fever, and night sweats. Constitutional symptoms are present in many types of infectious diseases, tumors, and other medical conditions ranging from the serious to the trivial. For people with HIV infection, constitutional symptoms may be a result of HIV infection itself or the result of such complications as pneumocystis pneumonia, tuberculosis, or widespread CMV infection.

Contagious: A disease that is *contagious* can be passed from one person to another. A disease that is *infectious* is caused by a microbe. All diseases that are contagious are also infectious; but some diseases, like toxic shock syndrome, are infectious and not contagious. HIV is both infectious and contagious, but is contagious only with specific types of contact.

Corticosteroids (also known as steroids, glucocorticosteroids, prednisone, and cortisone): Corticosteroids are drugs used to reduce the immune response. Numerous preparations are available that can be taken intravenously, by mouth, or in an ointment applied to the skin. Using high doses of corticosteroids for a long time can be dangerous: they reduce the immune system's defenses against certain infections. Corticosteroids are sometimes considered especially dangerous for people with HIV infection, whose immune defenses are already weakened. Nevertheless, many of the complications of HIV infection appear to result from an overly abundant but misdirected immune response. As a result, these complications of HIV infection respond well to corticosteroids, though the drug should be taken at the lowest doses for the shortest period.

Crixivan: See *Indinavir.*

Cryptococcosis: Cryptococcosis is an infection caused by the fungus *Cryptococcus neoformans.* This fungus can cause infection in otherwise healthy people. In people with HIV infection, however, it is especially severe, frequently causing meningitis. Common symptoms include headaches, fevers, vision problems, and seizures. The diagnosis is usually made by analyzing blood and cerebrospinal fluid obtained with a *spinal tap* (see below). The disease is treated with amphotericin B given by vein or fluconazole given by mouth; when treatment is stopped, the disease tends to recur so that long-term treatment is generally necessary.

Cryptosporidiosis: Cryptosporidia are parasites that infect the intestine and cause diarrhea. This infection, called cryptosporidiosis, can occur in otherwise healthy persons, but the diarrhea generally does not last long and is not severe. Cryptosporidiosis in people with HIV infection often causes devastating diarrhea that persists for months. People with cryptosporidiosis may lose large amounts of fluid and nutrients and, consequently, become severely malnourished. The diagnosis is usually established by simply examining the stool under a microscope to detect the parasite. There is no universally accepted form of treatment except to replace the lost fluids and nutrients. The best treatment is to recover the immune system with HIV treatments; the immune system then controls *Cryptosporidium* and may eliminate it.

Culture: A culture, in medical terms, is a medium in which microbes can grow. Most cultures in medicine are done to detect bacteria like strep and staph. Cultures have been done for over 100 years. A culture usually takes 24 to 48 hours, the methods are standard, and the cost is low. Viruses like HIV, however, are much more difficult to grow in culture and most labs don't offer this service. When necessary, specialized or research labs can get HIV to grow using cultures containing lymphocytes. The blood test to detect HIV antibody is a better, simpler, faster, and cheaper method of detecting HIV.

Cytokines: Cytokines are proteins secreted by cells of the immune system. They are the means by which these cells communicate with other cells of the immune system. They may stimulate (up-regulate) or suppress (down-regulate) various immune responses. For instance, a cytokine called IL-2 activates CD8 cells to attack infections. Most cytokines have multiple activities. For instance, IL-2 also up-regulates another cytokine called interferon gamma, and down-regulates still other cytokines called IL-10 and IL-4. Some of the activities are beneficial, some possibly harmful. Many cytokines can be produced in the laboratory and can be given as therapeutic agents. All must be injected because the digestive enzymes in the small intestine break them down. There are at least twenty-six cytokines known so far and probably a lot more to be discovered. Some of the main cytokines are the following:

CYTOKINE	MAIN ACTIVITY
Erythropoeitin (EPO)	Production of red blood cells
G-CSF (Neupogen)	Production of white blood cells
Interleukin-1 (IL-1)	Improves imflammatory response
Interleukin-2 (IL-2)	Stimulates CD8 cells to kill infected cells; promotes growth of B and CD4 cells; increases interferon gamma
Interleukin-4 (IL-4)	Growth of B and CD4 cells
Interleukin-10 (IL-10)	Reduces production of IL-2; reduces CD8 activity

Interleukin-12 (IL-12)	Stimulates CD4 cells to produce IL-2; produces interferon gamma
Interferon alpha (IFNα)	Inhibits HIV, stimulates certain immune cells called monocytes
Interferon gamma (IFNγ)	Kills certain pathogens; activates CD4 cells
Tumor necrosis factor (TNF)	Kills tumors; stimulates immune cells; causes fever and weight loss

Cytomegalovirus: See *CMV.*

d4T (stavudine, Zerit): A popular *nucleoside analog* (see below) that has few short-term side effects. Long-term side effects, however, include peripheral neuropathy (see below, *Neuropathy*), pancreatitis (inflammation of the pancreas with severe abdominal pain), *lactic acidosis* (see below), increased triglycerides, and the sunken-face look.

ddC (zalcitabine, HIVID): A *nucleoside* (see below) that seems to be relatively weak and toxic. Many physicians have stopped using it except in situations where no alternatives are available.

ddI (didanosine, Videx): A *nucleoside* (see below) that must be taken on an empty stomach. In many people, it causes stomach problems. Long-term use may cause pancreatitis (inflammation of the pancreas with severe abdominal pain), peripheral neuropathy (see below, *Neuropathy*), and *lactic acidosis* (see below).

Delavirdine (Rescriptor): An infrequently used *NNRTI* (see below)— infrequent because it is not very strong and must be taken 3 times daily.

Dementia: See *HIV-associated dementia.*

Diabetes: A common, sometimes inherited condition that is characterized by abnormal control of blood glucose, or sugar. Diabetes is relevant to people with HIV infection because protease inhibitors may cause it. The standard methods of controlling diabetes are diet, exercise, and weight loss. When these aren't enough, diabetes needs to be controlled with pills called oral hypoglycemics; and when pills aren't enough, you need injections of insulin.

Diarrhea: Loose and/or frequent stools that are a common medical condition in all people, but may be particularly common in people in advanced stages of HIV infection with CD4 counts below 200. It is important to tell your physician when the diarrhea is severe, persistent, or accompanied by weight loss, fever, or cramps. The cause may be side effects of medications, food poisoning, anxiety, gastro-enteritis, or some complication of HIV infection.

Dormant: See *Latency.*

Drug interactions: A drug interaction is the effect one drug has on another. Drug A might interfere with absorption of drug B, so that the levels of drug B in the body are lower than they ought to be. Or drug A might slow the body's metabolism of drug B, so that drug B lasts longer at higher concentrations and causes toxicity. Drug interactions are a big issue with most protease inhibitors. Make sure your doctor knows all the drugs you are taking.

Dysphagia: Dysphagia means difficulty with swallowing. The most common cause of dysphagia is an infection by *Candida albicans,* a fungus that can be easily treated (see *Candidiasis*). Less frequent causes are infections with herpes or CMV. In some people dysphagia has no readily apparent cause. For people with HIV infection and CD4 counts above 200, dysphagia is caused by the same things that cause it in people without HIV infection—the most common being gas-tro-esophagus reflux disease or GERD, treated with drugs to reduce stomach acid. The usual method of finding the cause of dysphagia is endoscopy, a procedure in which a tube is placed in the esophagus to visualize and biopsy the lesions. X-ray examinations are another means of viewing the esophagus. In many cases, neither of these tests is done, and the person is presumed to have a *Candida* infection if he or she also has *thrush* (see below) and if swallowing is painful.

Efavirenz (Sustiva): This is a nonnucleoside reverse transcriptase inhibitor that is highly effective against HIV when combined with two nucleosides. The main side effect is that it plays tricks on the brain, causing confusion, bad dreams, and a feeling of being disconnected. These side effects usually disappear after 2 to 3 weeks, but people must be aware of them and their effect on jobs, driving, etc. The drug is taken once daily, usually at sleep time so the person is not aware of the side effects when they are most severe. This drug, when taken in the first trimester of pregnancy, might cause birth defects. It should not be taken by pregnant women or women who may become pregnant. It is the only drug for HIV infection that clearly causes birth defects.

ELISA test: The ELISA (pronounced eelissa) is a blood test done to detect antibodies to certain microbes, among which is HIV. The ELISA is the first of two standard tests done together to detect antibodies to HIV. The test is extremely sensitive but not very specific. Sensitivity means that the test is able to detect HIV infection; specificity means that the test specifically detects a particular infection and no other. In other words, with ELISA, people who have HIV infection will rarely have a falsely negative test, but people who do not have HIV infection will commonly have a falsely positive test. As a result, the ELISA is used as a screening test, and those who are positive have a second test on the same blood sample called a *Western blot.*

The *Western blot test,* combined with an ELISA, is over 99.9 percent accurate in both sensitivity and specificity. The combination of tests is generally offered free of charge by most health departments and at a cost of $50 to $150 by commercial laboratories. The test offered may be *anonymous,* meaning that the person receiving the test cannot be identified, or *confidential,* meaning that privacy is honored but a record is kept identifying a specific person with the test result. The ELISA is easily performed, but the Western blot is more complicated and often done only by reference laboratories or on certain days of the week. For this reason, the results may not be available for several days. The test results are usually either positive or negative, but occasionally people have Western blots that cannot be clearly interpreted and the test results are considered indeterminate. The usual recommendation for people with indeterminate results is to have the test repeated in two or three months. People at a low risk for HIV and with indeterminate results almost never have HIV infection, and the cause of the indeterminate results is not known.

Emtricitabine (FTC, Emtriva): A nucleoside analog very similar to lamivudine. See *Lamivudine.*

Emtriva: See *Emtricitabine.*

Encephalitis: Encephalitis is an infection of the brain. (Meningitis, by contrast, is an infection of the meninges, the membrane surrounding the brain and spinal cord—see *Meningitis.*) Encephalitis commonly causes headaches, fever, seizures, and neurologic problems. The diagnosis is frequently made on the basis of the person's symptoms, combined with procedures to examine the brain such as *computerized tomography scan (CT scan)* (see above); *magnetic resonance imaging (MRI)* (see below); or electroencephalogram (EEG). Diagnosis can also be made by analyzing the cerebrospinal fluid obtained by a *spinal tap* (see below). In people with HIV infection, the usual causes of encephalitis are infection with HIV itself or such complications as CMV or toxoplasmosis.

Endoscopy: Endoscopy is a diagnostic procedure in which an instrument is passed through the mouth or rectum to examine an internal organ or to obtain a *biopsy* (see above). In people with HIV infection, the most common types of endoscopy are *bronchoscopy* (see above) to examine the lungs and endoscopies to examine the digestive system. Upper endoscopy of the intestine involves passing an endoscope through the mouth to examine the esophagus, stomach, or upper small intestine. Lower endoscopy of the intestine involves passing an endoscope through the rectum to examine the large intestine or colon. Endoscopes are flexible and can turn corners. Endoscopy requires the expertise of a specialist, can be done on an outpatient basis, and usually costs $1,200 to $1,800, except in New York City, where everything costs more.

Enfuvirtide (T20, Fuzeon): A drug that works against HIV by preventing it from attaching to and entering the CD4 cell. It is the first of a whole class of drugs that will work this way. It is used only when the standard drugs for HIV no longer work, usually because of resistance. It needs to be injected twice daily; the injections cause a predictable reaction with painful or itchy bumps. Most people learn to do their own injections with proper training. Adherence to this drug is actually better than to the drugs that are swallowed. But taking this drug also requires commitment. It must be taken with another drug or drugs against HIV; it can't succeed alone. It is also expensive—over $20,000 per year.

Enteritis: Enteritis is an inflammation of the small intestine; the most common symptom is diarrhea. In people with advanced HIV infection and CD4 counts of less than 200 and usually less than 50, the microbes that usually cause enteritis are *Cryptosporidium, Microsporidium, Mycobacterium avium* complex, and CMV. These microbes can be detected by examining stools under a microscope or with a biopsy of the small intestine done with an endoscope (see above, *Endoscopy*), a tube that is placed through the mouth and into the small intestine. Diarrhea in people with HIV infection and a CD4 count over 200 will often be due to medications, gastroenteritis (a self-limiting viral infection), anxiety, or food poisoning.

Epidemic: An epidemic is a disease that occurs in many more people than would be expected during a given time. *Epidemiology* is the study of the factors that determine the frequency and distribution of diseases.

Epivir: See *Lamivudine.*

Epzicom: A combination pill containing abacavir and lamivudine.

Erythropoeitin (EPO): A cytokine made in the body that stimulates production of red blood cells. EPO has been synthesized and can be taken as a drug. It has to be injected, it is expensive, and it has almost no side effects.

Esophagitis: Inflammation of a portion of the esophagus (the swallowing tube), which runs from the throat to the stomach. Common causes are *Candida albicans,* herpes simplex, CMV, and aphthous ulcers.

FDA: See *Food and Drug Administration.*

Fluconazole (or *Diflucan*): Fluconazole is used to treat fungal infections, primarily those caused by *Candida albicans* (thrush or candidal esophagitis) and *Cryptococcus neoformans* (cryptococcal meningitis). Fluconazole can be taken by mouth or by vein. Side effects are unusual; occasional problems are nausea, rash, or hepatitis.

Food and Drug Administration (FDA): The U.S. Food and Drug Administration, located in Rockville, Maryland, is the federal agency responsible for assuring that drugs (like penicillin and AZT), vaccines (like tetanus toxoid and the chickenpox vaccine), and devices (like artificial heart valves) are both safe and effective. Drugs cannot be sold in the United States unless the FDA has approved them. Approval is based on the drug's success or failure in clinical trials, which evaluate the drug's toxicity and effectiveness for a particular condition. The FDA also decides whether the drug can be sold over the counter (like aspirin), whether it requires a prescription from a physician (like all antibiotics), or whether it should be a controlled substance requiring a narcotic license (like morphine). In short, the FDA has broad regulatory powers. Some consider the FDA to be a bureaucratic nightmare—slow, demanding, and unresponsive to such critical needs as new drugs for HIV infection. Others consider that the FDA's awesome responsibility justifies its tedious but painstaking approval process. The FDA has always given a high priority to drugs for HIV, granting these drugs what is called an "expedited review." With expedited reviews, the requirements for approval are less stringent and after the studies are done, the review process is completed in a short time, often two to four months. The good news is that we get access to the drugs fast; the bad news is that we know less about them.

Fosamprenavir (FPV, Lexiva): A protease inhibitor that is usually boosted with ritonavir. Possible advantages compared to other PIs are that it can be taken once daily (though many take it twice daily), it can be taken with or without food, and it may have less effect on blood cholesterol than other PIs.

Ganciclovir (Cytovene): Ganciclovir is used to treat infections caused by cytomegalovirus and occasionally for infections caused by herpes simplex and other viruses. It is given intravenously. The most important side effect is a low blood count, especially neutropenia, which predisposes the person to bacterial infections (see *Blood count,* and neutropenia, under *Leukopenia*). If neutropenia is severe enough, the dose of the drug should be reduced, or the drug should be temporarily stopped. The drug is expensive.

G-CSF (Neupogen): A cytokine made in the body that stimulates the bone marrow to make white blood cells that fight infections. The drug must be taken by injection. Side effects are nil. The price is high.

Generic names: Most drugs have two names: a drug name and a trade name. For instance, atazanavir is the same as Reyataz: the first is the drug name, the second is the trade name from one drug company. Trade names are usually capitalized; generic drug names are not. When new drugs are discovered, they are patented, meaning that no one else can make them. So the company that made the discovery or owns the patent can charge whatever it can get. This arrangement can actually be good, because it keeps the pharmaceutical industry interested in discovering new drugs; it is the reason we now have more than twenty drugs for HIV. After seventeen years, patents run out and the drugs become generic. That's good too, because the drugs can then be manufactured by anyone and the price drops, sometimes to a small fraction of the original price. This decrease in price happened with ddI and AZT. The generic drugs must satisfy production requirements in order to be sold, providing assurance that the generic drug is as safe and as potent as the patented drug. We emphasize this point because some people think that generics are lesser drugs; they aren't. You should have no reservation about using them, providing they are licensed for sale in North America, Europe, or Australia. Many health insurance companies and managed care organizations or HMOs require that generic drugs be used when available. Physicians and medical journals tend to refer to drugs by generic names; patients tend to refer to them by trade names.

Gynecomastia: The medical term for breast enlargement in men that, in people with HIV infection, results from the redistribution of fat that is a side effect of long-term use of protease inhibitors. The enlargement may be generalized or nodular, and may be painful. Standard treatment when it is painful or cosmetically unpleasing is surgical reduction.

HAART (highly active antiretroviral therapy): HAART refers to the complex medical regimens of therapies directed against HIV that are likely to stop its replication and mutation. The goal of HAART is no progression of disease and no resistance to the virus. The progress in HIV therapy in the late 1990s is ascribed to the widespread use of HAART. The progress includes decreases in mortality, in the number of people with AIDS, in hospitalizations, in HIV-associated complications. HAART is also implicated in some of the newly recognized side effects, like *lipodystrophy* (see below).

HAD: See *HIV-associated dementia.*

Hemophilia: A person with hemophilia lacks a protein that helps the blood to clot. People with hemophilia bleed easily, even with a trivial cut; many have severe hemorrhaging into the joints and eventually get joint disease. Hemophilia is inherited, and only by men; the gene for hemophilia is carried by women, who do not get the disease but who can pass the gene on to their sons. Hemophilia has two forms, hemophilia A and hemophilia B; each form lacks a different clotting protein, called a *clotting factor.* Hemophilia is treated by substituting a commercial clotting factor for the clotting factor the blood lacks. The commercial clotting factor is extracted chemically from blood donated by hundreds or thousands of people. As a result, people with hemophilia are exposed to the blood of thousands of donors. Between 1978 and 1985, from the time HIV was introduced into the United States until the time the blood banks screened for HIV, people with hemophilia had a high risk of being infected with HIV. Approximately 70 percent of men with hemophilia A and 30 percent of men with hemophilia B acquired HIV infection from infected commercial clotting factors.

Since 1985, the risk of being exposed to HIV through clotting factors has dropped to practically nil. One reason is that donated blood is now screened for HIV; another reason is that clotting factors are heated and purified by detergents and biochemicals that kill HIV.

Hepatitis: Hepatitis is an inflammation of the liver. Many people have no symptoms and are unaware of having hepatitis. The symptoms, when people do have them, are loss of appetite, vomiting, yellow discoloration of the skin and eyes (jaundice), dark urine, sore stomach, and fever. Hepatitis is usually caused by viruses that are named alphabetically in their order of discovery, that is, hepatitis A through hepatitis E. Most important are hepatitis A, B, and C. Hepatitis A is caused by food poisoning; though it may be severe, it is always temporary. Hepatitis B and C are common in the general population, but more common in people with HIV infection. The reason is that HIV, hepatitis B, and hepatitis C are all transmitted by the same mechanisms: sex and blood. Both hepatitis B and C may cause persistent infection that lasts years or decades, cause chronic hepatitis, and may cause cirrhosis. The diagnosis of hepatitis is easily made with blood tests to determine liver function and to detect specific microbes, including hepatitis B, hepatitis C, and hepatitis A viruses. When the cause is unclear, it is sometimes helpful to obtain a biopsy of the liver.

For people with HIV infection who are also trying to manage chronic infections with the hepatitis B virus or the hepatitis C virus (two simultaneous infections referred to as coinfections), the following facts are important:

- All people with HIV and chronic liver infection need to avoid excessive alcohol, get vaccinated for hepatitis A, and avoid the drugs that are likely to injure the liver. If they haven't had hepatitis B, they need the vaccine to prevent it.

- All HIV drugs can cause liver disease; some are more likely to do so than others. Many HIV drugs are most likely to cause liver disease when the liver is already injured by chronic infection with, say, the hepatitis B or hepatitis C virus. We can't avoid the HIV drugs, but we can watch the liver closely by getting liver tests frequently and changing the drugs when necessary.

- Hepatitis B and hepatitis C are now treatable. The treatment for hepatitis C is a weekly injection with interferon (peg-interferon), which has substantial side effects; treatment usually continues for one year. Hepatitis C can actually be cured, but the rate of cure with an HIV coinfection is substantially lower. The treatment for hepatitis B will not cure it but will reduce its progression. Of the five drugs used for hepatitis B infection, three are also used for HIV. Coinfection with HIV and both forms of hepatitis makes treatment complicated. One reason is that the drugs used for HIV commonly cause liver disease. So before you can be treated for liver disease, your doctor must figure out whether the cause is hepatitis or the HIV drugs. Decisions about how to use these drugs with coinfection are tricky and best made by experts.

Hepatitis B virus: The hepatitis B virus is one of the microbes that causes hepatitis. Hepatitis B infection may be acute and cause serious symptoms that last up to a few weeks (see above, *Hepatitis*); it may be chronic with occasional symptoms and abnormal liver tests that last for months or years; or it may cause no symptoms at all and may only show up on a blood test. The tests for the hepatitis B virus are a little complicated:

1. The test might show that you have antibodies to the virus, which means either that you have been infected (but usually don't know it) or that you have already responded to the vaccine. In this case, you don't need the vaccine and you don't need to worry about hepatitis B.

2. The test might be negative, which means you have not been exposed to the hepatitis B virus. Most people with this test result and with HIV infection should get vaccinated.

3. The test might show that you have chronic infection with hepatitis B virus. This means you need to be evaluated for treatment for the virus.

About 5 to 10 percent of people with hepatitis B infection become chronic carriers of hepatitis B virus; they continue to carry the virus and can transmit it to others for years. People who are persistent carriers of hepatitis B virus may develop chronic hepatitis that over many years could eventually lead to cirrhosis or in rare cases, liver cancer. The frequency of chronic hepatitis B carriers is higher among people with HIV infection. The hepatitis B virus is transmitted the same way HIV is, by sexual contact or blood-to-blood transmission. The blood supply used for transfusions is screened for the hepatitis B virus and is therefore an unlikely source of this infection.

There is little evidence that chronic hepatitis B infection is worse in people with HIV infection than in people without HIV infection. In addition, the presence of liver damage or ongoing inflammation may complicate the use of certain drugs that require the liver for metabolism or that may occasionally cause further liver damage (see *Hepatitis*, above). Once infection takes place, treatment with interferon, lamivudine (3TC), adofovir, entecavir, or tenofovir can slow the hepatitis B virus, but the results are variable. Interferon has harsh side effects and the virus usually becomes resistant to lamivudine. It's better to prevent the infection with a vaccine. The vaccine is recommended for the people at risk for this infection: people who share needles to inject drugs, people who practice unsafe sex with gay men, family members who live in the same household, sex partners of people known to be hepatitis B carriers, and health care workers. Three injections are required, at a cost of about $150 to $200 for all three doses.

Hepatitis C virus: The hepatitis C virus, like hepatitis B, causes hepatitis. Hepatitis C is transmitted by blood, and far less frequently by sexual contact. The diagnosis is made by a blood test and sometimes by a biopsy of the liver. Unlike hepatitis B, hepatitis C cannot be prevented by vaccine. Most injection drug users and people with hemophilia have hepatitis C. Hepatitis C is quite different from hepatitis B in several ways: about 85 percent of the people with hepatitis C get chronic infection, meaning they carry this virus forever. Of the chronic carriers, about 20 percent develop cirrhosis over a period of 20 years, and about 4 to 10 percent die of liver failure or get a liver transplant. These odds are made much worse by alcohol abuse and by concurrent HIV infection. In fact, now that the prognosis with HIV infection is so much better, many people with both HIV and hepatitis C usually live long enough to get serious liver disease from hepatitis C. Hepatitis C can be treated with interferon and ribivirin. The treatment has many side effects, but about 30 to 50 percent of the people who get through the full 6- to 12-month course are cured of hepatitis C.

Herpes simplex virus: Herpes simplex is a virus that commonly causes infections of the mouth ("fever blisters" or "cold sores") and genitals ("genital herpes"). There are actually two different viruses: though similar in many respects, one kind (called herpes simplex no. 1) is most likely to infect the mouth and the other (called herpes simplex no. 2), the genitals. The symptoms of both infections are blisters on the mouth or genital area that first contain clear fluid, then become filled with pus, finally form scabs, and eventually disappear. Herpes simplex is a persistent virus: the virus remains dormant most of the time and then causes recurrent symptoms intermittently over a period of years. The initial infection with herpes simplex virus is often severe with large areas of blisters, occasional fevers, and pain and tingling in the area involved. Subsequent attacks are usually milder. The virus is transmitted to others by contact with the mouth or genitals, especially when the blisters are present.

Both the oral and the genital form of herpes are common infections in the general population; in people with advanced HIV infection, however, the blisters are more common, more severe, less likely to respond to standard therapy, more widespread over relatively larger areas, and persist for longer periods of time. Treatment with drugs like acyclovir, famciclovir, or valacyclovir makes the lesions heal faster, especially if taken early in the course of the infection. These drugs can also be taken continuously to prevent outbreaks. In addition, treatment reduces the risk of transmitting the virus to others. In people with HIV infection who have severe herpes infections, acyclovir may be given intravenously; once the infection is under control, the tablets are often given for extended periods to prevent recurrences.

Herpes zoster: Herpes zoster is caused by the same virus that causes chickenpox. The virus persists in the body and may cause symptoms decades after the original infection. Attacks after the first infection are called shingles, or herpes zoster. The skin sores with herpes zoster are similar to those of chickenpox and those of herpes simplex. With herpes simplex, the sores are on both sides of the body and usually on the genitals or mouth. With chickenpox, the sores are all over the body and don't hurt; with shingles, a crop of sores forms on one side of the body and *hurts*. The sores begin as red spots that become blisters filled with water; the blisters break down into sores with pus, finally scab over, and eventually disappear. Unlike herpes simplex infections or chickenpox, however, the later recurrences of herpes zoster are usually restricted to the area served by a single nerve. In other words, the blisters are restricted to one side of the body, usually in a band across the face, chest, abdomen, back, or leg.

In older people, herpes zoster is followed by post-herpetic neuralgia, a pain at the site of blisters that may persist for months after the blisters are gone. Post-herpetic neuralgia is fortunately infrequent among people with HIV infection. Herpes zoster is more common and more severe in people with HIV infection. It does not, however, necessarily mean that the immune system is weakening, and it clearly does not indicate AIDS. The diagnosis is generally made with a microscopic examination and culture of blisters, but the appearance of the blisters is usually all a physician needs to make a diagnosis. Acyclovir, famciclovir, or valacyclovir can hasten healing and reduce the most common complication of herpes zoster—severe pain.

Hickman catheter: People who require long courses of drugs given by vein will often have a tubing called a Hickman catheter. The catheter is inserted by a specialist, usually a surgeon, through the skin of the chest, and then tunneled under the skin to a vein in the chest. The end of the catheter comes out the chest wall above the breast. Drugs can be injected into the catheter as necessary. The advantage of a Hickman catheter is that it permits access to the vein without repeated needlesticks in the arms. Other devices are also available, including a type that is placed below the skin so that no tube comes out the chest wall.

It is important to know that the area around any catheter in a vein can become infected. Symptoms of infection of the area where the catheter is located are redness and pain, and sometimes pus. Symptoms of infection around the catheter inside the body are fever and chills; in most cases, the infection is inside the body and the skin around the catheter appears normal or feels slightly tender. Anyone with a Hickman catheter and these symptoms should tell a physician right away. Antibiotics should be given immediately, and sometimes the catheter needs to be removed.

Histoplasmosis: A fungus that is highly prevalent in the Ohio and Mississippi River valleys and is also found in other central, southwestern, and mid-Atlantic states. People with HIV infection are susceptible to it. The infection is often disseminated, that is, widely distributed all over the body. The disseminated form of histoplasmosis occurs in late-stage HIV infection when the CD4 count is under 100. Common symptoms are fever and weight loss. Treatment is with amphotericin B by vein and/or itraconazole by mouth.

HIV: HIV stands for the human immunodeficiency virus. HIV causes AIDS. There are occasional arguments that perhaps HIV does not cause AIDS, but at present, the great majority of scientific authorities accept HIV as the sole cause of AIDS. Several studies show that HIV reproduces rapidly and destroys CD4 cells, suggesting that the entire course of infection is similar to that of most other viral infections. HIV's uniqueness is that it takes a long time to make the person sick and that it attacks an unusual part of the body, the immune system.

HIV-associated dementia (HAD): HIV-associated dementia is the dementia that appears to result from HIV infecting the brain. Dementia means the loss of intellectual abilities, including the loss of memory, judgment, and concentration. HAD occurs in 20 to 30 percent of people with HIV infection, but usually only in the late stages.

Immune reconstitution: The term used to describe the return of the immune system when HAART (see above, *HAART*) controls HIV. Immune reconstitution is monitored by the CD4 cell count (see above, *CD4 cells*). Early studies questioned the competence of the CD4 cells that came back after HAART, but we now know that they work well. Even people with severe immune suppression and CD4 counts near 0 can have complete or near-complete recoveries. This means that people who took PCP prophylaxis for years can stop taking it when the CD4 count is above 250 for 3 months.

Immune reconstitution syndrome: In this syndrome, the immune system overresponds, usually to some opportunistic infection that is being treated at the same time HIV is being treated. When HIV is controlled, the immune system comes back and attacks the opportunistic infection with such vigor that the immune response itself causes symptoms. In most cases, the syndrome is managed by continuing to treat HIV, continuing to treat the opportunistic infection, and taking medication like cortisone to quiet the immune reaction.

Immune system: The human body is defended against a multitude of microbes by a complex system called the immune system. The principal components of the immune system are cells called *B lymphocytes, neutrophils,* and *T lymphocytes.* B lymphocytes make antibodies, the proteins that attack bacteria and viruses; neutrophils envelop and kill bacteria; and T lymphocytes provide communication between the parts of the immune system. Although these three components are somewhat interdependent, each takes primary responsibility for defense against certain types of microbes. For this reason, people deficient in different components are prone to infections with quite different microbes.

The cell type that is primarily affected in people with HIV infection is a type of T lymphocyte called a *CD4 cell* (see above). The most common infections encountered in people with few CD4 cells are caused by *Pneumocystis jiroveci,* cytomegalovirus, *Mycobacterium avium* complex, herpes simplex virus, herpes zoster, *Candida albicans, Toxoplasma gondii, Cryptosporidium, Cryptococcus, Salmonella,* and the bacterium that causes tuberculosis. People with immune systems weakened by HIV are not only subject to high rates of infections with these organisms, but the infections also tend to be severe, prolonged, recurrent, and often difficult to treat. At the same time, many other microbes that commonly cause infections in everyone do not appear to be unusually common or severe in people with HIV, presumably because the other components of the immune defenses remain relatively strong.

Incubation period: The incubation period of a disease is the time interval between infection with a microbe and the first symptoms of disease. For influenza and common colds, the incubation period is usually several days; for measles, chickenpox, mumps, and infections caused by many other viruses, the incubation period is two to three weeks. An unusual feature of HIV infection is that the first symptoms of a weakened immune system usually do not occur until several years after the infection takes place. Nevertheless, the *acute HIV infection* (see above) usually occurs at 2 to 4 weeks after HIV transmission.

Indinavir (Crixivan): A protease inhibitor that is usually taken with ritonavir (Norvir) twice daily. Indinavir may cause kidney stones composed of indinavir; the best way to prevent this is to drink large amounts of fluids.

Infectious: See *Contagious.*

Influenza vaccine: The influenza vaccine varies in effectiveness, depending on whether the strain of virus in the vaccine is related to the virus that is causing the influenza. The effectiveness of the vaccine changes every year. In most years, however, the vaccine probably prevents about 70 percent of the cases of influenza, and those who become infected despite having been vaccinated usually have less severe symptoms. Influenza is not known to be unusually common or severe in people with HIV infection. The main problem specific to people with HIV infection is that the symptoms of influenza can be confused with the symptoms of pneumonias such as pneumocystis pneumonia, which are caused by other microbes (see *Pneumocystis jiroveci*), a confusion it would be nice to avoid. Therefore, the CDC's Advisory Committee on Immunization Practices recommends that people with HIV infection routinely get the influenza vaccine every year.

Informed consent: Informed consent is a form of protection for people considering taking an HIV antibody test or undergoing certain medical procedures (like an operation) or considering participation in a clinical trial. Before taking the test, undergoing the procedure, or participating in the trial, the person or the person's representative must sign an informed consent form stating that he or she has been informed about the purpose, benefits, risks, and alternatives to the test, procedure, or trial, and that he or she consents to it. In the case of participation in a clinical trial, the informed consent form explains the purpose of the trial, what will be done, the risks of participation, the benefits of participation, what other treatments are available, and the right of the participant to leave the trial at any time.

Inoculum size: Inoculum size is a term used in the field of infectious diseases to describe the number of microbes necessary to cause an infection. In HIV infection, for example, a certain number of viruses is required before infection takes place. The specific number is not known. What is known is that the probability of transmitting HIV with the transfusion of one unit (or 500 milliliters) of infected blood is 80 to 90 percent (80 or 90 chances in 100). The probability of transmitting HIV with a needlestick injury, which injects only a fraction of a milliliter of blood, is 0.3 percent (1 chance in 300). The concentration of HIV in the fluid is another component of the equation. One milliliter of blood with a million HIVs (officially called *virus copies*) is much more likely to transmit HIV than a milliliter of blood with only 100,000 copies. This difference in the probabilities of transmission is due to differences in inoculum size. The definition of inoculum size actually includes both the volume of fluid and the concentration of viruses in it.

Intensification: The addition of 1 to 2 drugs to an antiviral regimen that's having a good effect, but not quite good enough.

Interferons: Interferons are proteins that cause cells to resist attack by certain viruses. Interferons are usually produced by the body, but they are also made artificially and used as medications. For people with HIV infection, interferons are mainly used to treat hepatitis B or hepatitis C. The drug works but only when given intravenously in very large doses, and the side effects may be severe. Most doctors now prescribe a special form of interferon, called peg-interferon, which needs to be injected only once a week. The major side effects of injected interferon are the achiness and fever that accompany flu: it is the interferon produced by the body that causes these symptoms during flu. Another important side effect is depression; less common side effects are nausea, vomiting, low white blood cell counts, rash, hair loss, and liver damage.

Invirase: See *Saquinavir.*

Isoniazid (INH): Isoniazid is the standard drug used to treat and prevent tuberculosis. Isoniazid is usually recommended for any person with HIV infection who has tuberculosis or who has a positive tuberculosis skin test. The usual dose is 300 milligrams, taken once a day by mouth. The most important side effect is hepatitis, including jaundice (yellowish skin and eyes), dark urine, nausea, and abdominal pain. This side effect is more likely in people who already have liver damage for other reasons, and in older people. People taking isoniazid and having these symptoms should stop taking the drug immediately and call their physicians. INH tends to cause a vitamin B6 deficiency, so INH and vitamin B6 are often given at the same time.

Itraconazole: An antifungal drug that is sometimes used to treat infections caused by *Candida, Aspergillus,* or *Histoplasma.* It comes as a capsule, a liquid, or in a form for intravenous administration. The capsule needs to be taken when there is food and stomach acid to permit absorption; the liquid form needs to be taken on an empty stomach.

Kaletra: See *Lopinavir.*

Kaposi's sarcoma: Kaposi's (pronounced kaposhee's) sarcoma is a tumor of blood vessels caused by a virus called *Kaposi's sarcoma herpes virus (KSHV)* or *herpes virus 8* because the virus is related to herpes. Approximately 20 percent of all people with AIDS have Kaposi's sarcoma, but the percentage is highest in gay men: for example, it is 20 times more common in gay men than in people with hemophilia. The symptoms of Kaposi's sarcoma are purplish nodules, usually a quarter of an inch to an inch in diameter, anywhere on the skin. The nodules are new, firm bumps; they aren't flat like a freckle. The nodules will grow in size and number. They sometimes occur on internal organs like the lung, brain, and gastrointestinal tract, though they often cause no specific symptoms at these sites. Some nodules are painful. The face and legs may swell if the lymph channels nearby are blocked. If Kaposi's sarcoma becomes extensive, people may have fever, weight loss, and severe fatigue.

The diagnosis can be established by a biopsy of the nodules. Biopsies are easy to do with nodules on the skin, but more difficult when the nodules are on internal organs. The main reason to do the biopsy is that the nodules might possibly turn out to be something other than Kaposi's sarcoma; and if they are Kaposi's sarcoma, they are an AIDS-defining diagnosis. Therapy depends on where Kaposi's is and what problems it causes. Skin bumps may only require cover-up makeup. Some lesions are treated with injections or irradiation. The serious form of Kaposi's is when there are over 25 spots, there is edema, or when the internal organs are involved. These conditions are often treated with chemotherapy like cancer.

Lactic acidosis: This is a complication of treatment with nucleoside analogs, primarily d4T, AZT, or ddI. The cause is toxicity to mitochondria, tiny particles inside cells responsible for the cell's metabolism. The result is an increase in lactic acid. The diagnosis is made by measuring the level of lactic acid in the blood. The symptoms are nausea, vomiting, stomach pain, weight loss, and shortness of breath. The symptoms occur in the context of taking one of these three drugs, usually for months. Lactic acidosis can be serious and, if advanced, even life threatening. We have no good treatment except to stop the drug responsible and provide support like intravenous fluids, dialysis, or a ventilator. Lactic acidosis takes a long time to clear up—weeks or months. Most people who have it can never use AZT, ddI, or d4T again.

Lamivudine (3TC, Epivir): A nucleoside analog that works powerfully against HIV, can be taken once a day as a single pill, can be taken with or without food, and has almost no side effects. A similar drug is emtricitabine (FTC, Emtriva). Nearly everybody who takes anti-retroviral treatment takes one of these two drugs. The two are never taken together because they are too similar. The one problem is that when the virus is not well controlled, it can get a mutation at codon 184 of the reverse transcriptase gene that reduces the action of both 3TC and FTC. This is the most common resistance mutation. After this mutation occurs, many people continue taking the drugs, which are still active against HIV even with the mutation. The two drugs are also effective against the hepatitis B virus (HBV) but for people with both HBV and HIV, taking the drugs can be tricky. For example, if the drugs are stopped for any reason, the hepatitis can flare up. Or the HBV may become resistant to these drugs after several months (as it is prone to do) so that the drugs no longer control it. Experts in hepatitis and HIV know how to deal with these issues.

Latency: Latency and dormancy (which literally means sleeping) mean the same thing: a microbe is in the body but is not actively reproducing, not invading any tissues, and not causing symptoms. Examples of microbes that are latent or dormant in many or most healthy people are: *Pneumocystis jiroveci, Toxoplasma gondii,* herpes simplex virus, the virus that causes herpes zoster, and cytomegalovirus. Once in the body, these microbes remain in the body. They remain latent or dormant until something tilts the balance in the immune system and permits them to become active.

Leukopenia: Leukopenia means a low number (or *penia*) of white blood cells (or leukocytes—*leuko* means white), the cells of the immune system that fight infection. Leukocytes include lymphocytes (cells that recognize foreign material) and neutrophils (cells that gobble up microbes). The normal leukocyte count is 4,000 to 8,000 per milliliter of blood. In people with certain infections, especially with bacterial infections, the leukocyte count is high (leukocytosis). In people with viral infections, including HIV infection, the leukocyte count is low (leukopenia). Having a low count of lymphocytes is called *lymphopenia;* lymphopenia is the expected result of HIV infection. A low count of neutrophils is called *neutropenia;* neutropenia can be caused by HIV itself or by some of the drugs—like AZT or trimethoprim-sulfamethoxazole (Bactrim or Septra)—commonly taken during HIV infection. Neutropenia becomes worrisome if the count is less than 750 per milliliter; if the count is less than 500 per milliliter, the person is prone to bacterial infections. Neutropenia is usually not a big problem in people with HIV infection; when it is severe, however, it can often be reversed with G-CSF (Neupogen) (see *G-CSF*).

Lexiva: See *Fosamprenavir.*

Lipoatrophy: This is the medical terms for fat loss. It is a side effect of d4T, AZT, and ddI. The fat is lost in the arms and legs, buttocks, and face. In the face, it causes a characteristic "sunken cheek" appearance and is usually a side effect of taking d4T—or, less commonly, AZT—for years. People don't like the change in the way they look, which they feel is stigmatizing. This fat loss has no medical consequences. When you stop taking d4T or AZT, the side effect may go away, but it may take years or may not happen at all. Some treatments with injections fill out the face. These treatments are often highly effective, but medical insurance does not pay for them.

Lipodystrophy: A complication of antiretroviral therapy that includes (1) high levels of blood fats, or hyperlipidemia, which predisposes the person to heart disease and stroke; (2) redistribution of fat on the body, resulting in a protuberant abdomen ("crix belly"), a collection of fat on the back of the neck ("buffalo hump"), enlarged breasts in women, thin arms and legs with prominent veins, and sunken cheeks; (3) diabetes; and (4) bone thinning or osteoporosis. Most people have one or two of these symptoms, not all four. The cause is not clear, but appears related to antiretroviral drugs.

Lopinavir/ritonavir (Kaletra): A combination of two *PI*'s (see below). One is lopinavir, which does the job against HIV, and the other is ritonavir, which is given only to increase the levels of lopinavir.

Lumbar puncture: See *Spinal tap.*

Lymph glands: The lymphatic system is a widespread network, like the blood circulation, of channels that carry lymph. Lymph is a clear fluid containing lymphocytes, or white blood cells (including CD4 cells), which are a part of the immune system. Lymph is manufactured in the lymph glands, clumps of lymphatic tissue that trap infecting microbes and are distributed widely throughout the body. When lymph glands are near the surface of the skin, they can be felt as bumps below the skin's surface. The usual locations where they can be felt are the back of the neck, below the jaw, under the armpits, and in the groin. Lymph glands are commonly swollen and sometimes painful and tender when they are infected. Many infections involve the lymph glands. In HIV infection, the lymph glands become infected early. The lymph glands are the sites where HIV concentrates most highly, where much of the destruction of CD4 cells takes place, and where much of the reproduction of HIV also takes place. Swollen lymph glands are likely to occur in three different circumstances: with *persistent generalized lymphadenopathy,* or *PGL* (see below), in which many lymph glands are swollen for months early in the course of HIV infection; with infection of the lymph glands by certain complications later in the course of HIV infection; and with lymphomas, which are tumors of the lymphatic system seen more frequently in people with HIV infection than in the general population. Swollen lymph glands may require diagnostic tests: the usual is a biopsy of the lymph gland or removal of the whole gland to permit microscopic examination of the lymphatic tissue.

Lymphadenopathy: Lymphadenopathy means swollen lymph glands. Swollen lymph glands are most common at the back of the neck, along the jaw, in the armpits, and in the groin. The lymph glands may feel like rubbery, discrete nodules that are rarely tender to touch and often pea-sized; glands of this description are common in everyone and in several conditions unrelated to HIV infection. If they are swollen to abnormal size for longer than a month in at least two different areas, they constitute *persistent generalized lymphadenopathy (PGL)* (see below).

Lymphoma: Lymphoma is a cancer of the lymphatic system. Lymphoma occurs most frequently in people without HIV infection, but people with weakened immune systems, including those with HIV infection, have lymphomas about forty times more frequently than normal. About 5 to 10 percent of people with AIDS have lymphomas, and for people with AIDS, lymphomas are classified as opportunistic tumors. Lymphomas are one of the few complications of HIV infection that appears to be increasing in the era of HAART, presumably because lymphomas are not so dependent on severe immune suppression—so immune reconstitution helps but not as much as with other HIV complications.

There are many types of lymphomas: some progress extremely slowly, cause few symptoms, and require minimal treatment; some are more severe. People with AIDS generally have lymphomas called non-Hodgkin's lymphomas of B cell origin. These lymphomas tend to be severe, and they also tend to involve unusual areas of the body like the brain, liver, kidneys, intestines, and lungs. The diagnosis is usually established with a biopsy. Treatment is variable and often requires the assistance of a specialist in cancer treatment using cancer chemotherapy or radiation treatment.

MAC: See *Mycobacterium avium complex.*

Magnetic resonance imaging (MRI): Magnetic resonance imaging is a technique used to make a three-dimensional image of the interior of the body. Though the technique is somewhat different from a CT scan (see *Computerized tomography scan*), the images are similar. The person getting an MRI is placed inside a large tubular structure and remains motionless for thirty to sixty minutes: the worst problems are boredom, noise, and claustrophobia. During that time, the person's body is bathed in a magnetic field, which causes the atoms in different tissues to give off tiny radio signals. The signals are different depending on the kind of tissue. An MRI is better than a CT scan at detecting diseases of the brain and spinal cord. MRI is painless, harmless, and does not involve exposure to radiation. MRIs are also expensive, from $500 to $1,000.

Managed care organization: An organization that takes financial and medical responsibility for its subscribers' health care. The best-known managed care organizations are called health maintenance organizations, or HMOs.

Marinol: The psychoactive component of marijuana. It is used to increase appetite in people with wasting. It is expensive, has psychological side effects, and most of the weight gain is fat, as opposed to a more useful protein. Whether or not marinol works as well as smoking marijuana cigarettes has not been studied.

Megestrol acetate (Megace): Megestrol is a female hormone that stimulates the appetite. The drug may cause reduced libido in men. Most of the weight gained is fat, rather than protein.

Meningitis: Meningitis is an infection of the meninges, the membrane that envelops the brain and spinal cord. The most common cause of meningitis in people with HIV infection is *Cryptococcus* (see under *Cryptococcosis*).

Methadone: Methadone is an opiate that is commonly used to control narcotic withdrawal symptoms and to maintain people addicted to morphine-like drugs, particularly heroin. Methadone maintenance is permitted only in programs approved by the Food and Drug Administration and the designated state authority. Methadone can be given by mouth or by vein. Side effects are those shared by all morphine-like drugs, which depress the central nervous system: dizziness, mental clouding, depression, and sedation. Methadone may cause physical dependence. If it is stopped abruptly after prolonged and regular use, it can cause withdrawal symptoms.

Metronidazole (Flagyl): Metronidazole is an antibiotic taken by people with HIV infection for common intestinal infections and common dental problems like gingivitis (inflammation of the gums) and periodontitis (infection of the structures that support the teeth). The drug is given by mouth or by vein. Side effects are unusual, primarily nausea and stomach pain. The side effects can improve if the drug is taken with meals or if the dose is reduced. Taking this drug for periods of months may cause pain in the feet that resembles the pain of HIV *neuropathy* (see below). The pain usually goes away when the drug is stopped.

Microbes: Microbes are organisms so small they require a microscope to be seen. They can be bacteria, viruses, parasites, or fungi. HIV is one example of a virus. Microbes cause infectious diseases. The microbes that commonly cause the infections that are complications of HIV infection are as follows:

Viruses: Cytomegalovirus, herpes simplex, herpes zoster, molluscum contagiosum

Bacteria: *Mycobacterium avium* complex, *Mycobacterium tuberculosis* (the cause of tuberculosis), *Salmonella, Nocardia,* pneumococcus, *Bartonella*

Parasites: *Toxoplasma gondii, Cryptosporidium, Isospora*

Fungi: *Pneumocystis jiroveci, Cryptococcus, Histoplasma, Candida albicans, Coccidioides, Aspergillus*

Mutation: A change in a gene that can in turn change certain of a microbe's characteristics: growth, appearance, sensitivity to drugs, ability to invade, and response to antibodies. HIV mutates extensively. Within a few years, the person infected with one strain of HIV has billions of different mutant strains in his or her body. If the person takes AZT, then evolution assures that HIV mutates to become resistant to AZT. Mutated strains of HIV also confound vaccine development because the immune system may not recognize them.

Mycobacterium avium complex (MAC): MAC is related to the bacterium that causes tuberculosis, though it is not contagious and is more difficult to treat. In the late stages of HIV infection, infection with MAC is spread widely throughout many organs in the body. It can cause fever, pneumonia, diarrhea, hepatitis, and many other complications. In a person with a CD4 count under 50, MAC most commonly causes prolonged fever and abdominal pain.

National Institutes of Health (NIH): NIH is a federal organization located in Bethesda, Maryland, that funds scientific research. NIH is the world's largest research organization. With a budget of over $10 billion a year, NIH is responsible for funding about a third of all research in the biomedical sciences, including research related to HIV infection, in the United States. About $1.8 billion is allocated annually to research on HIV. Some of the research sponsored by NIH is intramural; that is, it is conducted by the approximately one thousand researchers inside NIH; most of the research is extramural, at universities and medical schools throughout the country. Extramural research grants are awarded on the basis of priority, as determined by expert review of proposals. NIH is divided into fifteen different institutes, each with a different scientific specialty: the National Institute for Allergy and Infectious Diseases (NIAID) is responsible for most of the research into HIV infection. NIH is not related to the *Centers for Disease Control and Prevention* (see above), except that both are federally funded agencies with somewhat different roles in combating HIV and other diseases.

Funding for research into HIV infection from sources other than NIH comes from other federal agencies (Department of Defense, National Science Foundation, Veterans Administration, and the Centers for Disease Control and Prevention), pharmaceutical companies, local governments, and private foundations. Funding for this research escalated rapidly in the late 1980s until the total HIV research budget exceeded the funding for heart disease research at a time when heart disease was responsible for twenty times more deaths than AIDS was. Some view this as inappropriate, given the relative impact of the two; others feel AIDS research is underfunded, given its importance as a public health problem, its role as the major cause of death in Americans aged 24 to 44, and as a prototypic disease for many other conditions—that is, what we learn from HIV may be applied as well to such diseases as cancer, diabetes, and lupus.

Nelfinavir (Viracept): A protease inhibitor taken 2 times a day. The major side effect is diarrhea. This is the only protease inhibitor that is not "boosted" with ritonavir.

Neuropathy: Neuropathy is an illness involving the nerves. Nerves are responsible for (among other things) the movement of muscles and the sensation of touch, including the sensation of pain. The symptoms of a neuropathy can therefore be weakness of a muscle or pain and tingling. In people with HIV infection, the most frequent symptoms of neuropathy are painful feet and legs. There may be tingling as if the foot were asleep. Often the bottom of the foot is most affected, which may interfere with walking or require pain medication. Neuropathy may be the result of HIV infection or a side effect of some drugs, especially ddI, ddC, or d4T.

Nevirapine (Viramune): An *NNRTI* (see below) taken twice a day. The major side effects are rash and liver disease, usually in the first 8 to 16 weeks of treatment. Rash occurs in 15 to 20 percent of the people taking it and may be severe. A rash in the form of red splotches is usually not serious but should be checked out. Rashes are serious when they show blisters, involve the mouth or eyes, or occur with fever. The liver disease can be very serious; if you have severe stomach problems, a rash, or fever, you need immediate evaluation. You should report to your doctor any sickness during the first 8 to 16 weeks of taking nevirapine.

NNRTIs: Short for *nonnucleoside reverse transcriptase inhibitors* (see below).

Nonnucleoside reverse transcriptase inhibitors (NNRTIs): A class of drugs that inhibit reverse transcriptase but are not in the same class as nucleosides. Examples of NNRTIs are efavirenz, nevirapine, and delavirdine.

Norvir: See *Ritonavir.*

Nucleoside analogs: Nucleoside analogs, sometimes called just *nucleosides,* are a chemically related group of drugs used to inhibit HIV. Examples include the first drugs approved to treat HIV infection: AZT, ddI, ddC, d4T, ABC, 3TC, FTC, and TDF. Often these drugs are combined to reduce the "pill burden," the total number of pills you need to take. These combinations are AZT/3TC (Combivir), AZT/3TC/ABC (Trizivir), TDF/FTC (Truvada), and 3TC/ABC (Epzicom). They all work by the same mechanism, by inhibiting an enzyme called reverse transcriptase that is critical for HIV's survival. Nucleoside analogs often seem to have time-limited benefit, that is, after prolonged use they stop working. This happens because HIV develops resistance to a particular nucleoside analog. Nevertheless, HIV often remains sensitive to other nucleoside analogs, which can then be substituted or added.

Nukes or nucs: Shorthand for *nucleoside analogs* (see above).

Opportunistic infections: In all infectious diseases, the body's defenses are, for a while, inadequate to control microbial invasion. Many microbes can cause disease in people who are otherwise healthy. Other microbes, however, are fairly harmless and can cause disease only in people whose immune defenses are weakened. These microbes are called opportunistic microbes because the microbe takes the opportunity offered by a weakened immune system to cause disease. The opportunistic microbes that most frequently infect people with HIV infection are listed above, under *Microbes.*

Opportunistic tumors: Opportunistic tumors, like opportunistic infections, occur primarily in people with weakened immune systems. In people with HIV infection, the major opportunistic tumors are Kaposi's sarcoma, certain types of lymphoma, and cervical cancer. Two of these tumors and possibly all three are actually caused by viral infections.

Oral hairy leukoplakia (OHL): The symptoms of oral hairy leukoplakia are white (*leuko*) patches (*plakia*) on the tongue and elsewhere in the mouth. It usually produces no symptoms, but may distort taste or cause pain. It is caused by the same virus that causes infectious mononucleosis. These patches often appear similar to those of thrush; in fact, oral hairy leukoplakia is often diagnosed when people who appear to have thrush do not respond to the usual treatment. It can also be diagnosed with a biopsy of the patches. Oral hairy leukoplakia seems to occur exclusively in people with HIV infection. It generally indicates progressive weakening of the immune system. Most people have no symptoms, but when they do, the usual treatment is high doses of acyclovir.

Pancreatitis: Inflammation of the pancreas, an organ in the abdomen that makes insulin and digestive enzymes. Symptoms are abdominal pain, nausea, and vomiting. Pancreatitis is a potentially serious complication of alcoholism and of some drugs, like ddI or d4T, used to treat HIV infection.

Paromomycin: An antimicrobial drug used to treat cryptosporidiosis. It is taken by mouth and sometimes effectively reduces symptoms.

Pentamidine: Pentamidine is a drug used to treat or prevent pneumocystis pneumonia. Pentamidine is often used only when someone cannot take the best drug, trimethoprim-sulfamethoxazole. To treat pneumocystis pneumonia, pentamidine is given by vein for three weeks. To prevent pneumocystis pneumonia in people whose CD4 count is less than 200, pentamidine is given by aerosol directly into the lungs, at monthly intervals. When given by vein, pentamidine often has severe side effects, such as low blood pressure (causing fainting), low blood sugar, high blood sugar (diabetes), kidney failure, liver disease, low blood counts, or inflammation of the pancreas. These side effects are common when the drug is given by vein. They are rare or don't occur at all when pentamidine is taken as an aerosol, since so little of the drug gets into the system.

Persistent generalized lymphadenopathy (PGL): A diagnosis of PGL means that lymph glands are swollen for at least one month and at two different sites of the body, not counting the groin area. PGL often occurs early in HIV infection. Lymph glands are the location of HIV multiplication at a time when the patient feels well. (See *Lymph glands* and *Lymphadenopathy.*)

PIs: Shorthand for *protease inhibitors* (see below).

Platelets: Platelets are the component of blood that facilitates clotting. The number of platelets is often low in people with HIV infection—sometimes so extremely low that the person is prone to bleeding. The cause of the low platelet count may be HIV infection itself, or it may be the drugs that are used to treat people with HIV infection. The normal platelet count is over 150,000 per milliliter of blood; a count of 50,000 to 150,000 is low but usually causes no problem; a count of 10,000 to 50,000 is worrisome, and less than 10,000 is serious. These numbers are rough: some people do fine for years with counts of 5,000 to 15,000, while other people with counts of 30,000 have profuse bleeding.

Pneumococcal vaccine: The most common cause of bacterial pneumonia in people without HIV infection is a bacterium called *Streptococcus pneumoniae* or pneumococcus. Pneumococcus causes pneumonia about 100 times more frequently in people with HIV infection. Pneumococcal vaccine is recommended for people with HIV infection, since they are prone to frequent or severe infections by pneumococcus. It is best to take this vaccine relatively early in the course of the disease when the immune system is strong. This means having a CD4 count of over 200.

Pneumocystis jiroveci (formerly *Pneumocystis carinii*): This fungus commonly causes lung infection and pneumonia in people with HIV infection. *Pneumocystis jiroveci* pneumonia (PCP) is the most frequent serious complication in people with HIV infection. Pneumocystis pneumonia is the most common AIDS-defining diagnosis. The symptoms are cough without sputum, shortness of breath, and fever. These symptoms usually evolve over a period of weeks. The diagnosis is generally established by a chest X-ray or studies of lung function, combined with a microscopic examination of respiratory secretions to show the fungus. Treatment is with several drugs—most commonly trimethoprim-sulfamethoxazole, but also pentamidine, dapsone-trimethoprim, atovaquone (Mepron), or clindamycin-primaquine. Treatment is most successful when started relatively early in the course of the infection.

Pneumonia: Pneumonia is an infection of the lungs. The usual symptoms are cough, fever, and shortness of breath. The causes of pneumonia vary, and the treatment depends on the cause.

Polymerase chain reaction (PCR): Polymerase chain reaction is a method for multiplying some part of a microbe's gene to huge concentrations within hours. It allows for a very sensitive test, developed in the 1980s, for detecting many microbes, including HIV (see *Retrovirus*). Unlike the standard blood test for HIV infection, which detects antibodies to HIV, the PCR detects HIV itself. This test can now be used to measure the concentration of HIV in the blood, called the HIV viral load (see below, *Quantitative virology*). Concentrations usually range from 1,000 to 1,000,000 viruses per milliliter of blood. Concentrations are highest in the first few weeks of infection before the immune defenses have responded, and in the late stage of the infection, when the immune defenses have been destroyed.

Progressive multifocal leukoencephalopathy: Progressive multifocal leukoencephalopathy is a viral infection deep in the brain that is found only in people with severely weakened immune systems, including, occasionally, people with HIV infection. Progressive multifocal leukoencephalopathy has a distinctive appearance on CT or MRI scans of the brain, but a diagnosis can be established definitely only with a biopsy. The infection tends to be progressive, and no therapy is known to be effective. Among people with HIV infection, it occurs only in the late stage, when the CD4 count is under 50.

Prophylaxis: Prophylaxis is treatment to prevent a disease, as opposed to treatment to eliminate a disease already present.

Protease inhibitors (PIs): This class of drugs inhibits HIV by interfering with the enzyme protease, which is critical for assembling the complete virus after it has reproduced. Several drugs are in this class, including saquinavir (Invirase), ritonavir (Norvir), indinavir (Crixivan), fosamprenavir (Lexiva), lopinavir (Kaletra), atazanavir (Reyataz), tipranavir (Aptivus), and nelfinavir (Viracept). Initial tests show that PIs and the NNRTIs are the most potent drugs we have for decreasing the concentration of HIV. The initial effect is a decrease in viral load by 99 percent. To keep the viral load low without also developing resistance, PIs must be combined with nucleosides.

Protease paunch: Slang for the collection of abdominal fat that is a side effect of protease inhibitors. Another term is "crix belly," referring to Crixivan (indinavir), but the side effect can occur with any PI. It may disappear if treatment with the PI is stopped—for example, changing to efavirenz-based HAART—but the disappearance is very slow.

Pyrimethamine (Daraprim): Pyrimethamine is an antibiotic used to treat or prevent *toxoplasmosis* (see below). The full treatment usually combines pyrimethamine with a sulfa drug like sulfadiazine or clindamycin. Pyrimethamine is taken by mouth. The major side effect after prolonged use is anemia. To avoid anemia, another drug, leucovorin, is given at the same time. Other side effects include gastric intolerance, allergic reactions, and hepatitis. Many of these reactions are the result of the sulfa drug that is taken with pyrimethamine.

Quantitative virology: Quantitative virology is a method of determining the concentration of a virus in some part of the body, in this case, the concentration of HIV in the blood. "Viral load" and "viral burden" are synonymous terms for quantitative virology. Two different tests are usually used to measure quantitative HIV virology: *polymerase chain reaction* (quantitative RNA-PCR) (see above) and *branched chain DNA (bDNA)*. In both tests, parts of the virus serve as tags for that particular virus. These tags are multiplied to huge concentrations within hours so that the presence of that virus becomes obvious. Once the virus tags are detected, then the concentration of the tags is extrapolated backward to the original concentration of the virus. The concentration of HIV usually ranges from 1,000 to 1,000,000 viruses per milliliter of blood. Quantitative virology measures the amount of virus and appears to supplement the CD4 count to indicate the stage of disease, or the prognosis. Concentrations over 100,000 per milliliter usually indicate that the disease is progressing. Quantitative virology is also used to measure the response to therapy. Most drugs cause a decrease in viral concentrations within hours.

Randomized trial: A trial or experiment comparing treatments. Participants are assigned to take one treatment or the other. Which treatment they take is a matter of chance; their assignment is random. Random assignment is necessary if the trial is to be scientifically credible. See chapter 8.

Receptor: A docking site on a cell to which a molecule or microbe attaches before entering the cell. The receptor for HIV is the CD4 receptor, for which the CD4 cell is named.

Rescriptor: See *Delavirdine.*

Research: See *National Institutes of Health.*

Reservoir: A place, like the genital tract or the central nervous system, where HIV can hide from treatment.

Resistance: Resistance, when used in medicine, means that a drug is not effective because the microbe being treated has been able to change its chemistry so it is no longer susceptible to the drug (see *Mutation,* above). The result is either that the drug does not work in the test tube against this person's microbe, or that the person stops getting better; usually both results are found together. Resistance is usually qualitative; that is, HIV may be highly resistant or slightly resistant. Furthermore, the person with HIV infection has billions of genetically different HIVs. Some HIVs may be sensitive to one drug and not to another, some are sensitive to all drugs, and some are resistant to every drug. People with very resistant HIVs have usually had many different courses of antiviral drugs.

There are two methods of measuring resistance. One detects mutations that confer complete or partial resistance. These mutations occur at specific locations, called *codons,* on the relevant gene—the reverse transcriptase gene for nucleosides and NNRTIs, and the protease gene for PIs. An example: a mutation on codon 184 of the reverse transcriptase gene makes 3TC (lamivudine) ineffective. Many drugs require many mutations before becoming ineffective.

The other method of measuring resistance is with a phenotypic test, which simply measures the amount of the drug required to inhibit a particular strain of HIV. If the amount of drug to inhibit that strain is many times greater than the amount that inhibits untreated strains, then that particular strain is resistant.

Retinitis: Retinitis means an inflammation (*itis*) of the retina, the layer of cells at the back of the eye that collect and send images to the brain. Retinitis usually causes some loss of vision. The earliest symptoms are pain in the eye, "floaters" across the field of vision, or a blind spot, which is the loss of part of a visual field. In people with

HIV infection, the most common cause of retinitis is infection with *cytomegalovirus* (see above, *CMV*). CMV retinitis rarely occurs when the CD4 count is above 50.

Retrovirus: Retroviruses are a type of virus. Retroviruses do not have DNA, the molecule that holds the genetic code that cells use to reproduce themselves. Instead, retroviruses have RNA and an enzyme called reverse transcriptase, which turns RNA into DNA. When a retrovirus invades one of the cells of the body, it uses reverse transcriptase to turn its own RNA into DNA. This DNA then becomes part of the cell's DNA. When properly stimulated, the DNA then makes more retrovirus instead of more cells. Many different kinds of retroviruses infect many different kinds of animals. HIV is the most important retrovirus to infect humans; it causes disease in no other animal species except for certain types of monkeys. On the whole, it is not easy for retroviruses to pass from one species to another.

Reyataz: See *Atazanavir.*

Risk factor: A risk factor is a condition or behavior that makes it likely that a person with the risk factor will develop a condition—in this case, HIV infection. The major risk factors for HIV infection are needle-sharing with injection drug users and sexual contact with a person who has HIV infection. Another risk factor is having received blood products between 1978—when HIV infection was first known to exist in the United States—and April 1985, when the blood supply was first screened for HIV. Other risks that heighten the probability that HIV will be transmitted through sexual intercourse are multiple sex partners, failure to use condoms, sex with someone in the late stage of the disease (when the viral load is high), anal sex, and sex with someone who has a sexually transmitted disease, especially genital ulcers. The risk to an infant born to a woman with HIV infection is 20 to 35 percent if the mother has not taken drugs to inhibit HIV. A minor risk factor in terms of frequency is needlestick injuries in health care workers who care for people with HIV infection. Less than 1 percent of all people with HIV infection in the United States have no clearly defined risk factor, although many of these people either are too sick to provide adequate information or are providing information that is suspect.

Ritonavir (Norvir): A protease inhibitor commonly used with other protease inhibitors. The reason is that ritonavir increases blood levels of the other PI by inhibiting the enzyme normally responsible for getting the other PI excreted. Ritonavir can be used as a single PI, but many people have trouble tolerating the necessary dose.

Safer sex: Safer sex is a qualitative term. To be absolutely safe, sexual contact cannot involve an exchange of any body fluids—specifically, semen, blood, or vaginal secretions. The term safer sex recognizes the likelihood of human error and the inexactness of human knowledge. Safer sex refers to sexual intercourse using a condom, or sexual practices that do not involve exchange of body fluids.

Salvage therapy: Treatment against HIV after a previous treatment has failed and the viral load has increased.

Saquinavir (Invirase): A *protease inhibitor* (see above) that comes in two forms. The first form, introduced in 1995, was Invirase. Since the body absorbed only about 4 percent of the drug, it has now been augmented by giving it with ritonavir to "boost" its levels. The main side effect is stomach distress.

Seizure: A seizure is a convulsion, uncontrolled movements of the arms and legs accompanied by unconsciousness and inability to control urine or stool. The usual cause of seizures in people with HIV infection is an opportunistic infection or an opportunistic tumor of the brain, including toxoplasma encephalitis, cryptococcal meningitis, or lymphoma. Less commonly, seizures are caused by HIV itself, or result from an imbalance of electrolytes, or are a side effect of medications. Recurrent seizures can usually be controlled with drugs like Dilantin and phenobarbital. Anyone with recurrent seizures should be careful about his or her physical circumstances: be careful working on ladders, for instance, or driving. In many states it is illegal for a person with seizures to drive until seizures have been controlled for at least one year.

Seroconversion: The immune system usually takes several days or weeks to recognize a foreign substance like a virus and to produce antibodies to it. Six to twelve weeks after HIV enters the body, antibodies to HIV usually appear in the blood. Physicians call the appearance of antibodies in the blood *seroconversion.* That is, the result of a test for antibodies in the blood serum converts from negative to positive.

Shingles: Synonymous with *herpes zoster* (see above).

Sinusitis: The sinuses are air sacs next to the passageway from the nose. Sinusitis is an infection of the sinuses, usually as a result of a cold or an allergy. Anyone can get sinusitis, but people with HIV infection have it more often, it is more likely to affect many sinuses, and it is often more difficult to treat. Symptoms are pus drainage from the nose, headache, face pain, and fever. The usual treatment is with antibiotics taken by mouth, such as trimethoprim-sulfamethoxazole, amoxicillin, erythromycin, cephalexin (or Keflex), cefaclor (Ceclor), clarithromycin (Biaxin), azithromycin (Zithromax), ciprofloxacin (Cipro), or tetracycline. Some people do not respond to these drugs, and their sinuses need to be drained, a procedure done by a specialist called an *otolaryngologist* (ear, nose, and throat specialist).

Spinal tap: A spinal tap, also called a *lumbar puncture*, is a procedure for obtaining cerebrospinal fluid, the fluid that surrounds the brain and the spinal cord. The procedure involves inserting a needle into the middle of the back and into the meninges, a membrane that contains the cerebrospinal fluid. The cerebrospinal fluid is then analyzed for evidence of infection of the brain or spinal cord. Despite sounding unpleasant and risky, a spinal tap is a well-established medical procedure and is rarely associated with any important complications. The most common complaint is a headache following the spinal tap, a complaint made less likely by lying flat once the spinal tap is completed.

Statins: A class of drugs that lower blood cholesterol. Most protease inhibitors increase cholesterol, and statins are taken to correct the increase. The problem is that most PIs interfere with the metabolism of the statins, so taking the two kinds of drugs together gets complicated. They may cause muscle pain, which can be a serious complication. In general, PIs are never to be taken with lovastatin (Altocor, Mevacor) or simvastatin (Zocor). Other statins, such as atorvastatin (Lipitor) or pravastatin (Pravachol) are less problematic, but we still prescribe low doses and alert the person taking the drug.

Sustiva: See *Efavirenz.*

3TC (lamivudine): A nucleoside analog, like AZT, ddI, ddC, d4T, and abacavir, that acts against HIV by inhibiting the enzyme reverse transcriptase, which HIV uses to reproduce. 3TC also inhibits the hepatitis B virus. For HIV infections, 3TC is most commonly used in combination with AZT, TDF, or ABC. Side effects are rare.

T-helper cells: Synonymous with T4 cells, T4 lymphocytes, and CD4 lymphocytes. (See above, *CD4 cells.*)

T-suppressor lymphocytes: T-suppressor lymphocytes are another class of T lymphocytes (see above, *Immune system*). T-suppressor lymphocytes are synonymous with T8 cells, CD8 cells, and T8 lymphocytes. All T lymphocytes participate in the body's defenses. A small subset of the CD8 cells targets HIV and is therefore responsible for destroying the CD4 cells that harbor the virus and therefore the virus itself. During the initial illness, called acute HIV infection or acute retroviral syndrome, the concentrations of HIV are high. The CD8 response decreases the HIV concentration precipitously, and the symptoms of the initial illness accordingly disappear. The laboratory test called the T-cell subset analysis is a count of the various types of T lymphocytes.

Tenofovir (TDF, Viread): This drug is closely related to the nucleoside analogs but is a nucleo*tide*. It is highly active against HIV, has few side effects, and can be taken as a single pill once daily. It can cause kidney damage if taken in too high a dose—occurring if someone forgets to lower the dose when, for other reasons, the kidneys don't work well.

Testosterone: Many men with HIV infection have low levels of testosterone. This is especially true for men who take Megace, which is a female hormone. Testosterone may be important in the prevention and treatment of wasting, primarily in men with low testosterone levels. It is given as a patch or by injection at intervals of 1 to 2 weeks.

Thalidomide: A drug once abandoned because it caused birth defects when given to pregnant women. It is now available for people with HIV infection and is used to treat wasting and aphthous ulcers.

Thrombocytopenia: Thrombocytopenia is a low count (*penia*) of thrombocytes (or platelets), cells in the blood that facilitate clotting. The usual count of thrombocytes is 150,000 to 300,000 per milliliter of blood. Lower counts of 50,000 to 120,000 per milliliter are common in people with HIV infection. When the count is very low, from 5,000 to 25,000 per milliliter, bleeding problems may occur. People with HIV infection have thrombocytopenia because their bodies produce antibodies against their own platelets. Some people have no symptoms but must still be careful to avoid cuts or anything that could cause bleeding. Other people have excessive nosebleeds, excessive bleeding from cuts, bleeding into the stomach or intestines, and red spots the size of pinheads that come from tiny hemorrhages into the skin. Treatment is with drugs—*corticosteroids* (see above), *HAART* (see above), or gamma globulin given intravenously.

Thrush: Thrush is an infection of the mouth caused by the fungus *Candida albicans.* The symptoms are white patches along the gums, on the inside of the cheeks, on the roof of the mouth, or on the tongue. Thrush is extremely common in people with HIV infection, and is considered part of early symptomatic HIV infection. Thrush is easily treated with nystatin, clotrimazole, ketoconazole, or fluconazole.

Tipranavir (TPV, Aptiva): A protease inhibitor intended for people for whom prior treatment has failed. It must be boosted with ritonavir, and it can't be used with other protease inhibitors because of some harsh drug interactions. It interacts with many other kinds of drugs as well, and has a high rate of liver toxicity.

Toxoplasmosis: Toxoplasmosis is an infection caused by the parasite *Toxoplasma gondii. Toxoplasma gondii* is found in cat excrement and in rare meat, both of which are potential sources of infection. About 10 to 30 percent of all adults in the United States have *Toxoplasma gondii* in their bodies, but the majority are unaware of it. The carriers of *Toxoplasma* can be identified by a blood test for antibodies to the parasite. The parasite remains dormant (see *Latency*) and rarely causes disease unless the immune system is weakened. In people with HIV infection, the most common form of toxoplasmosis is an infection of the brain called toxoplasma encephalitis. The usual symptoms are headaches and fever, with a CD4 count below 100; many people have seizures, a weak arm, weak leg, or other neurologic symptoms. An MRI scan (see *Magnetic resonance imaging*) of the brain usually shows certain specific changes. Treatment is with a combination of pyrimethamine and either a sulfa drug or clindamycin. Toxoplasmosis can be prevented by taking *trimethoprim- sulfamethoxazole,* the same drug that prevents PCP (see below).

Trimethoprim-sulfamethoxazole (Bactrim, Septra): This is an antibiotic used to prevent and treat pneumonia caused by *Pneumocystis jiroveci.* Trimethoprim-sulfamethoxazole can be taken by mouth or by vein. Its advantage is that it treats or prevents many other infections as well. Its major disadvantage is that many people develop reactions to it—fever, rash, low white blood cell count, and hepatitis. Many people will tolerate the drug if they stop taking it for a while and then begin taking it again at a lower dose.

Triple therapy: The use of three different drugs to treat HIV, usually two nucleoside analogs and a protease inhibitor, either nevirapine or efavirenz. See *HAART.*

Trizivir (AZT + 3TC + ABC): One of the combinations of *nucleoside analogs* (see above) that are taken as one pill twice daily. The advantage is the reduction in "pill burden," which makes adhering to the drug regimen easier.

Truvada: A combination pill containing tenofovir and emtricitabine.

Tuberculosis (TB): Tuberculosis is an infection, usually in the lungs, that is over 100 times more frequent in people with HIV infection than in the general population. The bacterium that causes TB can either be dormant (inactive TB) or active (active TB). In active TB, the usual symptoms are fever, cough, weight loss, fatigue, and night sweats. People with either active or inactive TB may have skin tests that are positive for TB. In people with HIV infection, the skin test is less reliable, especially in the later stages of HIV infection, when the immune system is weakened. People with HIV infection and inactive TB should receive treatment to prevent active TB. People with HIV infection and active TB should receive a combination of four drugs that include isoniazid (INH), rifampin, pyrazinamide, and either streptomycin or ethambutol (Myambutol). A new form of tuberculosis is resistant to some or all of these drugs. This new tuberculosis occurs most commonly in people who do not complete the standard treatment and in people living in New York City.

Ultrasensitive: Describes a test for HIV that detects concentrations of the virus as small as 20 to 50 copies per milliliter. A newer ultra-ultrasensitive test will detect concentrations as low as 5 copies per milliliter.

Undetectable: Describes measurements of viral load that fail to detect HIV because HIV is in such low concentrations. What undetectable actually means differs according to the sensitivity of the test (see above, *Ultrasensitive*). Standard tests detect amounts of virus over 400 to 500 viruses per milliliter of blood; the "ultrasensitive" tests detect amounts over 20 to 50 viruses per milliliter of blood.

Vaccine: A vaccine is a substance, given by mouth or by an injection, that stimulates the immune system to form antibodies to some microbe. The polio vaccine, for instance, stimulates the immune system to form antibodies against the polio virus. These newly formed antibodies now protect the person against any subsequent exposure to that microbe. Some vaccines work better than others: with the polio vaccine, protection is nearly 100 percent; with the influenza vaccine, protection is about 70 percent. Vaccines for HIV infection are being tested in people with and without HIV infection. For people without HIV infection, a vaccine could hopefully work like any other vaccine, that is, it could stimulate antibodies that protect you if you are exposed to HIV. For people with HIV infection, a vaccine could hopefully stimulate the immune system to respond more effectively.

Vaginitis: Vaginitis is infection of the vagina. Symptoms are abnormal vaginal discharge, sometimes with severe itching. Vaginitis has three common infectious causes: (1) "yeast," or the fungus *Candida,* which is treated with antifungal drugs like Gyne-Lotrimin or fluconazole; (2) "trick," short for the parasite *Trichomonas vaginalis,* which is treated with metronidazole (Flagyl); and (3) certain bacteria also treated with metronidazole. The most common cause of vaginitis in women with HIV infection is yeast infection. This form of vaginitis is more likely to occur if you are taking antibiotics. Vaginitis is common in women without HIV infection, but those with HIV infection have it more frequently and it is more difficult to treat.

Varicella zoster: Varicella zoster is the virus that causes chickenpox (varicella) and herpes zoster (shingles). See above, *Herpes zoster.*

Vertical transmission: Medical lingo for the transmission of a microbe from a pregnant woman to her newborn baby.

Videx: See *ddI.*

Viracept: See *Nelfinavir.*

Viral load: Synonymous with quantitative HIV. Viral load is the concentration of HIV in the blood, which indicates the total amount of HIV in the body. The average viral load for an untreated person is 30,000 to 60,000, meaning 30,000 to 60,000 copies (viruses) per milliliter of blood. The usual goal of therapy is to reduce the viral load to *undetectable* (see above) levels, meaning less than 50 copies per milliliter.

Viramune: See *Nevirapine.*

Viread: See *Tenofovir.*

Virologic failure: Not the failure of the virus, but the failure of the treatment to inhibit the virus. The person taking treatment whose viral load falls only from 100,000 to 10,000 is said to have virologic failure, though this ten-fold decrease is nevertheless a 90 percent decrease in the amount of HIV. The person whose viral load returns to 100,000 despite treatment has complete virologic failure. The first goal of treatment is to decrease the virus ten-fold (or one log) within 1 to 4 weeks. The subsequent goal is to reach a viral load of less than 500 by weeks 8 to 16, and less than 50 at week 24. Despite virologic failure, life is still better than before treatment—presumably because the resistant HIV is injured and simply cannot do as much damage.

Virus: A virus is a tiny microbe that, unlike bacteria, can neither survive nor reproduce unless it lives in a cell. HIV is a virus that lives in CD4 lymphocytes in humans.

Wasting: Wasting is the term given—somewhat unfortunately—to the weight loss and malnutrition that often accompany HIV infection. The causes of wasting vary; they may include infections and tumors that are complications of HIV infection. Some people burn more calories because their metabolism increases, usually because of fever and common infections. These people may eat a lot and still lose weight. Other people have malnutrition due to starvation because of sores in their mouths, or depression, or apathy, or side effects of drugs that prevent them from eating. Many people in the late stages of HIV infection seem to have progressive weight loss with what is called *protein-calorie malnutrition,* which may be the result of the action of cytokines, proteins that regulate the immune system and can cause loss of muscle protein. Wasting can be an AIDS-defining diagnosis: according to the criteria of the Centers for Disease Control and Prevention, an unexplained loss of at least 10 percent of the usual body weight, accompanied by diarrhea or fever for 30 days, is diagnostic of AIDS. Treatment of wasting is varied and is tailored to the cause. Treatments include food supplements such as Ensure, Ensure Plus, Jevity, Criticare, Peptamen, or Perative; appetite stimulants such as Megace, Marinol, and thalidomide; and injections of growth hormone, testosterone, or anabolic steroids. Resistance exercise, like lifting weights, is also helpful.

Western blot: The Western blot is a test for specific antibodies, in this case, for antibodies to HIV. (See above, *ELISA test.*)

Wild-type HIV: Naturally occurring strain of HIV, that is, HIV with no mutations that may have conferred resistance. Some people use "wild-type" to mean the strain of HIV that's predominant in a community. In this case, the "wild-type" could conceivably be a resistant strain, if the particular community has extensively used antiretroviral drugs and has had *virologic failure* (see above).

Xanax: See *Benzodiazepines.*

Zerit: See *d4T.*

Ziagen: See *Abacavir.*

Zovirax: See *Acyclovir.*

Acknowledgments

This book owes a lot of its substance and spirit to the following people, who supplied information, answered endless questions, and read and reread drafts. We are grateful to Dr. Joel Gallant, director of the Moore Clinic at Johns Hopkins Hospital, for medical advice and for referring us to his extremely articulate patients; to both Linda Apuzzo, clinical research coordinator, and Jo Leslie, inpatient coordinator of the AIDS Service at Johns Hopkins Hospital, for highly informed advice on the social and emotional perspectives of the people who are their patients and the audience of this book; to Meg Garrett, senior attorney at the Johns Hopkins Health System, for advice and information on legal, financial, and insurance matters; to Susan Rucker, social worker and supervisor, Infectious Diseases, at the Johns Hopkins School of Medicine, for information on insurance matters and on the social service system and for advice on the emotional, familial, and social concerns of people with HIV infection; and to Heidi Hutton, psychologist, Johns Hopkins School of Medicine, Department of Psychiatry, for advice on the changing feelings and problems of people with HIV infection.

We are especially grateful to the people with HIV infection themselves, and to their caregivers, who told us with intelligence and in detail how to persist in living well.

We are also grateful to Jackie Wehmueller for close and concerned editing, for her unflappability, and for her iron fist in the velvet glove—especially for the velvet glove.

We thank, particularly, Jean Bartlett and Cal Walker.

Index